THE AMERICAN ACADEMY OF ORTHOPAEDIC SURGEONS

Instructional
Course
Lectures

Volume XX 1971

THE AMERICAN ACADEMY OF ORTHOPAEDIC SURGEONS

Instructional Course Lectures

Volume XX 1971

With 488 illustrations

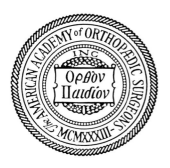

Saint Louis

THE C. V. MOSBY COMPANY

1971

5387

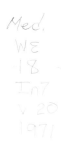

Contributors

Professor R. MERLE d'AUBIGNE, M.D.

Clinique Chirurgicale Orthopédique et Repatrice, Hôpital Cochin, Paris, France

FRANK H. BASSETT, III, M.D.

Associate Professor of Orthopaedic Surgery, Division of Orthopaedic Surgery, Department of Surgery, Duke University Medical Center, Durham, North Carolina

EUGENE E. BLECK, M.D.

Clinical Instructor, Stanford University School of Medicine; Orthopaedic Consultant, Children's Hospital at Stanford, Palo Alto; Orthopaedic Consultant, El Portal del Sol School for Orthopaedically Handicapped and Cerebral Palsied Children, San Mateo, California

EDGAR S. CATHCART, M.D.

Associate Professor of Medicine, Boston University School of Medicine; Head, Arthritis Clinic, Boston City Hospital, Boston, Massachusetts

ALAN S. COHEN, M.D., F.A.C.P.

Professor of Medicine, Boston University School of Medicine; Head, Arthritis and Connective Tissue Disease Section, University Hospital, Boston, Massachusetts

MARK B. COVENTRY, M.D.

Chairman, Department of Orthopedics, Mayo Clinic and Mayo Foundation; Professor of Orthopedic Surgery, Mayo Graduate School of Medicine, University of Minnesota, Rochester, Minnesota

A. JACKSON DAY, M.D.

Adjunct Associate Professor of Orthopaedic Surgery, Wayne State University School of Medicine; Chief, Orthopaedic Department, Children's Hospital of Michigan; Chief, Orthopaedic Department, Harper Hospital; Attending Orthopaedist, Detroit Orthopaedic Clinic, Detroit, Michigan

WILLARD E. DOTTER, M.D.

Orthopedic Surgeon, Department of Orthopedic Surgery, Lahey Clinic Foundation, Boston, Massachusetts

E. BURKE EVANS, M.D.

Professor of Surgery; Chief, Division of Orthopedic Surgery, Department of Surgery, The University of Texas Medical Branch, Galveston, Texas

CHARLES M. FRYER, M.A.

Director, Prosthetic-Orthotic Center; Instructor in Orthopedic Surgery; Northwestern University Medical School, Chicago, Illinois

JOHN GLANCY, C.O.

Assistant Professor of Orthopaedics; Chairman, Division of Orthotics, Indiana University Medical Center, Indianapolis, Indiana

J. LEONARD GOLDNER, M.D.

Professor and Chairman, Division of Orthopaedic Surgery, Department of Surgery, Duke University Medical Center, Durham, North Carolina

GEORGE HAMMOND, M.D.

Orthopedic Surgeon, Department of Orthopedic Surgery, Lahey Clinic Foundation, Boston, Massachusetts

WILLIAM H. HARRIS, M.D.

Associate Clinical Professor of Orthopedic Surgery, Harvard Medical School; Orthopedic Surgeon, Massachusetts General Hospital; Orthopedic Surgeon, New England Baptist Hospital, Boston, Massachusetts

MICHAEL HARTY, M.A., M.B., M.Ch., F.R.C.S.

Associate Professor, Department of Graduate Anatomy, School of Medicine and School of Allied Medical Professions, University of Pennsylvania, Philadelphia, Pennsylvania

ARTHUR J. HELFET, B.Sc. (Capetown), M.D., M.Ch. Orth. (Liverpool), F.R.C.S. (Eng.), F.A.C.S.

Professor and Director; formerly Chairman, Department of Orthopaedic Surgery, Albert Einstein College of Medicine, Yeshiva University, Bronx, New York

HENRY D. ISENBERG, Ph.D.

Attending Microbiologist, Department of Laboratories, Long Island Jewish Medical Center, New Hyde Park; Clinical Associate Professor, Department of Surgery, Division of Orthopaedic Surgery, The Downstate Medical Center, S.U.N.Y., Brooklyn, New York

JOHN J. JOYCE, III, M.D.

Assistant Professor of Orthopaedic Surgery, Department of Graduate Medicine, University of Pennsylvania School of Medicine; Chief of Orthopaedics, Germantown Hospital, Philadelphia, Pennsylvania

M. KERBOULL, M.D.

Clinique Chirurgicale Orthopédique et Repatrice, Hôpital Cochin, Paris, France

LEROY S. LAVINE, M.D.

Attending Surgeon in Charge of Orthopaedic Surgery, Department of Surgery, Long Island Jewish Medical Center, New Hyde Park; Professor and Head, Division of Orthopaedic Surgery, The Downstate Medical Center, S.U.N.Y., Brooklyn, New York

ROBERT E. LEACH, M.D.

Orthopedic Surgeon, Department of Orthopedic Surgery, Lahey Clinic Foundation, Boston, Massachusetts

HANS RICHARD LEHNEIS, C.P.O.

Director, Orthotics and Prosthetics, Institute of Rehabilitation Medicine; Instructor, Rehabilitation Medicine, New York University, School of Medicine and Post-Graduate Medical School, New York, New York

NEWTON C. McCOLLOUGH, III, M.D.

Assistant Professor, Department of Orthopaedics and Rehabilitation, University of Miami School of Medicine, Miami, Florida

KARL H. MUELLER, M.D.

Associate Clinical Professor, Department of Orthopedic Surgery, Medical College of Wisconsin, Milwaukee, Wisconsin

Professor M. POSTEL, M.D.

Clinique Chirurgicale Orthopédique et Repatrice, Hôpital Cochin, Paris, France

FRED P. SAGE, M.D.

Assistant Clinical Professor of Orthopaedic Surgery, University of Tennessee College of Medicine; Member of the Staff, Campbell Clinic, Memphis, Tennessee

ALAN DeFOREST SMITH, M.D.

Emeritus Professor of Orthopedic Surgery, Columbia University, New York, New York

WILLIAM R. TORGERSON, JR., M.D.

Orthopedic Surgeon, Department of Orthopedic Surgery, Lahey Clinic Foundation, Boston, Massachusetts

Preface

Volume XX of *Instructional Course Lectures* represents selective lectures given in the Instructional Course section of the annual meeting of the American Academy of Orthopaedic Surgeons held in Chicago in January of 1970. The selection of material has been determined considering past presentations by this Committee in the printed format. Emphasis has been on presenting well-rounded and diversified subject material representing many of the various spheres of the art and practice of orthopaedic surgery. Obviously this publication cannot cover all the courses presented. Many of these do not lend themselves to formal publication and others would be a reduplication of previously published material. The aim of the Committee in the presentation of the instructional courses, which is reflected in this publication, is to present the current state of knowledge in a given subject in as much depth as time will allow. Emphasis is on the tried and true rather than on innovations that have not had the experienced evaluation of time. This volume does not and should not attempt to be the sounding board of unproved techniques or theorems; rather it represents the expression of the state of the art as it is at the time of presentation.

We feel that the volume serves a definite purpose in providing a "packaged deal" where one can get a good analysis of a given subject, not just a brief abstract, and yet not be burdened with statistical analysis. The subject material does cover a wide sphere of orthopaedic involvement from basic science to pure clinical application and pertinent references serving as an additional source for those with a desire for further knowledge in depth.

Committee on Instructional Courses

William R. MacAusland, Jr., *Chairman*
Rocco A. Calandruccio
E. Burke Evans
William E. Snell
Warren G. Stamp

Contents

THE AMERICAN ACADEMY OF ORTHOPAEDIC SURGEONS

Instructional
Course
Lectures

Volume XX 1971

Chapter 1

Orthopaedic infections: their biologic role and clinical significance

HENRY D. ISENBERG, Ph.D., and LEROY S. LAVINE, M.D.
New Hyde Park, New York

The origin and clinical and therapeutic aspects of osteomyelitis have been reviewed periodically for many decades. The common denominator of these tomes is their singular preoccupation with the skeletal system. The impression these reports evoke is that the osseous structures of man are autonomous units totally independent from other organs, the body as a whole, and the environment in which the individual functions. Nevertheless, these limited views portray most aspects of the medical problems attending osteomyelitis. They reiterate that bone is a metabolically active tissue with a high rate of synthesis and resorption, depending on an adequate vascular supply. Thus acute osteomyelitis, hematogenously disseminated, affects rapidly growing bone most readily. They also underline the frequency distribution of the disease with respect to age. The various reviewers[3,15,16,18] have shown that 85% of reported cases of primary or hematogenous osteomyelitis have occurred in children 16 years of age or younger.

The accepted explanation for this age distribution as well as the predilection of hematogenous osteomyelitis for the metaphyses of long bone are based on the classic studies of Hobo[7] regarding the vascular state of the epiphyseal growth plate which encourages, by virtue of its characteristic distribution of capillaries originating from the nutrient arteries and the large sinusoidal veins, an ideal situation for seeding bacteria in this area during the retarded passage of blood through this system. In addition, the cellular defenses of both the afferent and efferent loops of the metaphyseal capillaries lack the usual active defensive cellular elements required to cope with the assault of potential purveyors of infectious disease. Trueta[15] has refined these considerations, further demonstrating, on the basis of local vascular anatomy, that conditions for initiating disease processes during childhood are most likely to start in the metaphyseal sinusoidal veins and, limited by the epiphyseal growth plate, can advance only laterally to involve the periosteum. In infants less than 1 year old the capillary bed still penetrates the epiphyseal plate and permits disease to proceed to that region, attended by septic arthritis and eventual destruction of the epiphysis. In this respect, conditions in the very young resemble those in the adult where, following anastomosis of metaphyseal and epiphyseal vessels after resorption of growth cartilage, the infectious process may spread to the subarticular space.

However, infectious disease of the bone as a primary consequence of hematogenous dissemination is but one aspect of the problem. In today's highly mechanized society, infectious disease secondary to trauma has assumed gigantic proportions. In addition, the advances of medicine and especially biomedical engineering have opened avenues for the introduction of microbial particles into body areas usually sterile and ill prepared to cope with residents essentially foreign to these parts.

At first consideration, little similarity between these different osteomyelitides seems to exist. Nevertheless, infectious disease viewed from the vantage point of advances in microbiology, host-parasite relation, chemotherapy, immunochemistry, etc. offers the opportunity to review the common aspects of all osteomyelitides and to consider infectious disease of the bone not as a disease or group of diseases peculiarly characteristic of a particular tissue but as part of the entire organism and its environmental interactions.

MICROORGANISMS AND DISEASE

Of course, infectious disease is defined traditionally as the result of microbial activities. But the microbial world is comprised of a staggering number of different orders and families, many of which are still practically unknown. Innumerable representatives are never encountered in the intimate environment of so-called higher forms, leaving a still overwhelming array of microorganisms forming a ubiquitous, dynamic biosphere around, in, and on the bodies of all other living organisms. Perhaps the least appreciated attribute of microbial life is that each minute microbial particle is indeed a complete organism, fulfilling within the confines of what is commonly called a cell all vital processes. Therefore microorganisms are distinguished by the total autonomy of each unit cell. All other organisms are composed of numerous cells specialized and organized to carry out specific tasks, the sum of which constitute the organizational level identified as the total organism. Thus microorganisms are acellular organisms, not subdivided into tissues composed of cells.

The human cognition of the living world has restricted all forms to two kingdoms: animals and plants. This grouping fails regularly at the level of microorganisms, which can display as individuals attributes representing each kingdom with impunity. Perhaps the cogent decision of nineteenth century scientists to regard the microbial forms as a separate kingdom—the Protista—deserves a more general acceptance, especially in view of the organizational complexities and differences that attend the procaryotic and eucaryotic expressions of life.[8] In other words, we should accept microorganisms or Protista for what they are and appreciate the artificiality of our present systems of classification, particularly at this so-called lower level.

Still we do recognize a semblance of categories that help in delineation of microorganisms of more obvious consequence with regard to human commerce, production, and, of course, health. The protistal kingdom can be divided conveniently into bacteria, a group that encompasses not only the classic representatives but the *Rickettsia*, *Mycoplasma*, and the large viruses known as *Chlamydia* or *Bedsonia*. In addition, there are the close bacterial relatives, the blue-green algae, the more complex yeasts and fungi, as well as that great array of microbial forms, the protozoa. The involvement of these protistal forms in the very nature of all

life on this planet is most impressive. But most pertinent to the intent of this discussion is the role of microbial forms in the human environment and in disease.

A certain segment of the Protista, mostly bacteria, some viruses and certain yeasts, fungi, and a few protozoa, have been described as pathogenic or virulent since the connection between microorganisms and disease became established. While the exact definition of pathogenicity and virulence as it pertains to these microbial particles has never been established, considerable experimental and theoretical efforts have led to alleged explanations of the manner in which these "dangerous" microorganisms achieve their end. Obviously, particular disease-producing agents must compete successfully with the resident or indigenous, sometimes referred to as autochthonous, microflora or microbiota of the human body.[9] They must gain access in some manner to one and all of the various body openings and coverings, be they skin, mucous membranes, or respiratory or gastrointestinal tracts, and possess the capacity to penetrate these structures and lodge themselves in the underlying, usually sterile tissues. It has been proposed that certain tissues or organs exert a selective influence on the microbial challengers, permitting certain particular offenders to remain unharmed. The microorganisms in turn can elaborate various injurious materials such as protein exotoxins or the peptide-lipopolysaccharide complexes, which constitute parts of their cell walls, or antigens with the pharmacologic property of endotoxins. Microbial enzymes may destroy or block the cellular defense mechanisms of the host, while other microbial enzymes may aid and abet their spread to various sites far removed from their point of entry. The protistal rate of growth is far greater than that of the host's cells and thus they abuse his hospitality by depriving him of essential nutrients while releasing the often harmful end products of their metabolism into their immediate microenvironment.

The connection between these microbial actions and infectious disease in man was established, rather tenuously and empirically, almost 100 years ago by Robert Koch. Simply stated, Koch postulated: (1) An organism is recovered from a lesion or pathologic process in a patient. (2) It is characterized by the laboratory. (3) It is introduced into an experimental animal where it initiates disease. (4) It is recovered from the animal. He concluded that a microorganism fulfilling these conditions is pathogenic. Generations of infectious disease experts have held to these rules in the strictest possible fashion despite the brilliant achievements of Smith,[14] Burnett,[1] and Dubos,[4] to name but a few. It is evident almost immediately that Koch's postulates are descriptive but that they do not explain infectious disease. One must conclude on the basis of these rules that disease production is a microbial characteristic, which should lead to a simple scheme permitting the classification of all Protista as either disease producers or harmless. Koch's postulates equate animal and human disease and ignore the portal of entry and number of organisms introduced, while designating that all Protista recoverable from lesions that can produce animal disease in the laboratory are pathogenic and denying this appellation to those failing to evoke such a response in other mammals.

Obviously, even this random sample of the many objections that can be leveled against this approach to an acceptable explanation of infectious disease leads to a very significant conclusion that there are few if any microorganisms whose presence in or on the human host leads invariably to overt clinical manifestations of infectious disease. The legion of Protista that constitute the human microbiosphere contain many components deserving the designation pathogenic on numerous occasions while still considered harmless under similar circumstances in other individuals or even in the same host but in different locales. Therefore the microbiota of man is composed almost exclusively of Protista, which are not only harmless most of the time but are actually beneficial to their host while still possessed of the potential to participate in, if not initiate, infectious disease. These microorganisms in our dynamic, though intimate, environment have been termed amphibionts by Rosebury,[12] the term suggesting their sometime pathogenicity as well as their ubiquity. What the recognition of this principle implies reinforces the pioneer work of Smith[14] and the modern work of Dubos,[4] who regard the ordinary healthy state with respect to the autochthonous microbiota as an equilibrium between all of the complex factors at the disposal of the host and equally complex attributes of the microbiota. Any disturbance of this equilibrium will lead to overt infectious disease. The outstanding difference between this view and the classic one exemplified by Koch's postulates is that the onus of disease production is removed from the microorganisms. Instead, the determinant role in the initiation and clinical manifestation of infectious disease is shared by the microbiota and the host, with the latter more often playing the decisive part. This is due in no small measure to factors acting on the host's health

which are totally unrelated to infectious disease but which, nevertheless, so affect his significant functions as to lower his capacity to maintain his equilibrium with the microorganisms present at that very moment.

HOST'S (PATIENT'S) DEFENSE MECHANISMS

It is thus the host's health and specifically his resistance that is of primary consideration in the sequences that lead to clinically overt infectious disease. Changes in the host's environment, the many and various stresses to which he is exposed, poisons, toxins, etc. all may contribute to lowering his resistance generally but especially locally. Trauma, anatomic abnormalities, or virus activity at a specific site may permit any microorganism present by chance to gain access to this point of lowest resistance and lead to the development of regional pathology. The host's capacity to respond to this incursion will be the decisive factor in the progress of clinical infectious disease.

Nonspecific mechanisms

A great many of the host's activities and mechanisms to ward off disease of any sort are still cloaked in ignorance. Little is known about the conditions described as normal[17]; to be sure, the few studies performed indicate considerable variation based on geographic location, age, experience, etc. We are aware that there are blood as well as tissue factors of a nonspecific nature in addition to the specific antibodies that contribute to that ill-defined host state, resistance. In general, resistance can be regarded as a combination of multifarious general and specific barriers, mechanical, chemical, and biologic in nature. Some of the most obvious defense barriers at the disposal of the human host are the skin and mucous membranes, the normal microbiota already mentioned, various "traps," removal mechanisms, and environmental selection. A detailed discussion of these first-line barriers as well as the other host mechanisms cannot be presented; the mere mention of some must suffice to convey the complexities as well as the intricacies of the host's armamentarium in the containment of microbial particles.

The skin and mucous membranes certainly offer a prodigious mechanical barrier that is not only difficult to penetrate but is constantly removing trapped microbial agents during desquamation. The adhesive properties of mucous secretions serve as traps for most particles they contact or which are impinged onto surfaces coated with this material. Lavage by saliva and tears as well as other secretions aids the process of removal of foreign objects, including microbial particles. These are also trapped by mucus-coated hairs and cilia. Expulsion of collected masses of intruders takes place during sneezing and coughing, while micturition and defecation eliminate microbial residents in the urethra and bowel, respectively.

There are many chemical barriers and defense mechanisms at the disposal of the human host, many of which are nonspecific in their action on Protista. The considerable acidity of the stomach guards against practically all potential microbial offenders present in food or swallowed at other times. A lowered pH acts as well against unwanted residents or survivors in the vagina of reproductively competent women, while unsaturated fatty acids as well as an unfavorable pH restrict the colonizing microbial population of the skin in general.

A special category of chemical agents, nonspecific in their selectivity at the protistan level but specific in terms of particular molecular arrangements present in their substrates, are the many enzymes of the host, whether extracellular or intracellular, confined to secretory glands, or universally distributed throughout the body. Some of these catalysts are produced apparently for the express purpose of injury to select microorganisms, while others have a wider range of activity. Perhaps the best-known species of enzymes with bactericidal activity are the lysozymes, present in tears, saliva, blood, and probably other body fluids. Another group, ill-defined chemically to date, are the granulocytic pyrogens which, released from polymorphonuclear leukocytes by endotoxins, some viruses, bacteria, and even tissue fragments, act on the hypothalamus to induce a rise in temperature. Leukocytic and local cellular glycolysis results in the accumulation of lactic acid in the microenvironment of a pathologic process, with the curtailment of growth of many bacteria that normally require a more neutral pH to initiate their proliferation and attain adequate numbers within a prescribed locus. Of course, practically all host cells contain lysosomes that harbor various carbohydrases, proteinases, peptidases, lipases, etc., all of which can act on the suitable substrates frequently offered by microorganisms. Blood contains several moieties, probably protein in nature, collectively known as phagocytin, which are required for the nonspecific phagocytosis of many bacteria. Tissues as well contain ill-defined proteins, histones, lipopeptides, and the like that display antimicrobial activities, as do certain histamine derivatives that convert, probably in an indirect fashion, enzyme precursors to active forms, displaying antimicrobial

properties exemplified by the kallikreinogen change to bradykinin.

The nonspecific biologic host defenses, of course, combine many if not all of the factors already enumerated and impart to them that special organizational character that leads to their designation as biologic. Foremost among these biologic nonspecific activities is the process of phagocytosis. The primary requirement for eliciting this response is the successful penetration of the host by a foreign particle. The classic inflammatory response ensues, consisting of the dilatation of surrounding blood vessels, increased vascular permeability, diapedesis, as well as vascular and tissue macrophage activities. Should local containment of the infectious process fail, reticuloendothelial macrophages in the proximal lymph nodes will attempt to retard the spread of the infectious disease. The failure of the lymphatic barrier permits the microorganisms access to the blood *via* the thoracic duct, which will expose the offenders to the phagocytic endothelial cells of the liver, spleen, and other organs as well as to the policing action of granulocytes and monocytes of the blood itself.

This veritable bastion of multilayered phagocytic defense systems is aided directly and indirectly by another multicomponent system—the complement of blood. Best known as a useful indicator system in the laboratory diagnoses of syphilis, studies of the role of these several serum proteins during the past 20 years have assigned them a significant place in the nonspecific curtailment of infectious disease as well as useful participants when specific host defense activities are applied. Classically, complement has been regarded as a four-component system. Complements 1 and 2 are known to be inactivated by heat (56° C.) but can be separated by dialysis against water at pH 5.0, which precipitates complement 1. Complement 4 is inactivated by ammonia or hydrazine. Complement 3 is a complex of at least five components, complements 5 through 9, all of which can be absorbed by certain preparations of yeast cell walls. All the complements are globulins. They do participate, that is, are fixed, during the formation of many but by no means all antigen-antibody interactions. The complements immobilize treponemas, lyse antibody-coated gram-negative bacteria and erythrocytes, and are involved in immune adherence, a process characterized by the adhesion of antigen-antibody complexes to nonspecific surfaces such as erythrocytes, platelets, starch granules, etc., thus assisting in the removal of inactivated debris. Complements 3, 5, 6, and 7 as well as antigen and antibody are involved in chemotactic leukocyte attraction. Histamine release by mast cells is thought to depend on the action of a polypeptide, anaphylotoxin, requiring somehow the action of complement 5 or 3 and possibly 4 and 2.

A third nonspecific biologic barrier to infectious disease has already been mentioned but deserves emphasis. Microbial competition plays a not insignificant role in preventing just any protist from establishing a foothold in any host. Many microorganisms produce in the laboratory and in nature a variety of materials that prohibit related or totally different Protista access to regions they inhabit. Antibiotics produced by fungi and certain bacteria are the best-known illustrations of such survival tactics. Bacteriophages or bacterial viruses may be associated with bacterial chromosomes and thus prove avirulent or attenuated toward these host organisms. The few vegetative viral particles produced under these circumstances can be virulent toward other variants of the same bacterial species or toward related species, generally leading to their destruction. The nutritional demands of Protista cover a very wide spectrum ranging from very simple fare to requirements of amino acids, vitamins, and other factors. Obviously, these requirements exert a selective pressure in addition to the metabolic end products produced by the multitudes of different Protista. On one hand, such end products may be injurious to certain populations, while others may be unable to exist unless other microorganisms initiated the decomposition of complex molecules or accumulated degradation products that serve as initial substrate for still other Protista. Undoubtedly, in certain densely colonized body areas a number of required factors may be limited, and the competition among competing microorganisms for such essential molecules as oxygen, carbon dioxide, or magnesium, to name but a very few, must be most decisive in selecting the kind and type of population established successfully in any area.

Specific mechanisms

In addition, the normal physiologic activities of a healthy host lead to transient bacteremias. For example, postprandial showers of intestinal bacteria are thought to occur with considerable frequency. These organisms are removed from circulation with great dispatch and without apparent harm to the host. This ready handling of microbial particles intruding on the host organisms is possible only if the microbial particles are established residents of the body, that is, if the host is acquainted with these microorganisms. This acquaintance is a very real factor based on the presence, within the host's blood, of protein defense factors directed specifically against these "old acquaintances," namely antibodies.

Antibodies are produced by the host in response to antigens or immunogens, which may be protein or polysaccharide in nature and in the case of microorganisms usually represent the outermost constituents of their cell walls, capsules, slime layers, or flagella. However, all antigens are not immunogens in all hosts. Briefly, antigenic properties are based on a number of conditions. Proteins are by far the best immunogens. To be antigenic, a protein should have a molecular weight greater than 10,000. Insulin, with a molecular weight of approximately 6,000, is a very weak antigen, while ribonuclease (molecular weight of 14,000) displays excellent antigenic activity. Certain amino acids seem to serve as determinant groups. These are tyrosine, phenylalanine, tryptophan, glutamic acid, lysine, and cystine. How these amino acids exert their determinant effect is not entirely clear as yet, but it seems to reside in their effect on the three-dimensional structure of the proteins. The polysaccharide antigens that figure importantly in microbial types, blood group substances, tissue types, etc., often as haptens or complex haptens, are composed of various hexoses (especially glucose and galactose), pentoses, methylpentoses, heptoses, octanoses, etc. They may be combined with proteins for greater antigenicity. Combinations with lipids as well seem not to enhance immunogenicity but increase the toxicity of the combination.

The reaction of the host to the immunogens is the production of specific antibodies. The very brief summary of these important proteins possible here cannot do justice to the significant role they play in the interaction of the host with his environment and in the protection of his integrity against all foreign materials, microbial as well as other. Antibodies may be divided into two groups, the humoral or soluble antibodies and the cell-fixed antibodies. The former figure much more prominently in the theme of this article. Antibodies have been purified and studied in a large variety of ways. But even in their most purified form, antibodies still represent a mixture or population of different molecules. They are heterogeneous despite their great specificity toward the antigen against which they were produced. This heterogeneity of antibodies may be intrinsic, that is, antibodies produced in different centers of the host. The different antibody-producing centers impart differences in structure determined by mendelian laws of inheritance. Since these antibody differences are inherited and independent of the antigens that stimulate their synthesis, they are considered intrinsic. Extrinsic heterogeneity depends on the variety of determinant groups presented by the antigen and by that part of the antigen "seen" by the antibody-producing cells.

There are several types of antibodies produced in response to the same stimulus or in response to the type of antigen presented. Best known of the immunoglobulins are (1) IgG, or γ-G, with a molecular weight of approximately 150,000, which travels as a γ_2-globulin electrophoretically, displays 7S behavior in the ultracentrifuge, and represents 71% of the immunoglobulins in man; (2) IgM, or γ-M, with a molecular weight of 1,000,000, electrophoretically moving as a γ_1-globulin, showing 19S behavior in the ultracentrifuge, and representing approximately 22% of the human immune globulin normally present; and (3) IgA, or γ-A, with a molecular weight of 300,000, electrophoretically moving as β_2- or γ_1-globulin, ranging in behavior in the ultracentrifuge from 9S to 11S, and representing about 7% of the immunoglobulins normally present in serum. Several additional immunoglobulins have been discovered to be present in minute amounts normally and functioning in ways that are even more obscure than the role of IgA. The functions usually associated with the immune response of the host are represented by the IgG and IgM moieties; this implies in no way that other immunoglobulins do not contribute significantly or decisively. It is merely a reflection of the still considerable lack of understanding that persists despite the many advances in this and related scientific disciplines.

A discussion of the specific host responses to the microbial challenge must include mention of the studies that have shed appreciable light on the structural complexities of the various immunoglobulins. Many different attempts to disassemble and resynthesize these particles failed. Understanding came through the study of myeloma proteins. In their simplest form, antibodies are dimers composed of two heavy or H chains and two light or L chains, each monomer consisting of a representative of each type of chain linked to each other by disulfide bridges. The monomers are joined, in turn, to form the functional dimer by the same disulfide bridge mechanism. Specificity of the immunoglobulins apparently resides in the light chains, which may be one of two types, κ or λ. The light chains are similar if not identical in all of the immunoglobulins, but the heavy chains differ so that IgG may be $\gamma_2\kappa_2$ or $\gamma_2\lambda_2$, while IgM has been described as a fivefold combination of the dimer

$\mu_2\kappa_2$ or $\mu_2\lambda_2$. The singular significance of these host proteins has been demonstrated most dramatically and variously during the past 5 years. It is their presence that leads to the ultimate rejection of transplants or, if the immunoglobulins are suppressed very efficiently over long periods of time, to overwhelming microbial disease.

Still, most of the mechanisms that control and depress host factors that may lead to clinically overt infectious disease remain unexplained if not unexplored. It is well known that circulatory disturbances such as local ischemia and generalized shock contribute to such a depression. Mechanical obstructions and nutritional deficiencies do so as well. Excessive application of alcohol, toxins, drugs used for anesthesia, and radiation tend to deprive the host of the capacity to muster an inflammatory response, but the exact mechanisms of action in which these agents or treatments accomplish this end remain mostly in the dark. Genetic disorders such as agammaglobulinemia and dysgammaglobulinemia are rare; the use of immunosuppressant therapy has helped to explain the end result of such genetic as well as induced states of lower defense potential in the host without clarifying the mechanisms accomplishing this end or revealing the means that would permit control. The vast number of chronic debilitating diseases and illnesses of viral etiology contribute to a general depression of host factors that impair the host's defense capabilities. Hormonal disturbances must also be considered functioning in this general area. On the whole, the complexities of the host matched by those of the Protista in his intimate environment have not been resolved sufficiently to enable us to construct a clear-cut picture of even the major events that lead to overt infectious disease. It is against such a background of uncertainty and an awareness of the shortcomings of even the most profound empiricisms that we must view the various aspects and manifestations of osteomyelitis.

OSTEOMYELITIS
Definition

Traditionally, osteomyelitis is considered in two categories: primary or hematogenously disseminated osteomyelitis and traumatic secondary osteomyelitis. There is a third distinct type of infectious disease of the bone. It is part of the second class of osteomyelitides, but differs so profoundly it must be considered apart. This type of osteomyelitis could be referred to as iatrogenic or nosocomial but is described most clearly as implantation-induced disease. The specific considerations of osteomyelitis must therefore encompass theoretical aspects, primary osteomyelitis, the two types of secondary osteomyelitis, modalities of treatment, and some clinical illustrations of the significant diagnostic and therapeutic criteria.

Mechanisms initiating osteomyelitis

The application of the preceding summary of the nature of infectious disease raises immediately the question of the mechanisms required to initiate microbial disease of bone. While the initiation of traumatic secondary osteomyelitis seems clear, the events that lead to the other disease manifestations are shrouded in mystery. The very early lesion of primary osteomyelitis cannot be or has not been detected. This suggests two possibilities. The one most readily accepted postulates that chance contamination of the proper region of bone by microorganisms in circulating blood serves as the nidus for the disease. There is the alternative that the innumerable lacunae of bone may be seeded prior to the earliest disease process; indeed, bone may harbor microorganisms normally; that is, these areas are not really sterile but have a resident nonproliferating microbiota delivered by chance after meals, exertion, etc. in the normal host. Survival of bacteria in tissues is, after all, not so uncommon. Thus an appreciable number of infectious disease specialists hold that the chronic state of some infectious diseases is the result of vegetative bacterial conversion to L-form microorganisms. This microbic phase, characterized by lack of complete cell wall production and intracellular existence of the Protista, does not permit ready detection unless laboratory attempts are made to ensure an osmotically proper environment for the isolation and proliferation of these more fragile stages in the microbial life cycle or spontaneous conversion to the vegetative phase of the microorganism takes place before the osmotic shock of ordinary laboratory media destroys the L-form of the organism.

However, vegetative phases of bacteria and bacterial spores have survived in certain tissues for an appreciable number of years and have led to the production of disease or the exacerbation of symptoms long after the initial presentation. Brill's disease, a recrudescent form of typhus, is an example of the latter, while the recovery of salmonellae from gallstones illustrates the former condition. Certainly, recurrence of primary osteomyelitis at the original site and with the same strain of staphylococcus, while not common, is encountered. Survival of the bacterium in bone is, therefore, more than a probability.

Unfortunately the detection of a single microorganism, especially in a tissue such as bone, is fraught with technical difficulties. Microbiology has very few tools and only a few preliminary successes in establishing the presence of resting nonproliferating Protista in tissues. The only reliable measure for the establishment of their presence in bone is growth on laboratory media under the prevailing, very unnatural conditions.

Preliminary experiments in our laboratory with samples of bone from the bone bank or from healthy bone at the time of surgery have not resulted in the recovery of microorganisms by the usual microbiologic methods for the cultivation of vegetative-phase Protista. No attempts have been made so far to isolate organisms that may be present as L-forms or strains not suited for ready cultivation under laboratory conditions.

Common microbial agents

Nevertheless, it is not inappropriate to consider the requirements a microorganism must meet in order to survive under conditions extant in bone. The microenvironment predominating in bone of all sorts demands primarily that microorganisms tolerate high osmolarity and a paucity of water. There are, besides spore-producing bacteria, two microorganisms in the human biosphere that meet this challenge: the staphylococci and the enterococci. The literature devoted to primary osteomyelitis makes it eminently clear that *Staphylococcus aureus* is by far the most common microbial agent involved in this disease. While the recovery of *Staphylococcus aureus* from primary osteomyelitis may be diminishing from a long-held high of 85% to 90% to the 50% encountered over the past 5 years on an active orthopaedic service in a large municipal hospital, it cannot be denied that this microorganism seems peculiarly suited to be involved in infectious processes in bone regardless of age group, but more prominently among children and young adults. No adequate explanation for the preferential selection of staphylococci by healthy or abnormal conditions in bones has been advanced. The bacterium, while well represented among the microbiota of the human host, is certainly not the most ubiquitous. It has no better access to the circulation that disseminates microbial agents to sites distant from the point of entry. The staphylococcal requirements for amino acids and vitamins are numerous, thus placing this bacterium at a disadvantage when compared to the very simple nutritional demands of most gram-negative rods. It may well be that such mundane staphylococcal attributes as ability to function in the presence of high salt concentrations, ability to survive under adverse environmental, especially dry, conditions without the assistance of spore formation, or proper seeding in appropriate locations because of the elaboration of extracellular enzymes acting on the coagulation mechanisms of plasma combine to establish the supremacy of *Staphylococcus aureus* as the most common microbial component of primary osteomyelitis. Of course, in view of the hemolytic, necrotizing, cell-destructive attributes of the major staphylococcal extracellular enzyme complex, a toxin, one would expect that this exotoxin might be a major factor in overt manifestations of primary osteomyelitis. Such a role has not been established for a toxin, and antibody production by the host against this moiety does not occur. The studies of Gladstone and co-workers[6] demonstrate an appreciable rise of antibodies against a toxin complex of staphylococci, the Panton-Valentine leukocidin, especially in osteomyelitis, an observation confirmed by Markham[11] and Lack and Towers.[10] While this specific antibody response may reflect the antigenic suitability of the leukocidin, it does reveal that in osteomyelitis the infectious disease processes are sufficiently retarded to permit the use of osteomyelitis as an exemplary model for the study of host-parasite interactions and, more significant, the development of diagnostic aids exploiting this particular attribute of the disease.

Elek's studies[5] to demonstrate and define differences in the physiologic activities of staphylococci from osteomyelitis as compared with those from other lesions or carriers were unsuccessful. Similarly, all serologic and bacteriophage types of *Staphylococcus aureus* have been encountered in primary osteomyelitis. The simplest attribute of *Staphylococcus aureus* is its ability to survive in high salt concentrations whenever it encounters such conditions; this milieu, however, appears to hinder the expression of certain staphylococcal disease-producing attributes, as exemplified by the rarity of staphylococcal disease in the nares or on the skin of cystic fibrosis patients. The enterococci, on the other hand, are very ready to become involved in secondary disease regardless of the environmental osmolarity. It may be a biased view, but survival without disease-promoting products by staphylococci in an osseous environment is a distinct possibility as long as no trauma or even a miniscule hematoma permits the initiation of rapid growth by the quasi-resting bacterium.

Streptococcus pyogenes used to occupy a place second

only to *Staphylococcus aureus* as an inciter of primary osteomyelitis. It is encountered rarely today despite the resurgence of streptococcal disease in the last decade. *Haemophilus influenzae* is also encountered more rarely, perhaps because of ecologic shifts in the microbiota of man. It is presently the vogue to associate certain hemoglobinopathies with salmonellal bone disease. This view obscures the occasional to moderate incidence of osteomyelitis by various serotypes of *Salmonella* in individuals without any indication of hemoglobin abnormalities in whom the septicemic stage of systemic salmonellosis provided the agents seeding bone. A variety of bacteria have been reported to be involved in the primary disease. *Staphylococcus aureus* remains the major microbial agent, but these reports should serve to remind the practicing orthopaedic surgeon that any microorganism can participate in osteomyelitic disease and that properly prepared smears and cultures in the hands of the professional microbiologists constitute a crucial part in the diagnosis and therapy of any particular case.

Traumatic secondary osteomyelitis

Secondary osteomyelitis following trauma may yield any and several microorganisms reflecting the microbial populations of the body surface as well as that of the external environment. The most effective antimicrobial treatment in such cases is the time-honored meticulous cleaning out of wounds, fractures, and adjacent areas. This mechanical debridement will remove physically the vast majority of microorganisms and deprive them of their nutrient milieu as well as the foreign bodies so essential for their survival and proliferation. Further bleeding and exudation within the affected site should be curtailed as much as possible.

Microbiologic monitoring of the surgical procedure attending trauma to bone can serve as a very useful guide for the orthopaedist. While not all of the microorganisms demonstrated in smears and cultures may become involved in disease production, their recognition and the knowledge of their antibiotic susceptibilities provide the clinician with the means of specific therapy at the local and the systemic level at the onset of clinical symptoms.

Nosocomial secondary osteomyelitis

The advances in medicine during the past decades have engendered another type of secondary infectious disease that affects, in no small measure, the outcome of surgical manipulations by the orthopaedic surgeon and that plays an important, though often ignored, role in the health of all patients who require prolonged stays in institutions. Nosocomial or hospital-acquired infectious disease is, of course, not limited to the surgical specialties but encompasses all manner of patients. It is a disease characterized by the nature of the microorganisms that are its purveyors and the nature of the patients affected, most frequently those who must reside in institutions for long periods, who are debilitated regardless of the underlying disease, who are exposed to chemotherapeutic agents and/or immunosuppressive drugs, as well as the individuals with various indwelling catheters or those who receive transplants or artificial implants. Perhaps the most striking feature of the disease is that no patient is admitted with the disease. It is a peculiar and particular feature of hospital life.

It is only proper that the clinician as well as the public should inquire into the causes of nosocomial disease and *a priori* implicate the institutions. But even before politicians and economists discovered the expediencies of environment and ecology, scientists have pointed to the selective pressures exerted by widespread and indiscriminate uses of any of the various new agents isolated or synthesized with the express purpose of curtailing harmful microorganisms. The selective pressures exerted by this uncontrolled usage have results that have become obvious to any and all interested in the dangers of unbridled interference with the natural ecologic order. Nosocomial disease is but another example of this disregard. The environmental pressures for the selection of antibiotic-resistant microorganisms, many of which were not found in man's intimate environment a few years ago but extant in today's institutions, is not solely or even to a large degree the result of the medical application of antibiotic drugs. The "wonder drugs" of two decades ago have found widespread use in the food-producing and food-preparing industries, where they serve to increase the yield of product per unit of feed, prolong the shelf life of produce, protect against spoilage, etc. Antibiotics have found their way into many products of the cosmetic industries and probably into some which have so far escaped detection. This continuous exposure of the total population to small amounts of antibiotic agents, coupled with the "enlightened" public's demand for antibiotic relief of minor infectious diseases not responsive to these medications, has effected a gradual change in the normal or indigenous microbiota of each individual. It has been stated earlier that the individual's very own microbial population is an essentially beneficial factor as long as good health prevails. Undoubtedly, even the antibiotic-

modified microbial population fulfills this role if there is no need for therapy. It must be quite obvious, on the other hand, that the contribution of patients to the institutional microbiota is composed, in part, of the resistant microorganisms harbored by each. These Protista in today's hospitals face higher doses and the most potent agents, in combination with sicker patients and a host of modalities designed and used without thought to their role as breeding places for highly resistant microorganisms with the capability to counteract these benefits.

We must also bring to this discussion, and for very serious consideration, the unfortunate realization that physicians and hospital personnel have forgotten the techniques that prevented the spread of contagious disease. Instead, a fervent, quasi-religious belief in antiseptic and antimicrobial molecules has been substituted. While successful originally, the advances on many medical fronts are threatened today by this neglect. Disinfectants and antiseptics are used improperly, that is, not in accordance with the manufacturer's prescription. Antibiotic and cytotoxic agents are applied without regard to their effects on other unrelated host systems and conditions. Even hand-washing and isolation techniques are no longer accorded the meticulous attention they deserve. Inhalation equipment is ignored as an important vector, along with the role of the various catheters and plastic implants as avenues for microorganisms that take full advantage of the host's initial reaction to a foreign body. In surgery the stress of anesthesia, blood loss, psychological strain, etc. adds further dimensions to this challenge. Thus it has been our experience, shared undoubtedly with many orthopaedic surgeons, that the implantation of any prosthetic device, whether metal or plastic, leads to infectious complications with mounting frequency. The reaction may not be immediate and can become manifest after years, unfortunately without providing the answer to the insistent query, were the organisms responsible left in situ at the time of surgery or implantation and carried dormant throughout this time period, or were the causative microbes sequestered serendipically from blood by the anomalous structure left in place? Still, many of the recent complications of implantation measures to correct orthopaedic defects regardless of their causes have been manifestations of microorganisms that must be considered hospital acquired. These are primarily bacteria which, as stated earlier, were unknown or unappreciated in the human environment and the human infectious disease process. They display a great deal of clinical and laboratory resistance to many, if not all, antimicrobial drugs, and in many laboratories and on many wards their role in the disease process is ignored. These nosocomially significant bacteria are a dynamic collection of various and varying taxonomic composition. Some are well known, such as certain bacteriophage types of *Staphylococcus aureus;* others are not. Thus we find not only several variants of *Pseudomonas aeruginosa,* still by far the most common, but also *P. fluorescens, P. maltophilia, P. stutzeri,* etc. They are joined by various species of the genus *Aeromonas* and *Flavobacterium* or by a group that has aroused much passion among the microbial taxonomists, the commonly called *Mima polymorpha, Herellea vaginicola,* and *Mima polymorpha* var. *oxidans.* The old and always ignored genus *Alcaligenes* has now been demonstrated as a contributor to the nosocomial scene. Indeed, the unsuspected genus *Aerobacter* has really gained notoriety in nosocomial disease under the new name *Enterobacter* and four well-defined species, *E. aerogenes, E. cloacae, E. liquefaciens,* and *E. hafniae,* in the company of a close relative and member of the tribe, pigmented and nonpigmented *Serratia.* Even old friends such as *Escherichia coli,* enterococci, anaerobic streptococci, and *Bacteroides* have emerged as bacteria isolated not infrequently from the various diseases acquired during hospital stays, including those persons with extensive orthopaedic repairs. Perhaps the most significant finding in our experience has been the isolation of *Proteus morganii* in over 80 of 100 cases of hip implantations in patients older than 65 years who developed secondary infectious complications. Of course, this experience is limited to one large municipal hospital, but *P. morganii* was not isolated from any other osteomyelitis patient present for as long and simultaneously with the elderly hip repair candidates.

Antibiotic therapy

All the bacteria recently complicating procedures share one feature, one characteristic: they are resistant to most available antibiotic drugs when tested by the usual laboratory procedures. It is significant that this aspect be quite clear. The usual laboratory test employed in most laboratories is the agar-diffusion or disk test that permits, using standardized and FDA-certified medicated paper disks, the evaluation of a bacterium's response to an antibiotic agent in concentrations that approach those in the human host following parenteral administration of the drug. The test ignores, of necessity, the pharmacologic and physiologic attributes that must be considered by physicians who prescribe the treatment. This state-

ment in no way diminishes the importance of laboratory guidance for the proper and specific treatment of bacterial infectious disease. It emphasizes the need to combine the laboratory results with each specific clinical application. This is especially significant when topical or local treatment can be used, as in the case of many orthopaedic situations. Here much higher levels of antimicrobial agents can be attained in the circumscribed and limited environment of involved bone. The laboratory guidance for such antibiotic uses should and can be tailored specifically to this need.

The effective use of antibiotic drugs is predicated on an appreciation of their action on the microorganism. The cardinal rule of antibiotic therapy is the recognition that antibiotic agents can act only on actively proliferating microorganisms. This is true of the bactericidal as well as of the bacteriostatic agents. It explains the ineffectiveness of chemotherapy in chronic infectious disease and the persistence of microorganisms in the host's tissues or cells, protected against the destructive action of antibiotics by the expedient restraint of growth. The size and possibly the life cycles of most Protista make their detection difficult if not impossible unless active growth takes place. In time this has come to mean that proliferation is equivalent to microbial life, nonproliferation to microbial death. This distinction obscures physiologic, nonproliferative activities of microorganisms and denies their survival over many years in tissues interrupted frequently or rarely by periods of activity that may become manifest as exacerbations of acute clinical symptoms.

Perhaps more significant is the fundamental lesson to be learned about the decisive role of the host in the eventual success of chemotherapy. Regardless of the advertised mode of action of the drug used, it is comparatively rare and only in the presence of very susceptible, actively growing bacteria that "cidal" levels of the antibiotic are achieved within the microenvironment of the actual disease process. In most instances the antibiotic content achieved is sufficient to prevent further increases in microbial particles. The various specific and nonspecific host factors can now catch up with the situation, which could have grown out of hand if the microorganisms had increased their numbers unchecked. The successful use of antibiotic agents is therefore based on the host's ability to deal effectively with the offending microorganisms.

Much has been made of the mode of action of antimicrobial chemotherapeutic agents. The reasoning that bactericidal drugs are to be preferred is logically, therapeutically, and theoretically sound, but frequently ignored by the very bacteria it ought to affect the most. The commonly used agents can be grouped together in the order that they achieve their inhibiting effects. The group that prevents the synthesis of cell wall constituents encompasses the penicillins, the cephalosporanic acid derivatives, and most of the drugs reputed to be bactericidal. Most other frequently employed agents such as the tetracyclines, the macrolides, the aminoglycosides, and chloramphenicol act by interfering with some stage or stages in the sequence of protein synthesis, most often at the level of ribosomal function. Some antibiotics such as the polymyxins have detergent-like qualities, while still others interfere by the competitive inhibition of enzyme reactions.

Unfortunately the microbial world did not hold still for the agents directed against them by man's ingenious exploitation of their fellow microorganisms' end products. Instead, it became quite obvious immediately that certain Protista were unaffected by certain antibiotics, that is, were "*naturally*" resistant to their action. Others, quite susceptible initially, displayed resistance eventually. Still others remained susceptible to the same agents over long periods. Several different and unrelated mechanisms account for these manifestations, not all of which are understood completely. It is obvious that a number of bacterial mutants display varying degrees of resistance to certain agents. In an environment containing such agents the mutant bacterium can proliferate and become established for as long as the selective pressure of the antibiotic is maintained. This situation also brings about the change in the qualitative composition of environmental microbiota, permitting microorganisms with natural resistance to various antibiotic agents to occupy the ecologic niches formerly occupied by antibiotic-susceptible groups. Resistance to several antibiotics resides in the ability of the mutant bacterium to elaborate enzymes that destroy or render ineffective specific agents. The classic example is penicillin and many of its derivatives, which are destroyed by penicillin-β-lactamase or penicillinase. Some other bacteria disarm the penicillins by elaborating a penicillin amidase that attacks the molecule at a different site. Chloramphenicol acetyl transferase is the enzyme involved in the resistance displayed to chloramphenicol. Similarly, the ability of resistant bacteria to acetylate or phosphorylate neomycin and paromomycin and adenylate or phosphorylate streptomycin gives evidence that the understanding of drug resistance is emerging from its dark ages and wild

guesses at mechanisms. More important, this comprehension may pave the way to measures that prevent the development and the selection of resistant organisms by manipulating the molecular arrangements of functional groups required for the action of these enzymes.

It is noteworthy that resistance to antibiotics can be communicated from one gram-negative bacterium to another by the transfer of an extra chromosomal piece of DNA, the resistance transfer factor (RTF). At this time this phenomenon involves the transfer of multiple resistance from donor to recipient cells without the need of exposure to the antibiotic agent. The selective pressures in the developed countries are such that these bacteria are maintained, although their chances of survival without the inhibition of the competing wild types may be slim. In gram-positive organisms, in which several of these mechanisms have not been demonstrated, transduction and lysogenization may account for the behavior of staphylococci vis-à-vis most antibiotics. In this process, bacteriophages carry the resistance marker to the recipient. If they are not virulent viruses with the recipient strain, the viral DNA becomes intimately associated with the bacterial DNA and imparts to the bacterium the capacity to resist antimicrobial agents.

It is not at all clear yet which of these mechanisms is the most common or if some others may not account for the rapid appearance of resistance. Whether mutational or infective, the problem of microbial resistance to the many agents in the clinician's armamentarium is real, pressing, and threatens the usefulness of the newest and latest agents, often before they become available to the public. The only present means of stemming the tide of antibiotic-resistant microbial populations is through the use of specific therapy, based on laboratory guidance, and administered in adequate doses over an adequate period of time.

Therapy without proper guidance

The practicing orthopaedic surgeon is justified, however, to register his disappointment that this discussion has not dealt with the practical situation he encounters frequently. No organism was isolated, often because no attempt was made to obtain a specimen for smear and cultural analysis. No other laboratory guidance data have been developed that would rule out certain bacteria and suggest, presumptively at least, others. The dilemma of choosing an antibiotic becomes very acute under these circumstances. There is, of course, no ready answer; no authoritative directive can be issued by anyone despite the conviction with which the use of certain agents has been touted as a panacea for all infectious disorders of bone. The only guide that can be offered is a series of educated guesses. Thus first consideration should be given to the most likely organism involved after the usual historic facts about the patient and his present illness have been established. If it is a primary osteomyelitis in an otherwise healthy young individual who has not been institutionalized recently, who is not sickly, and who has not had symptoms of food poisoning or other "minor" disorders, the chances that this patient's disease involves an ordinary staphylococcus are good, and penicillin therapy is indicated, monitored carefully with the usual laboratory examinations used to follow in an admittedly secondary manner the progress of the patient. The subacute or chronic osteomyelitic patient presents treatment problems that are almost insurmountable without some clue to the bacterium involved. It is at this juncture that the clinician must recall that the effectiveness of the antibiotic agent is limited to bacteria that proliferate actively, a circumstance unlikely in any chronic disorder. Long-term, adequate dosage treatment with a hopefully effective agent is the only choice. The possibility of L-form involvement, although never established satisfactorily, must be taken into account in deciding on the medication, and the macrolide agents or closely related drugs should receive serious consideration. These same agents— oleandomycin, erythromycin, and lincomycin—also deserve application when penicillin allergy is established or suspected in a patient.

The use of penicillin-β-lactamase (penicillinase)– resistant penicillins should not be entertained unless laboratory proof of the presence of penicillin-β-lactamase–producing organisms is provided or the history of the patient suggests the strong possibility that such bacteria may be involved in the disease process.

The increasing importance of gram-negative, rod-shaped bacteria has been mentioned already. No doubt, secondary osteomyelitis can be caused by these bacteria. They can be suspected to be involved in this disease, especially if the osteomyelitic process is secondary to surgical manipulation. Laboratory proof of this involvement is essential and should be obtained. Great care must be exercised in obtaining a proper specimen representative of the very nidus of infectious disease rather than of bacteria growing into the area from surrounding tissues and skin. The significant contribution of a smear to the clinical and microbiologic evaluation of the lesion must also be

reemphasized. Still, the concerned physician feels compelled on many occasions not to delay treatment while waiting for reports and wishes to initiate therapy, subject to change if laboratory guidance so indicates. In such cases, therapy with cephalothin, kanamycin, chloramphenicol, or gentamicin, not necessarily in this order, can be initiated. If an original inciter of the process cannot be obtained in the laboratory, therapy with high doses (100 million units/day) of penicillin or 14 Gm. of cephalothin can be administered with minimal toxic challenges to the patient.

General guide to treatment

The most practical guidelines for the treatment of osteomyelitis are rather simple.

1. The first requirement is systemic. Natural resistance and immunity must be enhanced by blood transfusion when necessary, in addition to the previously mentioned antibiotics, antisera, and antitoxins, so that any systemic disease can be brought under control and localized.

The second requirement is local treatment. The localized lesion must be dealt with along surgical principles that apply to the accumulation of infectious material anywhere. Incision, evacuation, and drainage is a time-honored surgical procedure. In many cases, saucerization and windowing of the bone are necessary. Adequate drainage must be maintained as long as reaccumulation of infected material requires it. Closed drainage (irrigation and suction) is one of the best means of effecting this treatment. We recommend the technique of Compere and associates[3] in which sterile Alevaire is used as the detergent. Alevaire, for which streptokinase or streptodornase may be substituted, is placed in normal saline solution and an appropriate antibiotic added. Systemic treatment is, of course, continued. Multiperforated plastic tubes are laid in the wound, each about ⅛ inch in diameter, and a ¼- to ½-inch outlet tube is attached for suction. We usually wash through 2 to 3 L. of solution in 24 hours, but this varies with the site and size of the area involved. The effluent is cultured daily. When it is negative for at least 3 to 4 days and all systemic symptoms have subsided, it is usually discontinued. We agree with Compere and associates that the detergent seems to enhance the effectiveness of the antibiotic and the mechanical debridement.

As part of the local treatment, we must not forget the importance of immobilization using casts, splints, and braces. By resting the part, healing is encouraged and spread of the lesion is minimized. Immobilization not only adds to the patient's comfort but helps avoid catastrophes such as pathologic fractures, with their subsequent morbidity and possible disabling deformity.

In chronic osteomyelitis the dreaded specter of amputation often appears. It may become necessary to amputate, not only because of malignant degeneration of a sinus tract, which fortunately occurs infrequently, but because some infections may become persistent and uncontrollable. Destruction due to infection may also be so extensive that, even after healing, part of the involved limb may become functionally useless.

2. Therapy should not be shorter than 6 weeks and preferably 12 weeks. Intravenous administration is preferable to the oral route, as is the intramuscular route, avoiding the hazards that accompany oral antibiotic therapy.

3. The patient's response should be monitored microbiologically, immunologically if need be, with specially devised tests and with the various other accepted laboratory examinations.

4. There is a great need to distinguish between microorganisms present originally in the lesion and those encountered later in or near the operative site, in drain tracts, and under casts. Unless there is irrefutable proof that a second microorganism has become established within the deep recesses of the bone and is initiating a disease process all its own, a rare occurrence, therapy need not be changed. Instead, care of the wound and cast should be reviewed and measures instituted to assure proper sanitation of the area. Even *Pseudomonas* acting as a secondary opportunist can be controlled with such simple measures as irrigation with 0.25% acetic acid under a cast or in the neighborhood of a wound.

5. Actual application or installation of the therapeutic agent into the area of the lesion through the drain is the most direct and successful way to cope with the offending microorganism. The high concentrations of drugs achieved in this manner are successful even with those bacteria shown to be resistant to them in the laboratory. The laboratory evaluation of antibiotic susceptibility deals with levels attainable by the oral or parenteral routes. It does not encompass the much higher values attainable by topical application. Cooperation between the orthopaedic and microbiologic services can lead to the evaluation of the drug effect on the organism in concentrations comparable to those applied directly. This modality of treatment is especially useful during the initial postoperative weeks when continuous or frequent application of the antibiotic is most efficient.

The effluent should be monitored for cells and bacteria. Many of the antibiotic agents not considered for parenteral administration or accompanied by undesirable side effects can be used in this manner since absorption from the site of irrigation is minimal.

Recently it has been suggested that hyperbaric oxygen treatment might have salutary effects on osteomyelitis. In very active osteomyelitis, antibiotics are certainly more effective. In the chronic phase, hyperbaric oxygen may injure or kill a few bacteria unable to cope with the increase in partial oxygen pressure, but it is unlikely that an adequate pressure differential can be achieved in bone. It may be that, as Sledge and Dingle[13] have proposed, hyperbaric oxygen increases lysosome activity, which may account for the observed response. Certainly at this stage more evidence is needed to recommend such therapy universally.

Perhaps the most significant suggestion for the orthopaedic clinician is to remind him of the dynamic state of infectious disease and to recommend that the only constant of the host-parasite interaction in osteomyelitis and any other infectious disease is the inconsistency of the parasites, the hosts, and the drugs. It may well be that this continuing challenge to the ingenuity of all involved in the care and treatment of these patients provides the basis for the perennial preoccupation of several professions with this disease.

REFERENCES

1. Burnett, F. M.: Natural history of infectious disease, ed. 3, Cambridge, 1962, Cambridge University Press.
2. Cawson, D. K., and Dunn, A. W.: Management of common bacterial infections of bones and joints, J. Bone Joint Surg. **49-A:**164, 1967.
3. Compere, E. L., Metzger, W. I., and Mitra, R. N.: The treatment of pyogenic bone and joint infections by closed irrigation (circulation) with a non-toxic detergent and one or more antibiotics, J. Bone Joint Surg. **49-A:**614, 1967.
4. Dubos, R. J.: The evolution and the ecology of microbial diseases. In Dubos, R. J., editor: Bacterial and mycotic infections of man, ed. 3, Philadelphia, 1958, J. B. Lippincott Co.
5. Elek, S. D.: Staphylococcus pyogenes, London, 1959, E. & S. Livingston, Ltd.
6. Gladstone, G. P., Mudd, S., Hochstein, H. D., and Lenhart, N. A.: The assay of anti-staphylococcal leucocidal components (F and S) in human serum, Brit. J. Exp. Path. **43:**295, 1962.
7. Hobo, T.: Zur Pathogenese der akuten haematogenen Osteomyelitis, mit Berucksichtgung der vital Farbungslehre, Acta Sch. Med. Univ. Imp. Kioto **4:**1, 1921.
8. Isenberg, H. D.: The origin of microbial life on earth and its implications for extra-terrestrial forms, Exobiology **19:**63, 1969.

9. Isenberg, H. D.: Indigenous and pathogenic micro-organisms of man. In Blair, J. E., Lennette, E. H., and Truant, J. P., editors: Manual of clinical microbiology, Bethesda, 1970, American Society for Microbiology.

10. Lack, C. H., and Towers, A. G.: Serological tests for staphylococcal infection, Brit. Med. J. **2:**1227, 1962.

11. Markham, N. P.: A haemagglutination test for staphylococcal antileucocidin, J. Clin. Path. **15:**54, 1962.

12. Rosebury, T.: Microorganisms indigenous to man, New York, 1961, McGraw-Hill Book Co., Inc.

13. Sledge, C. B., and Dingle, T. J.: Activation of lysosomes by oxygenation. Oxygen-induced resorption of cartilage in organ culture, Nature **205:**140, 1965.

14. Smith, T.: Parasitism and disease, Princeton, 1934, Princeton University Press.

15. Trueta, J.: The three types of acute hematogenous osteomyelitis: a clinical and vascular study, J. Bone Joint Surg. **41-A:**671, 1959.

16. Waldvogel, F. A., Medoff, G., and Swartz, M. N.: Osteomyelitis: a review of clinical features and unusual aspects, New Eng. J. Med. **282:**198, 1970.

17. Wilson, G. S., and Miles, A. A.: Topley and Wilson's principles of bacteriology and immunology, ed. 5, Baltimore, 1964, The Williams & Wilkins Co.

18. Winters, J. L., and Cahen, I.: Acute hematogenous osteomyelitis: a review of sixty-six cases, J. Bone Joint Surg. **42-A:**691, 1960.

Chapter 2

Orthopaedic management of hemophilia

A. JACKSON DAY, M.D.
Detroit, Michigan

The term "hemophilia" was apparently first used in 1820 by Johann Lukas Schönlein of Wurzburg to describe a disease of bleeding tendency, although the disease itself was known for hundreds of years previously. In the past 75 years there has been extensive research into the blood-clotting mechanism. To identify the deficiency in clotting, Roman numerals have been assigned to various factors such as fibrinogen, prothrombin, and thromboplastin. Almost all hemophiliacs may be divided into two groups, with 85% belonging to hemophilia type A, or factor VIII deficiency, and with 15% belonging to hemophilia type B, or factor IX deficiency, also known as Christmas disease. Hemophilia is a disease of the male carried by the female, although it is theoretically possible to have a female hemophiliac. The first sign of the disease often occurs following a bruise or bleeding after minor trauma or after extraction of teeth, epistaxis, circumcision, or tonsillectomy; occasionally hematuria may be the first sign. The appearance of the bruise in a hemophiliac is unusual and is characteristic in that the center point of impact causes general bleeding in a full circle outwardly and thus there is a choking off of the center area. The center area remains white and the discoloration occurs around the white center area (Fig. 2-1). Aside from bruising, there can be hematomas in the soft tissues of the extremities or of the trunk, and in the past some of these hematomas have been quite enormous.

There are many degrees of severity of hemophilia and this may be described as a percentage of the antihemophilic factor present, as measured against the normal amount. Thus the hemophiliac with a severe defect may have more frequent hemorrhages in more different locations than one with a milder case, and the methods of treatment and the results obtained should be discussed in terms of the severity of the disease.

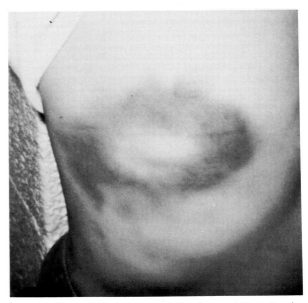

Fig. 2-1. Characteristic bruise of the hemophiliac showing the white center and pigmented periphery.

HEMATOLOGIC MANAGEMENT

It has been known for some time that blood plasma contained antihemophilic factor or anithemophilic globulin, often termed AHF or AHG. Such a large volume of blood plasma, however, is necessary to raise the titer of AHG that whole-blood plasma transfusion is not a practical therapeutic measure. The breakthrough occurred in 1965 when Judith Pool of Stanford developed the cryoprecipitated factor. This factor VIII material, however, has a half-life from 6 to 8 hours at ordinary temperatures and must be stored at −20° to −30° C. The cryoprecipitated plasma is now being produced in considerable quantity and there is no waste in its production because

15

the nonprecipitated plasma may be used for other purposes and also for the production of factor IX. Unfortunately the supply has not yet been adequate to meet the demands. There are also other plasma concentrates being produced commercially; the glycine-precipitated product is stable and dried, although as yet it is rather costly and also in short supply. In addition, factor IX concentrate is also available commercially. Since the commercial preparations are made from pooled plasma, there is a somewhat higher incidence of hepatitis than in the cryoprecipitated plasma.

The great advantage to the new plasma concentrates, however, is in the facility of treatment. If there is no other reason for hospitalizing a patient with a fresh hemorrhage, this patient may be treated on an outpatient basis, receiving the small amount of plasma concentrate in the office or clinic; and since there is an increase in the AHG titer in the blood from repeated injections of the concentrate, there is much better control of the disease and the orthopaedic complications are greatly reduced.

HEMARTHROSIS

Hemorrhage into joints is quite common in the hemophiliac, occurring in the knee, elbow, ankle, shoulder, wrist, and hip, the frequency being reduced in that order. When the hemorrhage distends the joint with blood, the joint becomes very painful and motion is greatly restricted. After the intravenous administration of AHG, it is assumed that the bleeding gradually stops and the blood is absorbed. If motion, and particularly excessive motion, should begin too soon after an acute hemorrhage, it is likely that the bleeding point will open and further hemorrhage may occur. It is advisable that the level of AHG be kept as high as possible with continued plasma concentrate therapy or injections for at least a day or two.

Management of acute hemarthroses

There is some difference of opinion concerning the orthopaedic management of acute hemarthrosis. In our hospital it has been the consensus of the hematologists and the orthopaedists that intermittent or continual distention of the joint with blood is detrimental to the health of the articular cartilage, and if this occurs over a protracted period of time, a nonspecific arthritis develops. It is believed that the elements of the decomposed blood deprives the articular cartilage of the normal nutrients so that a softening and breakdown of cartilage occur. There is a cellular infiltration of the synovium, and as the scarring takes place, a hyperplastic layer grows over the articular cartilage. Granulation tissue begins to replace subchondral bone and the resulting arthritis eventually resembles the changes of hypertrophic arthritis. Secondarily, the pain produced by these changes causes joint contractures and muscle atrophy (Fig. 2-2).

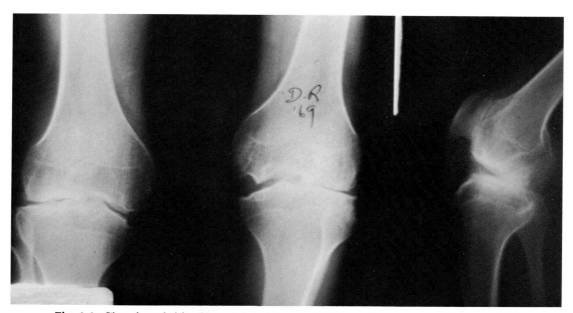

Fig. 2-2. Chronic arthritis of knee joint after repeated hemarthroses over a 10-year period.

In the treatment of acute hemarthrosis the orthopaedic management is directed toward the early aspiration of the joint as soon as the intravenous plasma concentrate has been given. Aspiration of the joint relieves pain and, as mentioned before, prevents the accumulation of the elements of the breakdown of blood that deprives the joint surface of nutrition. After the aspiration, in order to prevent motion in the joint, a so-called soft cast is applied. This consists of wrapping the extremity well above and below the involved joint with many layers of cotton cast padding such as *webril*. After five or six large rolls are applied, one outer layer of moderately stretched, elastic bandage is then applied. This large dressing allows only 5° to 10° of motion in the involved joint and makes the joint much more comfortable. After 4 to 7 days this soft cast is either removed entirely or reduced in thickness so that some increase in motion can be obtained. After a week to 10 days all external immobilization is discontinued and active exercising is started, but with a diminished amount of total activity. Thus for a weight-bearing joint the amount of walking is restricted and no running or jumping allowed until healing is complete.

It must be acknowledged that in some clinics aspiration of hemarthroses is not carried out. There has been no study found in the literature that actually compares these two methods of treatment. At our hospital we feel that the residual changes are much reduced by aspiration of the hemarthrosis.

Management of chronic hemarthroses

Hemophilia occurs with many degrees of severity. Some boys will have only an occasional hemarthrosis, whereas others will have many recurrences, the hemorrhages occurring in many different joints and often with little or no trauma. In this latter group, contractures have developed because of the repeated episodes of pain. Before a joint has regained its full range of motion after an acute hemorrhage, a second hemorrhage may occur, causing renewed pain and swelling, and over a period of time, fixed contractures develop. The most important therapy for the contracted joint is traction. For the mildly contracted knee joint, simple Buck's traction is very effective in overcoming pain and tightness and allows mobility at the same time. For contractures of more than 30°, Russell's traction is indicated because of the tendency for posterior subluxation of the tibia. Traction is also valuable for the hip and sometimes for the elbow. Bracing is better used as an intermittent device rather than continuously. For the knee, we use long cylinder braces with adjustable knee angles so that some pressure can be applied to straighten the knee, but these braces are worn only part time and are used in conjunction with active assisted exercise. Braces should be carefully aligned since a malaligned brace may be a factor in increasing the bleeding. Dynamic foot drop braces can be used at night to stretch contracted heel cords and overcome equinus deformities of the ankle. In some cases an acute hemorrhage oc-

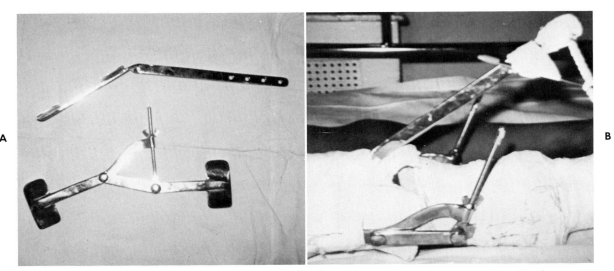

Fig. 2-3. A, Apparatus for the application of a Quengel cast to straighten a contracted and subluxated knee joint. **B,** Application of the Quengel apparatus to a cast to overcome the posterior subluxation of the tibia before twisting the windlass to correct the contracture.

curs in a knee joint that already has a flexion contracture. In these cases, after aspiration of the joint, a soft cotton cast is applied, and in the outer layers, anteriorly and posteriorly, medium corset stays are incorporated to exert a mild pressure to straighten the joint.

In some of our older patients who developed contractures prior to 1966, some knee contractures have been difficult to handle. As in any type of painful joint, the muscle spasm of the hamstrings produces a posterior displacement of the tibia on the femoral condyles and any attempt at correcting the deformity must be directed toward eliminating the subluxation before the straightening takes place. The Quengel cast developed by Momsen is a device for correcting the posterior placement of the tibia before any wedging is carried out to straighten the leg (Fig. 2-3). This is a tedious procedure and requires constant attention to small daily wedgings and subsequently managed physiotherapy to improve the range of motion and prevent recurrence of the contracture. Improper use of the Quengel cast may cause new hemorrhages and stiffness of the knee; therefore traction is a better method in the hands of the novice. In some of the chronic cases, ambulatory braces are worthwhile to correct contractures and these may be worn continuously or intermittently after episodes of hemarthrosis. Night splints or plaster shells may also be used to prevent injury and to avoid contracture, particularly in the juvenile patient.

Steroids

Steroids have been used in two ways in the management of hemophiliacs. It is reported that oral steroids have been used at the time of an acute hemarthrosis in addition to the use of concentrated plasma. Some benefit has been ascribed to this use of steroids, but there has been no explanation as to why it should be true since it has no effect on raising the titer of AHG or of even prolonging its half-life. Intra-articular use of hydrocortisone has been reported to be of some benefit. After the aspiration of an acute hemarthrosis, hydrocortisone may be instilled into the joint and this has tended to reduce pain and discomfort and perhaps speed the restoration of function.

SURGICAL PROCEDURES IN HEMOPHILIACS

Although surgical procedures such as appendectomy and operations to correct pyloric stenosis were done prior to the development of the plasma concentrates, elective procedures have now become a reality.

For any elective surgical procedure some preparation is made to have an ample supply of plasma concentrate available for postoperative use. Obviously, some surgical procedures would offer a greater hazard than others and an extensive supply of plasma concentrate should be available before surgery is undertaken. Elective surgery such as repair of hernias and extraction of teeth are now done when desired. Orthopaedic operations are being undertaken with more and more courage. Heel cord contractures can be overcome by Achilles tendon lengthening and posterior capsulotomy. Arthrodesis of the knee joint has been performed many times. Osteotomies near the knee have been done to correct fixed contractures, and some open reductions of fractures have been performed. Storti and associates[7] reported the use of synovectomy in some eleven cases, ten on the knee and one on the ankle joint. In our clinic we have not seen chronically swollen, boggy knees for which synovectomy would be indicated.

There has been no long experience with the hema-

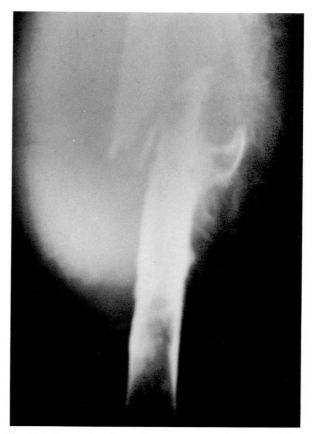

Fig. 2-4. Example of pseudotumor reported by Schneider.

tologic management for surgical procedures. If the AHG titer is kept at about 50% of the normal level during the first 2 or 3 days after surgery, it has been possible to reduce the amount of plasma and hold it at a 10% to 25% level during the next week or two. There have been reports of some bleeding occurring 2 weeks after an operation, but no firm rule can be established as to the length of the period of plasma therapy and this would certainly depend on the nature of the surgery also.

HEMOPHILIAC PSEUDOTUMOR

Mention should be made of the hemophiliac pseudotumor, a very unusual destructive disorder in bone that is believed to be started by hemorrhage that is either subperiosteal or within the bone and produces a pressure necrosis. Hemorrhage into the marrow space may cause bony sclerosis and destruction and new bone may be produced. Consequently, the x-ray appearance is misleading and may give the appearance of a sarcoma or of osteomyelitis (Fig. 2-4). Pathologic fractures are very common. An excellent review of pseudotumors was given by Bailey and co-workers[2] and a summary of the thirty-three cases reported in the world literature has been published by Schneider.[6] The treatment of this condition is, of course, plasma therapy and, for the developed pseudotumor, either excision or amputation.

SUMMARY

The treatment of hemophilia has been vastly altered and improved by the development of plasma concentrates containing AHG. Since it is easily given as an intravenous injection on an outpatient basis, it may be used prophylactically and in the very early treatment of any type of hemorrhage. The formation of large hematomas and extensive hemarthroses can be prevented. In the course of a few years the orthopaedic management has changed; there is now greater emphasis on mobilization of joints and prevention of deformities rather than on correction of contractures. It is probable that the number of severely arthritic hemophiliac joints will be much reduced and will be present only in the severe degrees of hemophilia. Elective surgical procedures may be undertaken whenever an adequate supply of plasma concentrates can be obtained for use during surgery and the projected postoperative course of treatment. One may predict that with the improved control of hemorrhage, few if any pseudotumors will be found in the future.

REFERENCES

1. Ahlberg, A.: Treatment and prophylaxis of arthropathy in severe hemophilia, Clin. Orthop. **53**:135, 1967.
2. Bailey, R. W., Penner, J. A., and Korte, G. J.: Successful excision of pseudotumor of hemophilia, Surg. Forum **16**:464, 1965.
3. DePalma, A. F.: Hemophiliac arthropathy, Clin. Orthop. **52**:145, 1967.
4. Ghormley, R. K., and Clegg, R. S.: Bone and joint changes in hemophilia, J. Bone Joint Surg. **30-A**:589, 1948.
5. Kisker, C. T., and Burke, C.: Double-blind studies on the use of steroids in the treatment of acute hemarthrosis in patients with hemophilia, New Eng. J. Med. **282**:639, 1970.
6. Schneider, J. R.: Hemophilic pseudotumor, Harper Hosp. Bull. **25**:270, 1967.
7. Storti, E., Traldi, A., Tosatti, E., and Davoli, P. G.: Synovectomy, a new approach to haemophilic arthropathy, Acta Haemat. **41**:193, 1969.

Chapter 3

Cerebral palsy

Part I
General principles

J. LEONARD GOLDNER, M.D.
Durham, North Carolina

Management of a child with cerebral palsy requires a thorough understanding of the many facets associated with this affectation of the neuromuscular system. The primary pathologic process is in the brain. Location of the particular lesions has been reasonably well documented by autopsy studies and by the work of Winders with a monkey colony. A physician caring for an infant or child with slow motor development, hypotonic extremities, slowness in the use of one extremity, or other aberrations of the musculoskeletal system must recognize pathologic reflexes and be aware of the developmental patterns of a normal infant and child as well as the genetic syndromes associated with multiple congenital defects characterized by a typical facial appearance and chromosomal aberrations.

The patient and the parents need special attention and should be aware in the beginning that cerebral palsy is an incurable condition that is nonprogressive. Improvement is usually slow and concomitant with the child's natural development. Treatment is justified and worthwhile. Many hours of particular kinds of therapy, however, are not always beneficial. Heavy bracing is usually unnecessary. Utilization of various forms of artificial stimuli have not proved successful.

The physician, in the initial assessment of the child with cerebral palsy, should know something about the patient's inherent intelligence, personality pattern, and learning ability and motivation. This requires an emotional, intellectual, and personality profile that allows definition of maximum and minimum therapy and provides the basis for future planning. The condition is nonprogressive and if noticeable changes occur in the musculoskeletal system that are regressive, then some other condition affecting the nervous system or the neuromuscular units should be suspected.

PATHOLOGIC REFLEXES
Persistence of pathologic reflexes

Certain reflexes present in the newborn infant persist for 16 to 20 weeks. These include the upward pull of the toes when the plantar surface of the foot is stimulated (Babinski's reflex), hyperactive tendon reflexes, and a neck-righting reflex. If pathologic reflexes persist, the prognosis for walking is bad.

Tests for infantile automatism

Moro reflex. The Moro reflex is tested by a sudden jarring of the table, dropping of the infant's head into extension 20° or 30°, or pinching the skin of the epigastrium. The classic reflex is sudden extension or spreading of the upper extremities (Fig. 3-1). This reflex appears by the age of 6 months but is usually absent in the normal child by 12 to 16 months. Extension is then replaced by adduction and flexion as the reaction to a sudden noise or surprise.

Head-turning reflex. The head-turning reflex is tested when the child is in the side-lying position. The head is tilted downward and rotated slightly toward the floor, and the lower extremity on the same side flexes at the hip and knee (Fig. 3-2). This involuntary reflex, if it persists, usually indicates that walking will be delayed or difficult.

Asymmetric tonic neck reflex. With the patient in the supine position, the head is rotated toward one side. If this is followed by extension of the upper and lower extremities on the face-turned side and flexion of the upper and lower extremities on the occiput side, the condition is abnormal (Fig. 3-3). The reflex usually disappears in a normal infant, if present, by 7 months.

Symmetric tonic reflex. The child is placed either in a quadriped position or in a prone position over the examiner's knee. Extension of the head causes

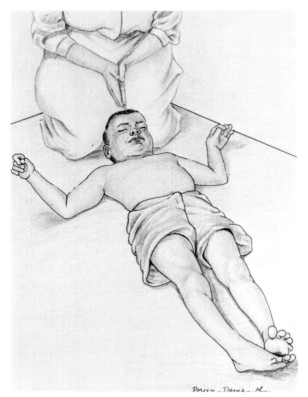

Fig. 3-1. Moro reflex. (Courtesy E. E. Bleck.)

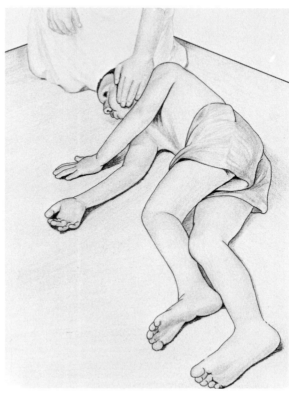

Fig. 3-2. Head-turning reflex. (Courtesy E. E. Bleck.)

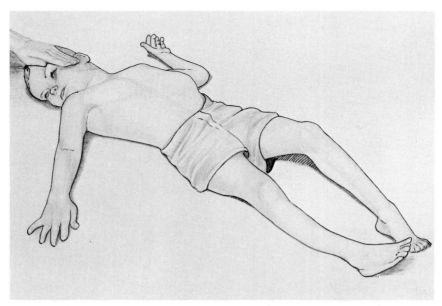

Fig. 3-3. Asymmetric tonic neck reflex. (Courtesy E. E. Bleck.)

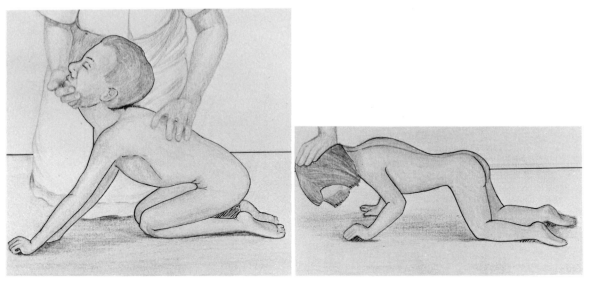

Fig. 3-4. Symmetric tonic reflex. (Courtesy E. E. Bleck.)

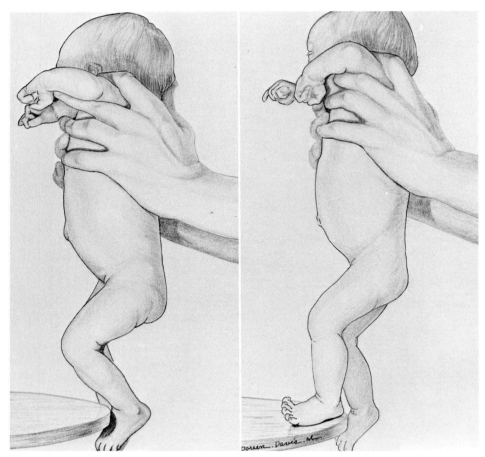

Fig. 3-5. Foot-placement reaction. (Courtesy E. E. Bleck.)

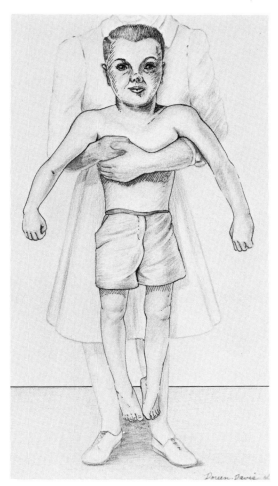

Fig. 3-6. Positive supporting reaction (extensor thrust). (Courtesy E. E. Bleck.)

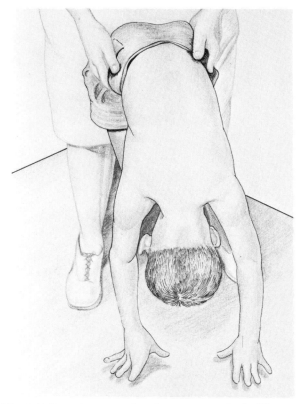

Fig. 3-7. Parachute reaction (space suspension). (Courtesy E. E. Bleck.)

extension of the forelimbs and flexion of the hind-limbs. Ventral flexion of the head causes flexion of the forelimbs and extension of the hindlimbs (Fig. 3-4). This reflex is normal up to the age of 4 to 6 months.

Foot-placement reaction. The child is held in vertical suspension with the examiner's hands under the patient's arms and lifted upward so the dorsum of the feet touch against the underside of the table. Normally one foot and then the other will be placed on the tabletop (Fig. 3-5). Occasionally both feet are placed on the table at the same time. The motor-retarded child will not place the extremities on the table, but the feet will remain under the edge of the table.

Positive supporting reaction (extensor thrust). When the child is placed in a weight-bearing position, the extremities extend at the ankles, knees, and hips and adduct and cross (Fig. 3-6). Extensor thrust is an abnormal reflex and is a bad prognostic sign for future unsupported walking.

Parachute reaction (space suspension). The child is held under the arms and tilted downward and forward. Normally an automatic extension of the upper extremities occurs, with the fingers spread as if ready to break the fall. If the head remains flexed and the upper extremities dangle, the child's motor development is obviously delayed (Fig. 3-7). This reflex appears at about the age of 9 months and persists throughout life. If the child older than 9 months does not have the parachute reaction, then neuromuscular development is deficient and the chances of walking are lessened.

Prognosis. If any two of the infantile automatisms are present or if the parachute reaction is absent, the prognosis for unsupported ambulation is bad. Sur-

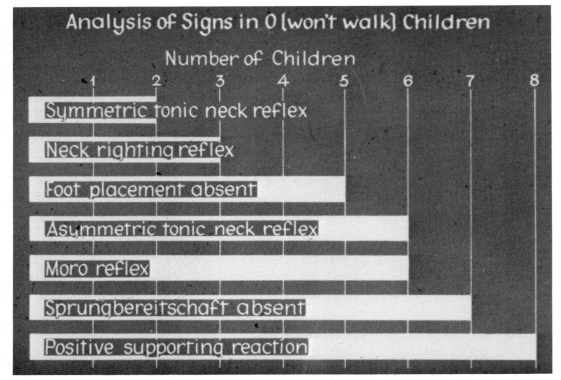

Fig. 3-8. Analysis of pathologic reflexes in children 1 to 8 years of age. (Courtesy E. E. Bleck.)

gery will not improve the child's chances of walking but will improve the ability to use side supports, diminish bracing, and increase endurance.

Bleck has carried out an analysis of pathologic reflexes in children ages 1 to 8 years. Fig. 3-8 shows the frequency of the abnormal reflexes and the comparative incidence of the signs that are significant as they appear in those children whose prognosis for walking is bad. The supporting reaction will be positive in all those children who will not walk, and the Moro startle reflex will be present in six out of eight. The symmetric tonic neck reflex persisted least frequently in the children who have a bad prognosis for walking.

ORTHOPAEDIC MANAGEMENT

The major orthopaedic involvement is exemplified in Fig. 3-9, which shows a patient with hemiplegic stance, adducted thigh, flexed knee, internally rotated hip, and equinovarus foot. Lordosis, mild scoliosis, and hip flexion contracture are part of this physical pattern also. These deformities affect gait, balance, stance, and coordination as well as speed and energy expenditure. The right upper limb is flexed at the elbow and wrist, the forearm is pronated, and the arm

is adducted. Function of this extremity, including the hand, is limited. The orthopaedic efforts are directed toward improving gait, diminishing permanent deformity, and increasing, if possible, the use and appearance of the right hand. The orthopaedist may be the team leader, a member of a group effort, or an isolated practitioner in a small community. He must establish communication with the family and other members of the medical team. Furthermore, as a part of his interest in a patient with cerebral palsy, the orthopaedist is obliged to increase and maintain his knowledge of the subject.

Knowledge of the basic principles of neuroanatomy and embryology is necessary in determining the localization of a lesion of the nervous system and in realizing the tremendous interrelationships among the systems affecting vision, balance, learning, walking, and coordination. A better understanding of the development and biochemistry of the nervous system is unfolding rapidly. Also, much useful information is obtained from those workers in the fields of child development and pediatric neurology and those who deal with the emotional conditions of both the normal and the handicapped child. Obviously, the musculoskeletal system is not the only area involved, although

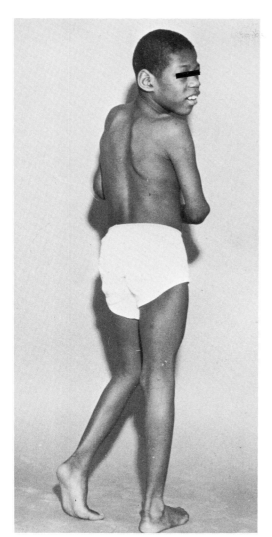

Fig. 3-9. Patient with pes equinus, knee flexion deformity secondary to equinus, and hip flexion secondary to knee position. Adduction and internal rotation are mild. The left upper extremity is also involved and is carried in the usual pattern of elbow and wrist flexion with thumb in the palm.

it may be the focus of interest for the orthopaedic surgeon. In addition to having medical and social information about the patient, the orthopaedist must have compassion for the patient and the family.

The physical assessment of the upper and lower extremities requires an understanding of the principles of gait, muscle testing, reflex determination, and the signs of spasticity. The muscle strength of an individual unit is tested by voluntary action of the patient and by the examiner palpating the muscle while motion is attempted and also applying resistance at the same time. Gross actions are determined

by observing the extremities as the patient walks, sits, stands, crawls, turns, and moves from a sitting to standing position. A muscle test is less reliable in a patient with cerebral palsy than one with flaccid paralysis. Nevertheless, information obtained from muscle testing is essential and the decision to carry out tendon transfers depends on this information. Results of the muscle test should be recorded for future reference.

The presence of spasticity is determined while muscle testing is being done or while range of joint motion is being determined. The evidence of the presence of spasticity include hyperreflexia, a stretch reflex, and clonus. All of these characteristics may not be detectable, but if all three are present, then spasticity exists without question. As the examination progresses, classification by the examiner is attempted and the extremities, hips, and spine are described as to how each relates to total body function. The patient is then described as a monoplegic with upper or lower involvement, hemiplegic, triplegic, tetraplegic (all four extremities involved), or spastic diplegic (both lower limbs affected). As a part of this total examination, a general impression is obtained concerning such characteristics as vision, hearing, speech, intelligence, and emotions, and specialized members of the team are asked to concentrate on these aspects of of the patient's condition at the appropriate time.

After the physician submits a diagnosis and recognizes obvious deficiencies and the effect of systemic problems on development and ability to sit, walk, stand, and function, a general plan for immediate care is outlined and a prognosis concerning growth and development through maturity can be hypothesized. The latter is of help to the therapist and to the family. This, of course, can be altered as progress occurs or regresses. The entire program requires the cooperative efforts of the orthopaedist, physical and occupational therapist, pediatrician, psychiatrist and psychologist, anesthesiologist, orthotist, nurse, school teacher, social worker, and other members of the group who conscientiously devote their careers to aiding the severely handicapped. Examples of patterns of management based on age of the patient will be discussed.

Newborn to 1 year of age

After the diagnosis is established, a program of external stimulation, minimal splinting, moderate stretching, and frequent observation is started. The wrist should be protected from a position of constant flexion, the foot should not be in equinus, and the thigh should be abducted if possible. The family should be made aware of the immediate deficiencies as well as any progress that occurs. The child needs handling, love, and attention.

Ages 1 to 2 years

Tremendous growth occurs during this time and tendon lengthening may be necessary if equinus or wrist flexion cannot be easily controlled. The decision depends on motor activity, progressive change, the patient's intelligence, and family cooperation. At this

age a myotomy and localized neurectomy of a superficial branch of the obturator nerve may prevent a femur from dislocating by diminishing pelvic obliquity. Balance and walking efforts will be improved if the foot is at right angles, the thigh is not adducted, the pelvis is level, and the extremities are relatively the same length. The other aspects of the program already established prior to 1 year of age are continued.

Fig. 3-10, *A*, shows a 3-year-old child with adducted

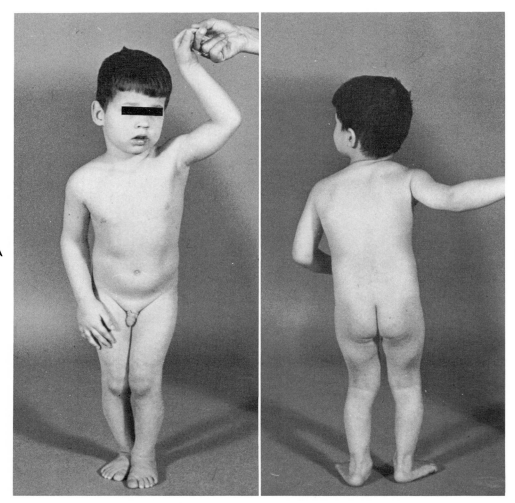

Fig. 3-10. A, A 3-year-old child with cerebral palsy who is classified as a spastic diplegic. The upper extremities are normal, the intellect is good, and the lower extremities are in equinus with the knees flexed, hips flexed, and thighs adducted. Balance is good for sitting. There is persistence of extensor thrust. In order to assist the child in walking, the contractures were released at the hips, knees, and feet. **B,** Posterior view shows valgus of the feet, overaction of the spastic peroneals, adduction of the thighs, and flexion of the knees. Treatment included subtalar arthrodesis of both feet, mild heel cord lengthening, and lengthening of the peroneal tendons. He was able to wear braces and use crutches. Unassisted walking or walking without side supports is not likely.

thighs, flexed hips, equinus feet, and severe spasticity in all the involved muscle groups. He could not stand alone. Walking required external support and great effort. He moved from one place to another by sliding on his buttocks. Children of this age are not interested in laborious walking or extensive bracing because it tends to slow them down. They should be allowed to move around on the floor in order to establish independence and ego. This child's deformities were becoming more severe as growth occurred.

Fig. 3-10, *B*, illustrates the equinovalgus feet, contracted calf muscles, prominent talar heads, and thigh adduction. A decision to release the contractures was made in order to improve standing balance, produce a wider stance, diminish hip flexion contracture and spinal lordosis, and make application of braces easier. Energy expenditure while walking would also be diminished. Treatment included recession of the iliopsoas on both sides, myotomy of the adductor brevis, and neurectomy of the superficial branch of the obturator nerve, all procedures being done through the same medial incision. The knee contracture was diminished by lengthening of the semitendinosus and biceps tendon bilaterally, but no tendon transfer was done. The feet were treated by heel cord lengthening at a point where the incision would not be compressed by the shoe counter, lengthening of the peroneus longus and brevis proximal to the lateral malleolus, and a subtalar arthrodesis (Grice-Green procedure) using homologous bone. The child wore bilateral long leg casts with spreader bars for 8 weeks and was then placed in long leg braces with a pelvic band while walking reeducation was started. He wore the braces intermittently for a year and they were gradually discarded as his gait improved to the point where he could balance and control himself with crutches only. His pattern of walking indicates that he will always need some external support. He is up and about all day long. Simultaneous treatment of the hips, knees, and feet is a reliable approach provided that overtreatment or undertreatment is avoided.

Ages 2 to 4 years

If walking has not occurred by this time, then the possibility of obtaining a functional gait should be questioned. If there are pathologic reflexes such as abnormal steppage, absence of righting reflexes, or persistence of other reflexes that usually disappear at 6 to 12 months of age, then the likelihood that the child will walk without side support or walk at all is minimal. If walking is unlikely, then lower extremity

treatment insofar as surgery is concerned is performed to prevent hip dislocation and severe equinus. The child with monoplegia or hemiplegia should always be treated since walking is usually possible. Other questions can be asked, and probably answered, during this same age period.

Will one or two crutches be necessary? Many patients develop a functional gait so long as they continue to use axillary crutches. These side supports provide poise, confidence, rhythm, and security, conserve energy, and make walking with or without braces possible.

Will the 4-year-old child who requires braces and crutches for walking continue to walk in later years? If the effort is tremendous at 4 years of age, even if contractures and deformities have been corrected, functional walking at 8 or 9 years of age is unlikely. A wheelchair is easier. Every effort should be made to keep the child moving, but insufficient balance, muscle weakness, excessive spasticity, recurrence of deformity, and tetraplegia all affect the walking pattern.

What is done for the 5-year-old child who is not likely to walk? A circular walker with a seat in the center allows movement from one place to another provided that the home or institution is large enough for this apparatus. A wheelchair with minimal attachments is also helpful. The measurements and size should be compatible with the child's age and size.

How much and what types of surgery can be done when the child is 4 or 5 years old? Surgery, if indicated, can include tendon lengthening, myotomy, localized neurectomy, tendon transfer, osteotomy, arthrodesis, or combinations of any or all of these. Surgery of the hips, knees, and feet can be done as isolated procedures or in a coordinated approach on all three areas. Simultaneous surgery on both lower extremities has proved to be a logical and satisfactory approach to the problem. The accuracy of preoperative assessment, the experience of the surgeon, the availability of two operating teams, and the patient's ability to tolerate extensive surgery are the limiting factors in determining how much and which surgery should be done at a single stage.

Ages 4 to 8 years

Learning ability and motivation are primary considerations in this age group. The management of the physical deformities follows a pattern similar to those already mentioned for the younger child. Side supports are used if necessary; bracing is added to augment weakened invertors or evertors of the feet or to maintain the feet at right angles. If the thigh muscles and hip muscles are inadequate for joint support, then external assists are desirable. Bracing, if needed, will aid in development of a walking pattern. Effort should be directed toward elimination of the daytime brace whenever this is practical.

Surgical treatment of this age group is directed toward muscle balance and stabilization of feet, knees, hips, and spine, and the specific operative procedure depends on the kind of deformity and the presence or absence of contracture.

Decisions for surgery

The usual questions of the surgeon are what should be done, when is the operation to be done, and how should it be performed? The pattern of operative procedures will be determined by a careful analysis of alterations about the feet, knees, and hips and will necessarily include information about muscle strength, roentgenographic appearance of the bones and joints, total body balance, and the other characteristics that have been discussed. If the surgeon is in doubt about tendon lengthening as compared with tendon transfer, then the lengthening is safer than the transfer. Before an arthrodesis or osteotomy is carried out, soft tissue surgery such as tendon transfer or tendon lengthening should be attempted if there is a chance that balance and stabilization will be maintained. For the foot, stability is the goal, and if soft tissue fixation and tendon transfers done early do not allow persistent correction, then osteotomy or fusion can be done at a later time.

The ultimate goals of treatment are as follows:
1. Maximum independence
2. Full utilization of available strength
3. Prevention of joint dislocation
4. Avoidance of excessive soft tissue deformity
5. Walking with minimal external support and minimal energy expenditure
6. Cosmetic improvement

Decisions concerning treatment are affected by the patient's growth, development, and individual variations. Soft tissue contractures occur during rapid growth. Hypermobile joints contribute to genu recurvatum, equinovalgus, or subluxation of the hip. Paralysis of certain muscle groups exists because of the brain area involved in the initial pathologic process (area 4, paralytic; area 6, spastic). The condition of the muscle groups influences the final decision for treatment.

Fig. 3-11, *A*, shows the extremities of a 14-year-old girl with slight atrophy of the right calf. She could place her foot on the floor provided that her knee was in moderate extension. As she walked, the foot assumed the position of equinus and inversion (Fig. 3-11, *B*). She had been wearing a brace at night for 10 years and had been able to maintain sufficient soft tissue stretch during periods of rapid growth. In order to give her the best possible gait and to eliminate the inverted appearance of the foot as she walked, a mild heel cord lengthening was done through a 1-inch posterior incision, and the anterior tibial tendon was transferred under the dorsal retinacular ligament to the second cuneiform bone. These procedures did not weaken her calf strength, caused no atrophy, allowed weight bearing without backknee, and provided a consistent, uniform, and active dorsiflexion. The anterior tibial tendon was controlled voluntarily and not by a mass reflex between the hip and the foot. Individual differences alter treatment decisions and lead to variations in end results of certain operative procedures.

A successful tendon transfer in one patient might not function the same in another because of hypermobility of knee or foot joints. Tendon transfer alone may correct the deformity, whereas another patient with a seemingly similar deformity may require joint arthrodesis. The multiplicity of influences on the deformities such as spasticity, ligament hypermobility, bone growth, and muscle weakness influence the end result of a group of operative procedures or a particular reconstructive operation. Thus the surgeon must be familiar with the biomechanics and particular characteristics of musculoskeletal deformities. Examination must be complete and detailed in order to recognize the existence of contractures and joint deformities.

The calf muscle is examined and tested when the knee is flexed, the foot is inverted, and forcible dorsiflexion is applied. This maneuver determines the length of the soleus muscle and gives information, although inconclusive, about the tension or contracture of the gastrocnemius. The knee is then extended and the foot held in the same position. If the gastrocnemius is contracted, the foot will be forced into equinus and the severity of the contracture can then be determined by the position of the foot. The importance of the inverted foot position while testing the length of the calf muscles needs emphasis. The calcaneocuboid joint must be blocked by adducting the forefoot, the sustentaculum tali is placed under the talus by inverting the hindfoot, and the navicular is localized on the medial side of the head of the talus as the entire foot is inverted and dorsiflexed.

The hamstring muscles are tested for strength with the patient prone, the knee flexed, and the examiner

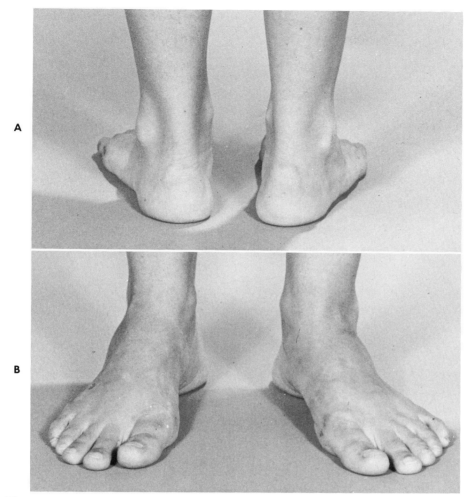

Fig. 3-11. A, The right calf in this 14-year-old girl with spastic hemiplegia is moderately smaller than the left calf. She has worn a night brace for many years and has minimal equinus and inversion. The deformity is sufficient to warrant treatment. Heel cord lengthening should be mild, and transfer of the anterior tibial tendon will diminish inversion. **B,** Anterior view shows mild cavus and inversion. The static appearance of the foot is satisfactory, but during gait the foot inverts and there is moderate internal rotation of the tibia. The deforming muscle is the anterior tibial muscle. Heel cord lengthening was performed and the anterior tibial tendon was moved to the dorsum of the foot and reinserted into the base of the second cuneiform. Balance was reestablished.

applying resistance while the patient is told to voluntarily flex the knee. The presence of contracture is determined with the patient supine, the hip at a right-angle position, and the tibia extended. The residual angle is then noted. The hip is then extended as much as possible, the tibia again extended, and the difference in knee position recorded. Tension on the gracilis is determined by abducting the thigh, flexing the hip, and extending the tibia. The contracted gracilis can be palpated medially.

Hip contracture is determined by locking the pelvis by rotating the opposite femur in external rotation. The involved thigh is then internally rotated, adducted, and extended, and the range of motion observed and determined. The initial position of the head in the acetabulum allows fixation by the anterior ligament of the hip joint and prevents the femur from gliding into external rotation. If this occurs, then the contracture is masked. With the femur fixed in internal rotation and adduction, the distance between origin and insertion can then be determined as extension is attempted.

The strength of the gluteus medius is determined with the patient in a side-lying position. The extremity is placed in maximum extension and abduction with the femur internally rotated. The gluteus medius is palpated as abduction action is attempted voluntarily and resistance is applied by the examiner. The gluteus maximus is tested in a similar way with the patient in the prone position.

Anterior tibial muscle function is determined by asking the patient to dorsiflex the foot. The anterior tibial muscle, if functioning voluntarily, can be readily palpated on the medial side of the ankle as the patient makes a voluntary effort to elevate the foot. If voluntary action is not possible, then a mass reflex or a confusion pattern is elicited. The patient is asked to voluntarily flex the hip while the examiner applies pressure on the anterior thigh. As this is done, the anterior tibial muscle will automatically dorsiflex the foot if this muscle is functioning. Fig. 3-12, *A*, shows the foot of a 17-year-old girl who, when the knee was flexed, could put her foot on the floor. As she walked, however, her foot inverted involuntarily, causing the outer border of the forefoot to strike the floor before heel-strike. This indicates a spastic equinus with inversion. Fig. 3-12, *B*, shows the patient attempting to elevate the foot by voluntarily contracting the anterior tibial muscle. Even with the knee flexed, the foot could not be elevated to right angles. Treatment consisted of a mild heel cord lengthening and transfer of the anterior tibial tendon to the second cuneiform. Treatment prevented equinus, eliminated inversion during swing phase, and resulted in a more stable and graceful gait.

The same patient's upper extremity demonstrated

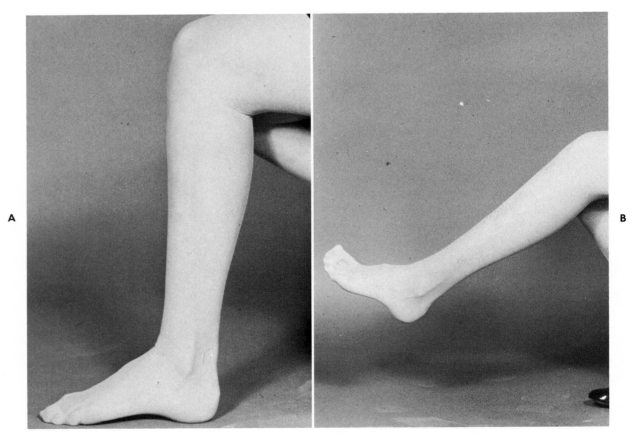

A   B

Fig. 3-12. A, With the knee flexed, the foot is at right angles and the relationship between the foot and leg is essentially normal in this 17-year-old girl. **B,** With the knee partially extended, equinus occurs and mild spasticity of the gastrocnemius is evident. Extension of the toes is attempted because anterior tibial function elevates the foot only via a confusion reflex that requires hip flexion simultaneously with knee and foot elevation. The claw toes were corrected by transferring the flexor tendons to the extensor mechanism. The anterior tibial tendon was transferred to the second cuneiform and a mild heel cord lengthening was performed.

thumb-in-palm deformity and spasticity of the flexor digitorum profundi and flexor digitorum sublimis muscles. Also, there was overaction of the wrist extensors as the fingers were closed. Treatment was directed toward both the upper and lower extremities, which is frequently the program. The surgeon can make a logical decision concerning a particular method of treatment if he has an understanding of muscle function, joint mechanics, and the action of spastic muscles. The effects of these muscles on joint position and strength are also considered when a decision is being made as to the way a contracture should be managed. Treatment might include the following procedures:

1. Myotomy-fasciotomy and/or neurectomy
2. Release of a muscle origin and transfer of the origin to a different location
3. Lengthening of the tendon proximal to the insertion or at the musculotendinous junction
4. Transfer of the insertion of the tendon

Certain principles of treatment have proved to be effective during the past 25 years. The principles of multiple operative procedures on more than one extremity has proved beneficial to the patient, has diminished the number of visits to the operating room, and has allowed earlier development of a gait pattern that is more uniform and less awkward and energy consuming. Careful preoperative assessment is necessary. Overtreatment, moreover, must be avoided. The procedures in the young child should be nondestructive and usually reversible.

The following surgical principles have proved to be reliable and effective:

1. Tenotomy in the infant and child with the potential for walking or not walking may be helpful. Regeneration occurs and bridges a mild defect.
2. Tendon lengthening is done at any age. Overlengthening should be avoided. Improvement in joint motion usually results.
3. Tendon transfer is reliable if the strength of the muscle-tendon unit is good, if an excessive number of transfers are not done simultaneously, and if balance is established between the agonists and antagonists.
4. A subtalar arthrodesis is reliable in maintaining the calcaneus under the talus and preventing forefoot abduction. This is usually done for equinovalgus but can be used in equinovarus deformities to prevent recurrence. Tendon lengthenings and tendon transfers, as indicated, should accompany the subtalar arthrodesis.
5. Calcaneal osteotomy through the posterior beak of the bone is reliable if the deformity is not excessive and if muscle-tendon imbalance is corrected.
6. Triple arthrodesis is a useful procedure in correcting a foot deformity in an older child (10 years of age or older) who has had no prior treatment or has had uncontrollable structural changes in the foot.

Fig. 3-13 shows a 17-year-old boy with untreated spastic equinovarus with structural change and severe contractures. The foot was treated by calf muscle lengthening, a posterior ankle capsulotomy, lengthening of the toe flexors and posterior tibial tendon, and a pantalar arthrodesis, including ankle and tarsal bones, in order to put the foot in a satisfactory weight-bearing position. Other procedures that have proved to be reliable are as follows:

1. Pantalar arthrodesis
2. Osteotomy of the proximal femur for correcting anteversion and coxa valga (diminishes dislocation of the hip)

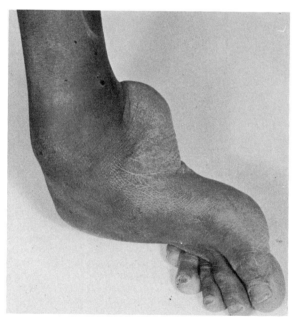

Fig. 3-13. A 17-year-old boy with spastic hemiplegia who had never been treated. His intellect is impaired, and although he is not educable, he is trainable. Because of the severe equinus of the talus and the changes that had occurred within and around the joint, a pantalar arthrodesis was performed so that a conventional shoe would fit the foot and so that the plantar surface of the foot could be put in a satisfactory weight-bearing position. There has now been a 3-year follow-up. Fusion has occurred, there is no pain, and the gait is satisfactory.

3. Osteotomy of the ilium or acetabular region as an adjunct to soft tissue release, iliopsoas tendon transfer, and femoral osteotomy, either for correction or prevention of dislocation of the hip

QUESTIONS AND PROBLEMS

The general principles have been mentioned. Certain questions have been asked frequently during the presentation of the *Instructional Course Lectures* concerned with cerebral palsy. Some of the answers will be found in the following material by Drs. Bassett, Evans, and Bleck. I am listing some of these questions so that the reader will recognize certain objectives of these authors.

Foot and ankle deformities

1. *Gastrocnemius-soleus lengthening:* When is the tendon lengthened by a heel cord step cut, a musculotendinous junction lengthening, a gastrocnemius origin release from the femur, or neurectomy?
2. *Talipes equinovalgus:* When are the peroneal tendons transferred to the dorsum of the foot? When are the peroneal tendons rerouted anteriorly without detaching the insertion? When is osteotomy of the body of the calcaneus indicated? When is osteotomy of the calcaneus in the region of the subtalar joint done? When is subtalar arthrodesis preferable to osteotomy? When is external support for day and/or night use prescribed?

A 6-year-old boy with an equinovarus deformity of the foot and a secondary or dynamic flexion deformity of the hip and knee was seen for treatment. The right upper extremity was flexed at the wrist, showed limited extension of the fingers, and a thumb-in-palm deformity was present. Treatment was directed toward both the leg and the hand. A step-cut heel cord lengthening restored foot position and balance without weakening the calf noticeably; the knee and the hip corrected actively after the equinus was eliminated. Upper extremity reconstruction was carried out simultaneously with improvement in hand and finger position and function.

3. *Talipes equinovarus:* What are the indications for anterior tibial tendon transfer? When are the posterior tibial tendon and heel cord lengthened simultaneously? What is the indication for re-routing the posterior tibial tendon anteriorly, leaving the insertion attached to the navicular and plantar surface of the foot? What are the indications for subtalar arthrodesis in the child with equinovalgus or equinovarus foot deformity? What are the indications for osteotomy of the calcaneus? What are the indications for triple arthrodesis in the management of talipes equinovarus?
4. *Foot and ankle equinus:* When is lengthening of the triceps surae sufficient rather than tendon lengthening, posterior ankle joint release, and triple arthrodesis? What are the indications for pantalar arthrodesis in the management of the spastic foot?

Management of knee deformities

1. Lengthening of the hamstring tendons may include one, two, or all three tendons. How is this decision made?
2. What is the indication for transfer of the semitendinosus tendon to the lateral aspect of the distal femur?
3. When is the gracilis tendon lengthened or transferred?
4. Flexion contracture of the knee may require osteotomy of the distal end of the femur. What is the indication for this procedure?
5. Quadriceps muscle reinforcement implies muscle weakness and knee contracture. How is the quadriceps tested prior to making this decision?
6. Patellar tendon advancement is utilized less frequently now than in the past. What are the reasons for this change?
7. When should the knee retinaculum be released both medially and laterally?
8. What are the indications for transferring hamstring tendons, and how many should be transferred to the lower femur?
9. If genu recurvatum results from hamstring transfer, how should this deformity be corrected?
10. When else does genu recurvatum occur and how is it treated?

Adduction of the thighs

1. When should myotomy of the adductor muscles be done, and how many muscles should be included?
2. Is there an indication for a unilateral myotomy when both sides are involved?
3. What are the indications for extrapelvic and intrapelvic obturator neurectomy?

4. What are the indications for transfer of the origin of the adductor muscles to the ischium?

Hip flexion contracture

1. What are the indications for lengthening or transfer of the rectus, sartorius, tensor fasciae latae, or iliopoas muscles?
2. How is a contracture of the iliopoas muscle detected?
3. With a known contracture of the iliopoas, is the rotational limitation of the femur external or internal?
4. What technique is used to determine if the iliopsoas is contracted or spastic?
5. Do roentgenograms assist in determining the presence of fixed lumbosacral lordosis? What angle between the upright femur and the sacrum is normal and what angle is greater than normal?
6. After the iliopsoas is transferred to the greater trochanter, how does the patient actually flex the hip?
7. When is a subtrochanteric osteotomy desirable in correcting flexion contracture of the hip?

DIFFERENTIAL DIAGNOSIS

Cerebral palsy is suspected when an infant shows abnormal central nervous system development or musculoskeletal abnormalities with increased or decreased muscle tone and reflex alterations. Several conditions are considered in the differential diagnosis.

Primary muscle *hypotonia* is characterized by excessive relaxation of the extremity and trunk muscles, hypermobile joints, and diminished muscle tone. The reflexes may be present or diminished. The infant moves the extremities, but the musculoskeletal system is floppy. If a pathologic condition such as a primary neuropathy or myopathy is present, other studies, including muscle biopsy and enzyme determination, would suggest the proper diagnosis.

Primary mental deficiency may accompany slow motor development of the infant. Hypotonicity and slow motor response are observed frequently. As the child develops, the usual signs of spasticity or athetosis do not appear. Walking is usually delayed and coordination is deficient.

Occipital-cervical abnormalities (basilar depression) affect the upper cervical spine or cerebellum and compress the corticospinal tracts, causing spasticity in the extremities. Such abnormalities may simulate changes that occur in cerebral palsy, but the onset is usually late. Limited neck motion, a low hairline, and a short neck are frequently associated with occipital-

cervical abnormalities. Roentgenograms will aid in making the diagnosis.

Diastematomyelia may cause lower extremity neurologic change, but the onset is usually after birth and slowly progressive.

Hydrocephalus, with or without myelomeningocele, may result in muscle weakness or spasticity because of brain damage. The combined changes resulting from increased intracranial pressure and a lesion of the lumbar and sacral nerve roots may cause a syndrome that has many of the characteristics of cerebral palsy.

Inborn errors of metabolism such as phenylketonuria, abnormalities of glucose metabolism, or dysfunction of protein synthesis can be suspected and diagnosed if certain blood and urinary tests are positive. These infants are usually slow in development and do not show signs and symptoms compatible with the usual findings seen in the patient with cerebral palsy.

Developmental variations such as hypermobility of joints, delayed onset of walking, toe walking in an otherwise normal child, or alterations in the vestibular or optic systems suggest pathologic conditions that might be similar to that seen in the child with cerebral palsy. Frequent and careful examination and the pattern of progress will usually aid in the differential diagnosis.

A hemiplegic infant or child with a mild deformity may go undiagnosed for several months. The child may be considered as awkward or clumsy. A stretch reflex, mild muscle spasticity, and hyperactive reflexes as well as the gait and posture will usually result in an accurate diagnosis.

DIAGNOSTIC AND TREATMENT PROGRAM

Once cerebral palsy is suspected, diagnostic studies should be initiated. If the presence of the condition is reasonably certain, the parents should receive detailed counseling concerning future expectations, a program of observation and treatment should be instituted, and a differential diagnosis made. False optimism should be avoided, but total pessimism should not exist. The family should receive a reasonable and realistic explanation of the child's condition frequently. Many parents tend to follow a program of wishful thinking and block out unpleasant information. Group orientation of the parents is helpful. These parents, in particular, are comforted by communicating with other parents who have children with cerebral palsy. Medical and paramedical personnel must aid in establishing security and direction for these families.

Each child with cerebral palsy is given a detailed

examination and the information recorded accurately. The muscle test should be carried out even though the results are not as accurate in cerebral palsy as in poliomyelitis. The Vineland Social Maturity Test provides information for those working with the child as to intelligence, motivation, and intellectual status. Other psychological tests are given at the proper time in order to provide an index of basic information for future education.

Vision and hearing are examined and speech is assessed. A deficiency in any of these may affect the interpretation of basic intelligence. Other deficits such as condition of teeth, diet, anemia, or particular illnesses are diagnosed and treated.

The physical treatment program is initially directed toward preventing or correcting contractures and providing activities that encourage the child toward assuming an upright position. Sitting, crawling, and then standing are attempted, and information is obtained concerning the patient's reactions to external stimuli in both the upper and lower extremities. A physical therapy program should be planned in a realistic way, with emphasis on the patient's abilities, potential, and progress. Maturation of the nervous system permeates the program.

Sensation in both the upper and lower extremities should be assessed. If upper extremity function is reasonable but sensation is only fair or poor, then the parents should know this. After the accumulation of data is completed, the physician should communicate with the occupational and physical therapists so that each knows that whe other is doing and planning, and each one records in the patient's record appropriate observations and suggestions for treatment. The therapists should be assured that a child's progress is not necessarily related to the degree of enthusiasm and the ability of the therapist. If the child's progress is slow, the therapist is not to blame.

The patient's family is advised that improvement and regression will alternate, that emotional responses of the child will vary, and that behavior will change occasionally. These are part of the growth and development pattern.

The ultimate goal is an independent adult, physically, emotionally, and intellectually. Unfortunately, these goals are not always attained.

REFERENCES

1. Adams, J. P., editor: Current practice in orthopaedic surgery, St. Louis, 1966, The C. V. Mosby Co., vol. 3.
2. Baker, L. D.: A rational approach to the surgical needs of the cerebral palsy patients, J. Bone Joint Surg. **38-A:**312, 1956.
3. Banks, H. H., and Green, W. T.: Adductor myotomy and obturator neurectomy for the correction of adduction contracture of the hip in cerebral palsy, J. Bone Joint Surg. **42-A:**111, 1960.
4. Bassett, F. H., III, and Baker, L. D.: Equinus deformity in cerebral palsy. In Adams, J. P., editor: Current practice in orthopaedic surgery, St. Louis, 1966, The C. V. Mosby Co., vol. 3.
5. Bleck, E. E.: Personal communication, 1969.
6. Bleck, E. E.: Management of hip deformities in cerebral palsy. In Adams, J. P., editor: Current practice in orthopaedic surgery, St. Louis, 1966, The C. V. Mosby Co., vol. 3.
7. Eggers, G. W. N.: Surgical division of patellar retinacula to improve extension of the knee joint in cerebral spastic paralysis, J. Bone Joint Surg. **32-A:**80, 1950.
8. Eggers, G. W. N.: Transplantation of hamstring tendons to femoral condyles in order to improve hip extension and to decrease knee flexion in cerebral spastic paralysis, J. Bone Joint Surg. **34-A:**287, 1952.
9. Evans, E. B., and Julian, J. D.: Modifications of the hamstrings transfer operation. Presented at the annual meeting of the American Academy for Cerebral Palsy, New York City, 1964.
10. Fiorentino, M. R.: Reflex testing methods for evaluating CNS development, Springfield, Ill., 1963, Charles C Thomas, Publisher.
11. Grice, D. S.: Further experience with extra-articular arthrodesis of the subtalar joint, J. Bone Joint Surg. **36-A:**246, 1955.
12. Keats, S.: Operative orthopaedics in cerebral palsy, Springfield, Ill., 1970, Charles C Thomas, Publisher.
13. Muster, W. T.: A follow up study of iliopsoas transfer for hip and stability, J. Bone Joint Surg. **41-B:**289, 1959.
14. Paine, R. S.: On the treatment of cerebral palsy, Pediatrics 29:605, 1962.
15. Paine, R. S.: Evolution of partial reflexes in normal infants in the presence of chronic brain syndromes, Neurology **14:**1036, 1964.
16. Paine, R. S.: Early recognition of cerebral palsy and prognostic signs, Instructional Course Lecture, The American Academy for Cerebral Palsy, Cleveland, 1965.
17. Paine, R. S., and Oppe, T. E.: Neurological examinations of children, Clinics and Developmental Medicine, 20/21, London, 1966, The Spastic Society in association with William Heinemann, Ltd.
18. Phelps, W. M.: Long term results of orthopaedic surgery in cerebral palsy, J. Bone Joint Surg. **39-A:**53, 1957.
19. Pollock, G. A.: Surgical treatment of cerebral palsy, J. Bone Joint Surg. **44-B:**68, 1962.
20. Seymour, N., and Sharrard, W. J. W.: Bilateral proximal release of the hamstrings in cerebral palsy, J. Bone Joint Surg. **50-B:**274, 1968.
21. Silver, C. M., and Simon, S. D.: Gastrocnemius muscle recession (Silfverskiöld operation) for spastic palsy, J. Bone Joint Surg. **41-A:**1021, 1959.
22. Steindler, A.: Postgraduate lectures on orthopaedic diagnosis and indications, Springfield, Ill., 1951, Charles C Thomas, Publisher, vol. 2, p. 69.

Part II
Deformities of the feet due to cerebral palsy

FRANK H. BASSETT, III, M.D.
Durham, North Carolina

When the muscles of the leg are affected by brain damage in cerebral palsy, and smooth, coordinated movement is lost, function is impaired and deformities occur. Loss of function results from ineffective neuromuscular control, but often the impaired action is made worse by muscle imbalance and related deformities. The goal of orthopaedic management of the affected extremity is to achieve maximum function. Since little can be done to improve central nervous system control of the affected muscles, therapy is aimed at establishing muscle balance in order to correct or prevent deformities.

The primary factor in the development of a foot deformity is a spastic muscle or group of muscles overpulling less spastic, normal, or flaccid antagonists. If allowed to persist, secondary adaptive soft tissue and skeletal changes occur that lead to structural deformity. A specific foot deformity in the patient with cerebral palsy will show wide variation in the degree of severity. This depends on the age of the patient, the degree of muscle spasticity, prior therapy, and the maturity and rigidity of the deformities. Therapy is individualized but always aimed at restoring muscle balance and aligning the bones and joints in a weight-bearing position that will allow the patient to assume an erect position.[2] If the child has the potential for walking, therapy to correct deformities of the feet are indicated. If walking, even with braces and side supports, is unlikely, then surgery should not be done. Thus the physician must have guidelines to determine the prognosis for walking.

EVALUATION OF DEFORMITIES

In the order of decreasing frequency, foot deformities in the patient with cerebral palsy are equinus, equinovalgus, equinovarus, and toe flexion and other toe deformities due to the involvement of the intrinsic muscles of the foot. Calcaneovalgus deformity is rare. Occasionally a child will have a foot deformity only, and diagnosis and treatment are relatively simple. Usually involvement of the extremity is diffuse and deformities about the knee and hip accompany those

of the foot. Appraisal is then directed toward determining whether the foot deformity is primary, secondary to one of the other deformities, or a double primary deformity exists. Another possibility is that the foot deformity is a result of overflow, which is the involuntary contraction of one muscle group caused by stimuli resulting from voluntary contractions of another muscle group. When multiple joints are involved, the observer, in order to evaluate dynamic integrated muscle function, should have the patient walk or attempt to walk with help.[9] In this way the trunk and both lower extremities can be assessed as a functional unit. Keen observation of the neuromuscular dysfunction of each segment of the lower extremity is required, first as an integral unit and then as separate segments.

The child is placed on the examining table, and the examiner determines whether the deformities are due to muscle contracture or to spasticity without true shortening. Systematic appraisal of each muscle and muscle group will help confirm which deformities are primary, which are simple adaptations by the child to assume erect posture, or which are the result of overflow. For instance, a child who scissors and tiptoes while walking but who has little spasticity and no contracture in the triceps surae on the examining table probably tiptoes as the result of overflow from spastic adductors or quadriceps muscles.

Muscle analysis must also include tests for strength, muscle length, clonus, tension, rigidity, resistance to rapid passive stretch, and resistance to stretch by slow, steady pressure. This information must be recorded for future comparison.

Actual muscle strength is difficult to assess in cerebral palsy. The standard tests used to determine muscle power in poliomyelitis are less accurate in cerebral palsy. The reasons for this difficulty are threefold. (1) Stimulation of a spastic muscle by stretching or active contraction often produces a contraction of unpredictable degree. Clonus or repetitive rhythmic contractions may occur. (2) The degree of spasticity in a muscle does vary from time to time. Emotional excitement, a strange environment, or crowds often aggravate tension or muscle tonus. (3) In children with a brief attention span the cooperation necessary for accurate muscle testing is often lacking. Nevertheless, a complete study of the agonist and antagonist muscles is a prerequisite to rational therapy, and an effort at grading will provide useful information.

Equinus results primarily from overactivity in the triceps surae, which is an antigravity muscle that is

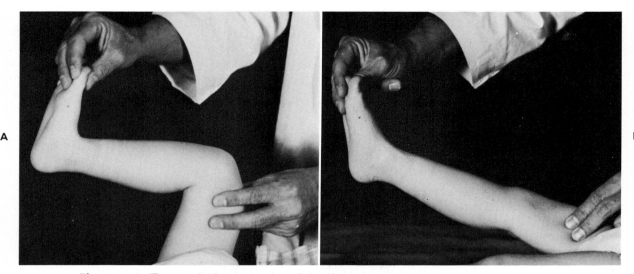

Fig. 3-14. A, To test whether an equinus deformity is correctable and to examine the triceps surae for resistance to stretch, the foot is dorsiflexed passively. In this instance the triceps surae is tested with the knee flexed in order to lessen the effect that the gastrocnemius has on the equinus deformity. The foot dorsiflexes beyond 90° with ease, indicating that the soleus muscle does not have a contracture. **B,** The leg is tested in a similar way with the knee in extension, thereby testing the gastrocnemius as well as the other muscles of the leg that may participate in producing equinus, particularly the soleus muscle. In this instance the foot cannot be passively dorsiflexed beyond a right angle, indicating that the gastrocnemius is the primary offending muscle producing the equinus.

more powerful than the antagonist dorsiflexor muscles. In a strength analysis of the triceps surae the gastrocnemius and soleus muscles should be tested separately. The soleus muscle is tested with the knee flexed (Fig. 3-14, *A*). Since the gastrocnemius portion of the triceps surae originates from the femoral condyles, it is partially relaxed when the knee is flexed and is eliminated from the test for the soleus muscle. The soleus should be tested for strength and resistance to stretch. The gastrocnemius strength and resistance to stretch is tested with the knee extended and the foot dorsiflexed (Fig. 3-14, *B*). If equinus is present and not affected by knee flexion, then a state of contracture exists. The peroneal, posterior tibial, and toe flexor muscles are plantar flexor muscles in addition to their other functions. Power from these muscles for plantar flexion is limited, but they can cause equinus. Failure to recognize the part that any of these muscles may play in the production of equinus will occasionally result in a poor response to therapy or recurrence of equinus deformity.

A varus or valgus position of the heel is often associated with an equinus deformity. Equinovalgus is more common and usually results from the bowstring effect of the heel cord on the ankle and subtalar joints.

Because of restricted dorsiflexion of the foot by the tight heel cord, the calcaneus rotates posterolaterally beneath the talus. If severe enough, the sustentaculum tali and the plantar calcaneonavicular ligament lose their normal supporting position for the anterior portion of the talus, and a rocker-bottom deformity results. The hindfoot stays in equinus. The apparent dorsiflexion occurs at the midtarsal area. Spastic peroneal muscles contribute to this deformity and, when overactive, tend to stand out as a tight band behind the lateral malleolus.

Overactive posterior tibial and toe flexor muscles contribute to equinovarus deformities. When equinovarus results from involvement of a posterior tibial muscle, the posterior tibial tendon can be palpated as a tight band behind the medial malleolus when the foot is dorsiflexed. If the toe flexors are involved, the toes curl into flexion when the foot is dorsiflexed.

TREATMENT
Equinus without fixed contracture

A mild equinus deformity due to spasticity in the triceps surae without contracture or actual shortening can usually be corrected passively with ease. Gentle stretching of the muscle in a plaster cast, followed by a night splint of plaster, molded plastic, or a brace may be all that is necessary to control the deformity. For ambulatory purposes a short leg brace, preferably of the Klenzak style, will allow adequate push-off and help maintain muscle balance. However, if firm resistance is met with passive attempts to correct the deformity or if correction cannot be maintained by nonoperative means, surgical correction may be necessary. When the involvement is primarily in the gastrocnemius portion of the triceps surae, surgery should be directed at lengthening only this portion of the muscle complex. The procedures described by Baker,[2] Bassett and Baker,[7] and Strayer[18,19] are both effective. When the involvement includes the soleus muscle as well as the gastrocnemius, lengthening of the Achilles tendon by any of the commonly used methods is the procedure of choice.[5,10,12,13]

In the young preambulatory patient a Denis Browne type of splint with a 90° outrigger is useful in controlling equinus while maintaining the thighs in abduction. To help develop strength and standing balance, the outrigger should be removable so the child can stand in the splint.

Severe equinus without fixed contracture

Deformities of a severe nature are difficult to correct by nonoperative means. If one cannot achieve correction by surgical lengthening procedures, additional surgery in the popliteal area, either recession

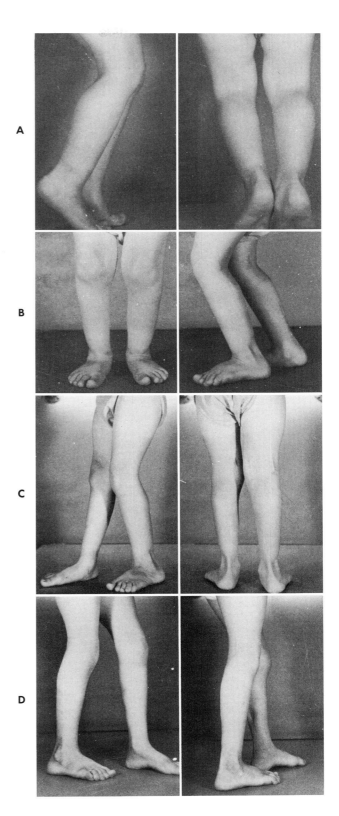

Fig. 3-15. A, Initial photographs of a 2-year, 8-month-old spastic paraplegic with equinus deformities and a tendency toward depression of the longitudinal arches. The child had a reciprocal gait and the potential for ambulation. Two weeks following the initial photographs a bilateral mid-third lengthening of the gastrocnemius aponeurosis was carried out. Proximal surgery included bilateral adductor myotomy, rectus femoris tenotomy, and gracilis tenotomy. **B,** Photographs taken 11 months after the initial surgery demonstrate bilateral calcaneus deformities, the result of overlengthening of the gastrocnemius aponeurosis. Care should be taken to avoid this complication of surgery for the correction of equinus. It weakens push-off and prolongs gait therapy. **C,** Photographs taken 2 years, 2 months following initial surgery demonstrate recurrence of equinus with eversion of the heel and pronation of the foot. Occasionally after surgical correction in a young child, equinus recurs due to growth. **D,** Appearance of the lower extremities following bilateral relengthening of the gastrocnemius aponeurosis, rerouting of the overactive peroneals, and lateral open-wedge osteotomy of the calcaneus. Note the restoration of the longitudinal arches and the position of the rerouted peroneal tendons. The child is presently brace free. He ambulates independently using bilateral axillary crutches for balance.

of the gastrocnemius origins as described by Silfverskiöld,[14,15] modifications of this procedure,[1] or neurectomy of the motor branches to the gastrocnemius and/or soleus, may be required.[17]

Equinus with fixed contracture

Lengthening of the gastrocnemius aponeurosis or the Achilles tendon may not allow adequate correction of equinus when the deformity is of long standing and passive correction is not possible. A posterior capsulotomy of the ankle is occasionally necessary.

Equinovalgus without fixed contracture

A valgus deformity commonly is associated with equinus, particularly in the patient with a tendency toward relaxed joints. When a tight heel cord restricts easy placement of the heel on the floor, the motion of the subtalar joint is such that the calcaneus tends to displace laterally and posteriorly. When mild, correction of the equinus component of the deformity may correct the valgus deformity as well. Usually the peroneal muscles are overactive, however, and contribute to the deformity. Therefore lengthening of the peroneal tendons may be necessary to achieve inversion-eversion balance. Baker and Hill[4] prefer to reroute the peroneal tendon anterior to the lateral malleolus to minimize the influence of the spastic peroneal muscles in the production of the equinovalgus foot (Fig. 3-15).

When the valgus deformity is severe enough, the calcaneus rotates beneath the talus to the point that the anterior portion of the calcaneus no longer provides support for the head of the talus. As the sustentaculum tali displaces laterally and posteriorly, the talus drops into more equinus. In such cases, neither correction of the equinus nor soft tissue surgery of the peroneal tendons will maintain correction of the deformity.

To maintain the foot in the desired position, triple arthrodesis is considered to be the procedure of choice if the patient is over 12 years of age. In the younger child this operation is not necessary. When passive correction of the heel restores the longitudinal arch of the foot by placing the talus and calcaneus in normal relationship, lateral open-wedge osteotomy of the os calcis, as described by Baker and Hill,[4] easily maintains the desired talocalcaneal relationship (Fig. 3-16). Silver and associates[16] prefer to change the weight-bearing alignment by a more oblique, posteriorly placed calcaneal osteotomy. Extra-articular talocalcaneal fusion (Grice procedure) produces equally gratifying results (Fig. 3-17).[3,11]

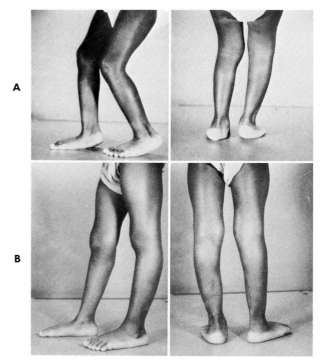

Fig. 3-16. A, A 3-year, 4-month-old patient with severe spastic paraplegia. When first seen, the patient was able to ambulate only with help. The gait was complicated by scissoring, equinus deformities of the feet, abduction of the forefeet, and clonus in the triceps surae. On the examining table the knees extended easily with the feet in plantar flexion. No tightness in the hamstrings was noted, indicating that the knee flexion was due primarily to involvement of the gastrocnemius muscles. Note the equinus and rocker-bottom deformities. **B,** Appearance of the lower extremities 9 months following bilateral midthird lengthening of the gastrocnemius aponeurosis and open-wedge osteotomies of the calcaneus. Note the correction of the knee flexion deformities, the equinus, and the rocker-bottom soles. The patient is presently brace free but because of poor balance uses a walker.

Regardless of which procedure is to be used, the surgeon should not forget to achieve muscle balance by appropriate soft tissue surgery, to avoid overcorrection, and to correct the deformity with the surgery and not rely on postoperative plaster correction.

Equinovalgus with fixed contracture

When passive correction of the foot cannot be achieved and the deformity is fixed, lengthening or rerouting of the peroneal tendons must be accompanied by appropriate capsulotomies of the joints of the hind- and midfoot as needed to correct the deformity. To maintain correction, extra-articular

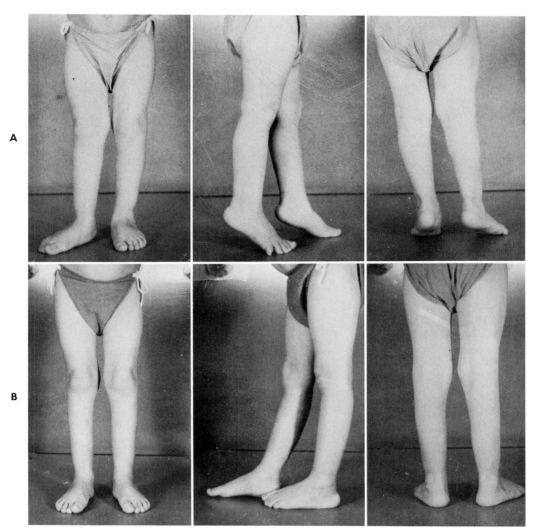

Fig. 3-17. A, A 3-year, 5-month-old spastic paraplegic who walked on his toes without aid. Note the mild pronation of the feet. Although the peroneal muscles were slightly overactive, it was not believed that they contributed to the pronation. A midthird gastrocnemius aponeurosis lengthening corrected the equinus deformities. Three months following surgery the longitudinal arches remained depressed, indicating that correction of the equinus deformity was not sufficient to overcome this portion of his original deformity. Therefore bilateral extra-articular subtalar arthrodeses were done 8 months after the original surgery. **B,** Four months following the Grice procedures. Note the restoration of the longitudinal arches. Equinus remains corrected and the extremities are in good weight-bearing alignment. The patient is presently brace and crutch free and ambulates independently.

subtalar fusion is usually necessary in the young child. When the patient is over 12 years of age, stabilization by triple arthrodesis should be done with appropriate lengthening of the Achilles and peroneal tendons.

Equinovarus without fixed contracture

Muscles whose tendons pass behind the medial malleolus usually contribute to this deformity. When the deformity is mild and easily corrected passively, plaster immobilization to stretch out the involved muscles and permit the overstretched peroneals to gain strength may help in reestablishing muscle balance. Usually such conservative management does not result in permanent correction. Long periods of bracing with an outside T strap may control the deformity, but if the need for bracing can be eliminated by

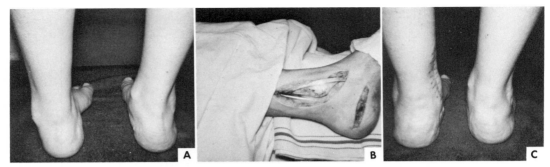

Fig. 3-18. A, Child with spastic hemiplegia. Note inversion of the heel on the involved side. **B,** Photograph taken at surgery demonstrates rerouted posterior tibial tendon. The plantar intrinsic muscles were released from their origin on the calcaneus through the incision located on the medial aspect of the heel. **C,** Position of foot 7 months after surgery. (Courtesy Dr. Ronald Losee, Montana State Training School and Hospital, Boulder, Mont.)

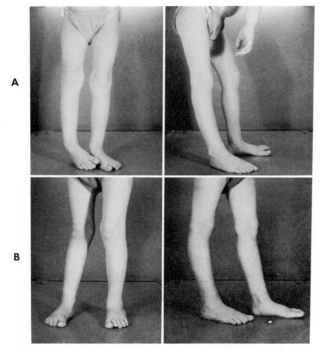

Fig. 3-19. A, A 5-year, 7-month-old patient with athetosis and spastic quadriplegia with widespread weakness of a flaccid nature. Note the supination of the right foot associated with equinus. On the examining table the deformities could be corrected with ease, indicating minimal involvement of the leg muscles associated with some overflow. For fear of excessively weakening push-off power in the presence of athetosis, surgical correction was limited to rerouting of the posterior tibial tendon and lengthening of the toe flexors on the right. The triceps surae was not lengthened. **B,** Six months following surgery. Note that the right foot is in better balance. Due to the athetotic movements, the position of the foot alternates unpredictably from calcaneus to equinus with ambulation. At present the child is ambulating with one crutch. He is brace free.

surgery, then surgery should be considered. Rerouting or lengthening of the posterior tibial tendon is effective (Fig. 3-18). When the toe flexors are involved and contribute to the deformity, they should be lengthened (Fig. 3-19).

Equinovarus with fixed deformity

Even when fixed contracture is present and permanent bone and joint changes have occurred, the deforming force should be eliminated. The same operative principles and techniques should be used as when the deformity is not fixed. Appropriate capsulotomies also may be needed in the younger patient. A laterally based, closed-wedge osteotomy of the calcaneus, posterior to the subtalar joint, has been helpful in aligning the heel. In the older child, triple arthrodesis may be necessary.

Supination deformity

When supination of the mid- and forefoot is associated with the swing phase of the gait due to "overpull" of the anterior tibial muscle relative to the power of the peroneus longus and brevis, peroneus tertius, and lateral toe extensors, balance of the foot can be achieved successfully by a transfer of the anterior tibial tendon to the midfoot, usually in the region of the third cuneiform. Each foot must be analyzed individually, however; the exact location for the transfer will depend on the mobility of the foot and the relative strength of the involved muscles.

Forefoot deformities

A variety of deformities of the forefoot can be produced by spasticity of the intrinsic muscles or by muscle imbalance of those muscles that insert into the toes. Hallux valgus is such a deformity. Often it is due to spasticity in the adductor hallucis muscle. On the other hand, it can result from improper shoeing or abnormal weight distribution on the great toe in a child with an equinovalgus deformity of the foot. If the deformity is due to spasticity in the adductor hallucis muscle, the deformity can be temporarily relieved by local anesthetic block of the adductor muscle. When the deformity is relieved by nerve block, sectioning of the tendon often will result in permanent correction.

A hallux varus deformity due to spasticity in the abductor hallucis muscle has been reported by Bleck.[8] When infiltration of the abductor muscle by a local anesthetic agent eliminates the deformity, permanent correction can be obtained by surgical release of the overactive muscle near its insertion.

Postoperative care

Deformities of the feet should be corrected by surgery and not by postoperative plaster casts. Plaster casts are needed only to maintain the correction. The casts should not be overpadded and should not be applied directly over the heels. Even when the plaster is well molded, uncontrollable movement by the patient may cause a friction sore over the heel. Such a lesion prevents the comfortable fitting of shoes and prolongs postoperative gait training.

The postoperative use of braces, night splints, or posterior plaster splints should not be forgotten. Premature removal of such appliances may lead to a recurrence of the deformity, particularly when surgery is done in the very young child and recurrence due to growth is likely.

Postoperative therapy is aimed at restoration of joint function, improvement in muscle strength, and gait training.

SUMMARY

When the function of a child with cerebral palsy is hindered by deformities of the feet and the child is ambulatory or has potential for walking, efforts should be aimed at restoring muscle balance, correcting deformities, and aligning the joints of the lower extremity so the child can achieve erect posture. Only by achieving these goals can maximum possible function be achieved.

REFERENCES

1. Baker, L. D.: Triceps surae syndrome in cerebral palsy, Arch. Surg. **68:**216, 1954.
2. Baker, L. D.: A rational approach to the surgical needs of the cerebral palsied patient, J. Bone Joint Surg. **38-A:**313, 1956.
3. Baker, L. D., and Dodelin, R. A.: Extra-articular arthrodesis of the subtalar joint (Grice procedure), J.A.M.A. **168:**1005, 1958.
4. Baker, L. D., and Hill, L. M.: Foot alignment in cerebral palsy patient, J. Bone Joint Surg. **46-A:**1, 1964.
5. Banks, H. H., and Green, W. T.: The correction of equinus deformity in cerebral palsy, J. Bone Joint Surg. **40-A:**1359, 1958.
6. Bassett, F. H.: The foot in cerebral palsy. In Giannestras, N. J., editor: Foot disorders; medical and surgical management, Philadelphia, 1967, Lea & Febiger.
7. Bassett, F. H., III, and Baker, L. D.: Equinus deformity in cerebral palsy. In Adams, J. P., editor: Current practice in orthopaedic surgery, St. Louis, 1966, The C. V. Mosby Co., vol. 3.
8. Bleck, E. E.: Spastic abductor hallucis. Presented at the annual meeting of The American Academy for Cerebral Palsy, New Orleans, 1966.
9. Eggers, G. W. N., and Evans, E. B.: Surgery in cerebral palsy, Instructional Course Lectures, The American Academy of Orthopaedic Surgeons, J. Bone Joint Surg. **45-A:**1275, 1963.
10. Green, W. T., and McDermott, L. J.: Operative treatment of cerebral palsy of spastic types, J.A.M.A. **118:**434, 1942.
11. Grice, D. S.: Extra-articular arthrodesis of the subastragalar joint for correction of paralytic flatfeet in children, J. Bone Joint Surg. **34-A:**927, 1952.
12. McCarroll, H. R.: Surgical treatment of spastic paralysis, Instructional Course Lectures, The American Academy of Orthopaedic Surgeons, Ann Arbor, 1949, J. W. Edwards, vol. 6, p. 134.
13. McCarroll, H. R., and Schwartzmann, J. R.: Spastic paralysis and allied disorders, J. Bone Joint Surg. **25:**745, 1943.
14. Silfverskiöld, N.: Reduction of the un-crossed two-joint muscles of the leg to one-joint muscles in spastic conditions, Acta Chir. Scand. **56:**315, 1924.
15. Silver, C. M., and Simon, S. D.: Gastrocnemius muscle recession (Silfverskiöld operation) for spastic equinus deformity in cerebral palsy, J. Bone Joint Surg. **41-A:**1021, 1959.
16. Silver, C. M., Simon, S. D., Spindell, E., Litchman, H. M., and Scala, M.: Calcaneal osteotomy for valgus and varus deformities of the foot in cerebral palsy. A preliminary report on twenty-seven operations, J. Bone Joint Surg. **49-A:**232, 1967.
17. Stoffel, A.: The treatment of spastic contractures, Amer. J. Orthop. Surg. **10:**611, 1913.
18. Strayer, L. M., Jr.: Recession of the gastrocnemius. An operation to relieve spastic contractures of the calf muscles, J. Bone Joint Surg. **32-A:**671, 1950.
19. Strayer, L. M., Jr.: Gastrocnemius recession, J. Bone Joint Surg. **40-A:**1019, 1958.

Part III
Knee flexion deformity in cerebral palsy

E. BURKE EVANS, M.D.
Galveston, Texas

Knee flexion deformity in cerebral palsy is either a primary or a secondary phenomenon—possibly, even probably, more often the latter.

Among spastic infants a common postural pattern is that of ankle equinus, knee extension, and hip adduction. This pattern is seen frequently enough to be included in the early diagnostic features of spastic cerebral palsy, and it is elicited by holding an infant aloft by his axillae. Although it is apparently an extensor pattern, the hips will tend to be in that amount of flexion imposed by contracture, and knee extension may not be complete. When these same children are in time required to bear weight or when they do so voluntarily, a strong plantar thrust, hip flexion, or both may cause the knees to be further flexed. Insofar as he is able, the child will do what he must to achieve vertical alignment—flexing the knees and/or extending the back. But however positive the interrelation of ankle, hip, and knee deformity, the sequence of change is not easy to predict. A child may accommodate to a tight heel cord or strong plantar thrust by toe walking, by backknee, by knee flexion if the gastrocnemius is the prime offender, or eventually by breakdown of the foot. If the hip flexors are tight, the child may either flex the knees and keep the back straight or in flexion, or he may lean forward with the knees straight, compensating by means of lumbar lordosis for the forward tilt.

Accepting the fact that knee flexion contracture in patients with cerebral palsy is often a secondary phenomenon, we must in addition recognize that knee flexors can be the primary offender and that hip flexion, at least, may be secondary to the knee flexion.

In considering the patterns of accommodation to the upright or weight-bearing position, it is tempting to assume that the relative strength and spasticity of the various muscle groups determine whether the knees will be extended or flexed. Of course, sitting postures promote, accentuate, and perpetuate existing contractural patterns and create others, and thus influence standing posture. Severe knee flexion contractures occur in children who have never stood or walked. It is thus possible that the final pattern is less related to measurable contracture, peripheral strength, weakness, or spasticity than to cerebral dictation—or even to chance.

Those muscles that may cause a knee flexion contracture or create a crouch stance by their overaction, are as follows:
1. Hamstrings
2. Iliopsoas
3. Gastrocnemius and soleus
4. Tensor fasciae latae
5. Hip adductors
6. Rectus femoris

And it follows that for correction of knee flexion, whether of a primary or secondary nature, the offending muscles must be compromised. If we are dealing essentially with muscle imbalance in spastic cerebral palsy, then the improvement of skeletal alignment should not be difficult provided we are able to assess the problem accurately.

ASSESSMENT OF MUSCLES

We should try to determine at least three things about a muscle or group of muscles: (1) the strength, (2) the degree of spasticity, and (3) the amount of contracture. The relationship among these three is not always positive and the best determination is often an estimate. In general, the strength of spastic muscles is best tested by positioning the part at or near the point of maximum passive excursion for the muscle or group of muscles to be tested. The patient is then asked to resist pressure. The quality of spasticity is extremely variable among patients, but it is consistent in the individual, whereas intensity of response to stretch may vary from one group of muscles to another in the same person. In all testing the abrupt passive motion gives an indication of spasticity. The slow continuous motion reveals more about contracture.

One of the most telling points of assessment has to do with the patient's ability to respond readily to a command to move a part or parts. The greater the time lag between command and execution, the poorer the candidate for surgery.

The strength of the quadriceps can be estimated by observing the standing posture and gait of the patient. If a child who walks in a crouch can appreciably correct knee flexion on command and can do so repeatedly, his quadriceps are of good quality (Fig. 3-32). If he cannot correct the sag but tends to sink into a deeper crouch when walking or standing, the strength of the quadriceps may be assumed to be fair (Fig. 3-30). The quadriceps are checked with the child on his

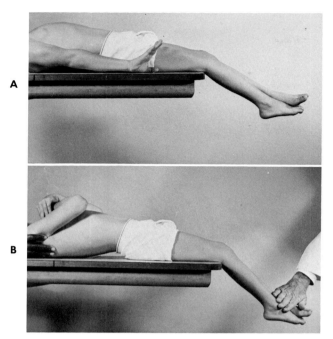

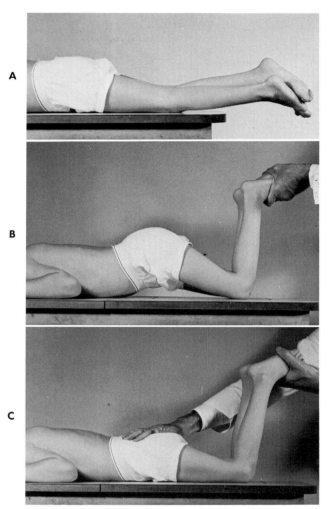

Fig. 3-20. **A,** The quadriceps are checked with the patient on his back and his legs hanging off the table. **B,** He is asked to straighten both legs and to hold as resistance is applied to both extremities. The test is as effective with the trunk supported in slight flexion to relieve the back, but it cannot be performed with the patient sitting up.

Fig. 3-21. **A** and **B,** In the prone rectus test, if both knees are flexed at once, the buttocks will rise sharply. **C,** The patient will usually relax somewhat from this position if pressure is applied to the buttocks.

back and with his legs hanging off of the table, both extremities being tested simultaneously (Fig. 3-20). Resistance is applied at the extreme of extension. The most troublesome isolated quadriceps contracture is that of the rectus femoris. This muscle may be tested with the patient recumbent also, either unilaterally as in testing for hip flexion contracture (Fig. 3-24) or bilaterally (Fig. 3-25). In the unilateral test the amount of restriction of knee flexion on the free side can be determined with some degree of accuracy. If in this position the knee is forced into flexion, the hip will flex or the back will arch. The prone test for rectus femoris tightness incites mass reflex hip flexion, but firm continuous pressure on the buttocks after the knees are flexed will reduce hip flexion to that amount which more nearly reflects the degree of rectus femoris contracture (Fig. 3-21).

Hamstring strength is most easily checked with the patient sitting. The incompetence of these muscles with the hip extended is as real in the child with cerebral palsy as in the normal child, plus the fact that with spasticity there is greater quadriceps resistance. Hamstring contracture is best demonstrated

with the patient recumbent. We have two ways of measuring hamstring contracture. (1) The "absolute" contracture is that amount of flexion which persists in recumbency when the patient's hips are extended maximumly (Fig. 3-22, *A*). (2) The "measurable" contracture is that which is present when the patient's hips are flexed at 90° (Fig. 3-22, *B* and *C*). In both of these measurements, however, the examiner may be deceived because of the presence of hip flexion contracture. If in the presence of a measurable hip flexion contracture the knees extend in recumbency to within a few degrees of full extension, hamstring extensibility may be considered to be adequate. For

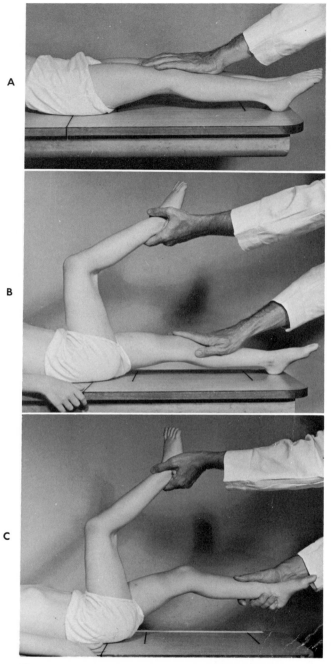

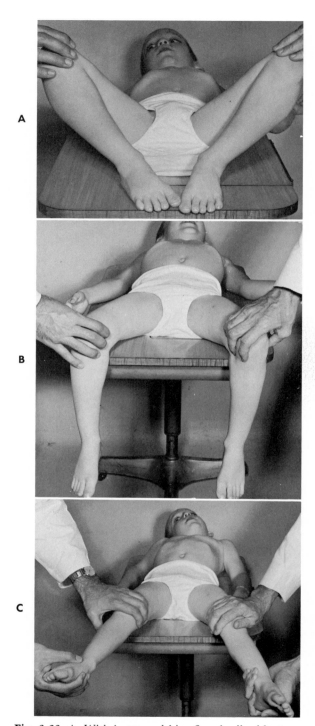

Fig. 3-22. A, In this patient the absolute hamstring contracture is 15°. Part of the resistance is due to the hip flexion contracture. **B,** Classically, to measure hamstring contracture, the opposite extremity is held with the hip and knee in extension so as to stabilize the pelvis. The extremity to be tested is flexed to 90° at the hip before the knee is extended. The contracture measures 65° in this patient. **C,** As would be expected, stabilizing the pelvis with the opposite hip in sufficient flexion to accommodate to its contracture allows more knee extension on the opposite side. The contracture now measures 55° in this patient.

Fig. 3-23. A, With knees and hips flexed, all adductors are maximumly relaxed and the thighs may be most widely abducted. **B,** With hips extended and knees flexed, the gracilis and semitendinosus remain relaxed and the single articulation adductors are tested. **C,** With knees extended, the gracilis and the medial hamstrings now restrict abduction. The difference in the amount of hip abduction obtainable with the knees flexed and with them extended is not always striking, but it is always measurable.

measurement of degrees of contracture, it is easier to flex the hip at 90°, with the opposite hip in extension or flexed sufficiently to accommodate to its contracture (Fig. 3-22, *B* and *C*).

The role of the hamstrings in adduction may be checked with the patient recumbent by abducting the extended hips with the knees flexed at 90° to relax the hamstrings and with the knees extended as much as possible to put the hamstrings on a stretch. This maneuver tests also the most offending adductor—the gracilis (Fig. 3-23). The hamstrings are enough involved in thigh rotation that in extending the knee on the flexed or extended hip the examiner will frequently be aware of an internal rotation pull, which is due to medial hamstring tightness.

Hip flexion contracture is tested in the routine manner (Fig. 3-24). It is often helpful to see how much

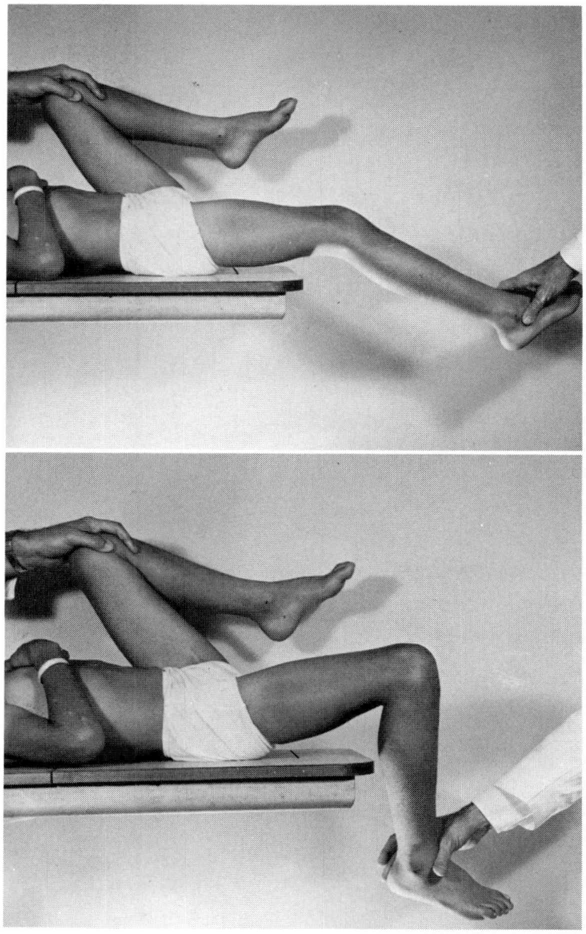

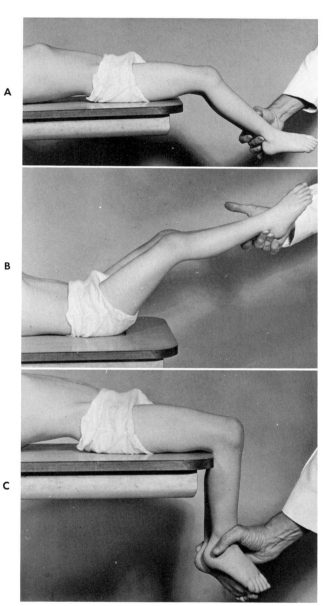

Fig. 3-24. A, In the standard test for hip flexion contracture the lordosis is corrected by flexing both hips and the pelvis is stabilized by holding one extremity in flexion while the opposite extremity is extended. Knee flexion, as shown here, is restricted by quadriceps tightness. **B,** Forced flexion of the knee causes the hip to flex because of tension on the rectus femoris.

Fig. 3-25. A, With thighs parallel to the table and extremities simply supported, there is a visible lordosis. **B,** The lordosis is corrected by flexing the hips to 45°, a measurement approximating the hip flexion contracture. **C,** The lordosis is accentuated by flexing the knees on the extended hips. This maneuver puts tension on the rectus femoris.

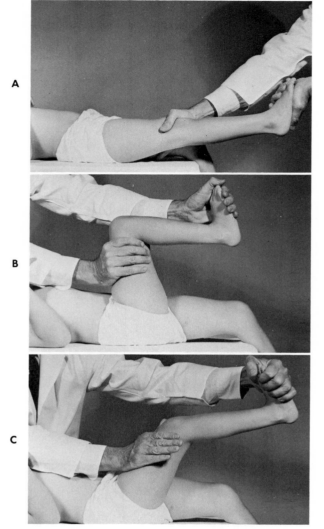

Fig. 3-26. A, With isolated gastrocnemius contracture, the knee can be extended if the ankle is in equinus. **B,** When the knee is flexed, the ankle can be dorsiflexed a few degrees above neutral. **C,** If the ankle is held firmly in dorsiflexion, the knee cannot be extended.

flexion of both extremities is required to flatten the back (Fig. 3-25). Perhaps the most consistently offensive hip flexor is the tensor fasciae latae. Not only does it cause hip flexion but, through the fascia lata, knee flexion as well. It is an offender in internal rotation. The prone "rectus" test may provoke a tensor response. But tensor tightness is palpable. The Ober test is of little use if there is contracture of hip flexors other than the tensor. The iliopsoas may be assumed to be tight in all patients with crouch stance of long duration, often independently imposing a prominent

lordosis. It cannot be isolated from the tensor fasciae latae in testing if there is an adduction contracture.

The effect of a tight gastrocnemius on the knee is easy to demonstrate. If the hamstrings are not tight, the knee can be passively fully extended so long as the ankle is in equinus (Fig. 3-26, *A*). If, on the other hand, the ankle is held firmly in dorsiflexion with the knee flexed (Fig. 3-26, *B*)—the classic test for gastrocnemius tightness—the knee cannot then be fully extended (Fig. 3-26, *C*). Thus the patient with gastrocnemius tightness may walk on his toes with his knees reasonably straight, or he may sink to his heels with his knees in flexion (Fig. 3-27). If the soleus is equally involved, knee position does not affect the equinus.

SURGICAL PROCEDURES

Thus it is possible by examination to determine what muscles or groups of muscles are responsible for the flexed knee posture and the quality and extent of this responsibility. If the hamstrings are not themselves offenders, then we can relieve the knees by surgically weakening the gastrocnemius (Fig. 3-27), the hip flexors (Fig. 3-28), or both by various means. My preference is tendo Achillis lengthening for equinus (I use the White procedure) and simple division of offending muscles for hip flexion. Division or posterior transfer of adductors may relieve knee flexion by release of the gracilis as a knee flexor and by obviating the patient's need to flex the knees in order to stand with adducted extremities.

A truly isolated knee flexion contracture, that is, one due to contracture of the hamstrings alone, is rarely observed in a patient who has neither hip flexion contracture nor equinus. And yet if there *is* true hamstring contracture, with or without contracture at other levels, something must be done surgically to relieve it.

Hamstrings may be weakened surgically by means of release at either end, by lengthening, by transfer, or because there are so many of them, by a combination of these procedures. As it turns out, the means of compromise is probably far less important than the degree. In dealing with the hamstrings it should be an inviolable rule that surgery be held to a minimum and only the amount necessary to obtain knee extension be performed. And there is one other somewhat opposing rule which is as well inserted here—it is *not* necessary to obtain full knee extension surgically, particularly if the quadriceps are of good quality.

All procedures that weaken the hamstrings have three common ill effects. (1) They reduce posterior

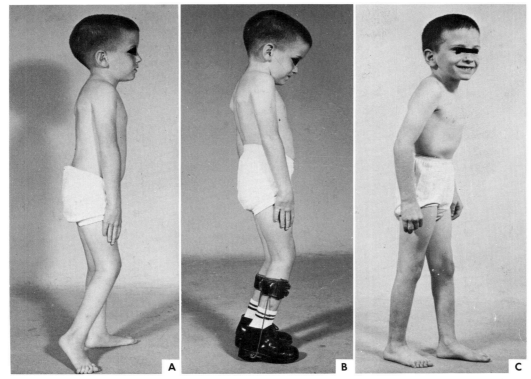

Fig. 3-27. A, A 5-year-old boy with spastic diparesis. Bilateral gastrocnemius contracture is more marked on the right. The left foot is severely pronated. **B,** Braces control equinus, but the tight gastrocnemius muscles prevent knee extension. **C,** Equinus and crouch stance have been corrected by bilateral heel cord lengthening. Note improvement of the position of the left foot.

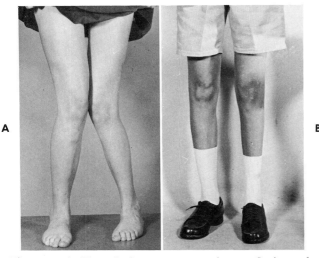

Fig. 3-28. A, Knee flexion stance secondary to flexion, adduction, and internal rotation contracture of the left hip. The diagnosis is asymmetric spastic diparesis. **B,** Correction of crouch has been achieved by means of extensive unilateral hip release, including adductor, iliopsoas, and rectus femoris tenotomies and tensor fasciae latae myotomy.

pelvic stability, giving an excessive degree of lumbar lordosis if it does not already exist or accentuating that which does exist. (2) They decrease knee flexion power. (3) They produce backknee (Fig. 3-29). The degree to which each of these conditions occurs, or whether or not they occur, depends upon the extent of the hamstring surgery and upon the pattern and severity of involvement.

Considering briefly the Eggers hamstring transfer, since it is this procedure with which we are most familiar, there is little resemblance between the present and the original practices. The last full hamstring transfer and retinaculum release was performed in 1963 on an 11-year-old boy who had so severe a contracture that he literally sank to and walked on his knees (Fig. 3-30, *A*). The result was satisfactory (Fig. 3-30, *B*), though he required subsequent hip releases and rotational tibial osteotomies.

Since 1953 the hamstring procedure has been variously modified to fit the different degrees and patterns of involvement. It was determined to my satisfaction that the semitendinosus was, as a rule, the most offen-

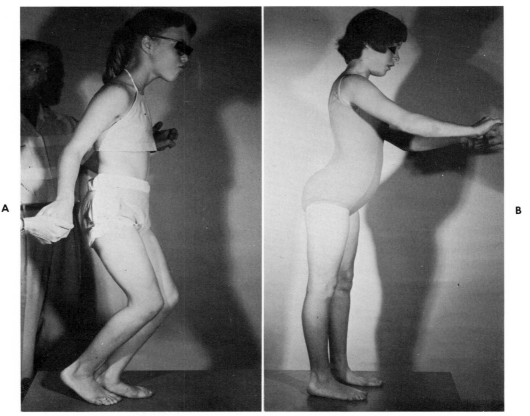

Fig. 3-29. A, A 12-year-old girl who has spastic diparesis with hip and knee flexion contractures. **B,** Two years after complete hamstring transfer, the hip flexion contracture persists. There is marked lordosis and marked knee flexion weakness. This deformity, 5 years later, is unchanged.

sive of the hamstrings and the biceps femoris the least; and I became convinced that the gracilis served no essential purpose.

The semitendinosus and gracilis have the advantages of parallel fibers and good leverage. When the hamstrings are simply divided, these two muscles may retract as far as the upper one third of the thigh. Functionally, the gracilis and semitendinosus are muscles of speed and excursion. The other two muscles have the bulk to make them powerful but sufficient anatomic encumbrance to reduce their excursion. The semimembranosus is bipennate and the relatively short diagonal fibers of its two sections incline distally toward a longitudinal septum. The insertion is into the tibia at the joint margin and into the capsule itself. The ischial portion of the biceps receives the femoral portion in the distal one third of the thigh, and it is this femoral portion that restricts the excursion. Because the semimembranosus and biceps femoris cannot, due to their anatomic restriction, participate in knee flexion contracture to the extent

that the semitendinosus and gracilis do and because tests usually seem to indicate they are less involved than the other two muscles, there is seldom reason to do more than an aponeurotic lengthening. In current practice my minimum procedure is gracilis tenotomy with resection of a 5 cm. section and semitendinosus lengthening or transfer, usually to the ipsilateral condyle. The maximum procedure includes gracilis tenotomy, transfer of the semitendinosus, and aponeurotic lengthening of the semimembranosus and biceps femoris, a section of the aponeurosis being removed from the latter. Thus what was originally a total transfer procedure has become a combination of tenotomy transfer and lengthening.

The change came after observing, particularly in the early postoperative phase, excessive lumbar lordosis and excessive backknee. Functionally, however, the most important ill effect was the loss of knee flexion power.

It is clear, from the experience of other surgeons and more recently from our experience at The Uni-

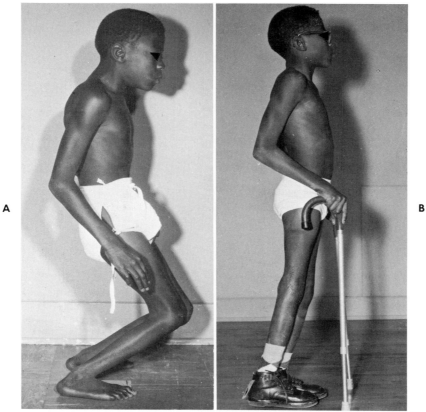

Fig. 3-30. A, An 11-year-old boy with severe knee flexion contractures. He walked most often on his knees. The quadriceps took minimum resistance. **B,** Fourteen months after complete hamstring transfer and retinaculum release bilaterally his knees are straight and the quadriceps have good strength.

versity of Texas Medical Branch, that simple lengthening may suffice for all tendons. We resect a portion of the gracilis because we do not wish it to function again below the knee; we transfer the semitendinosus for the same reason, but we wish, if possible, to retain it as a pelvic stabilizer. If the semitendinosus, because of its greater leverage and excursion, is the most offensive of the hamstrings in the knee flexion deformity, it may be for the same reasons the most important pelvic stabilizer; and I suspect that even the slightest degree of weakening of the semitendinosus will result in a corresponding accentuation of lumbar lordosis. It seems reasonable thus, in transferring the muscle, to place it in the femoral condyle under some degree of tension, but this is more easily proposed than executed. When the semitendinosus is transferred, it is placed in the condyle under a small flap of periosteum and cortex in much the same fashion previously described.[1] Others simply secure it at the adductor tubercle to the tough soft tissue available there. (Our incisions are now simple, short, vertical ones paralleling the gracilis medially and the biceps laterally.)

Transfer of the hamstrings to the femoral condyles might, in theory, improve hip extension. But in the transferred position the muscles are in effect lengthened; their resting length is altered and their strength diminished, so that although extension of the free thigh on the pelvis may be improved, extension of the pelvis and trunk on the fixed thigh probably is not.

What the hamstring transfer offers, which no other procedure does, is permanency of correction. Patients with the transfer require only long leg bracing to control backknee. Over the long course, that is, 2 to 5 years after surgery, we have seen the backknee disappear and the lumbar lordosis improve (Fig. 3-31). However, though the transferred hamstrings may eventually reattach below the knee, good knee flexion power is seldom restored. In the more severely involved, knee flexor weakness is probably a functional

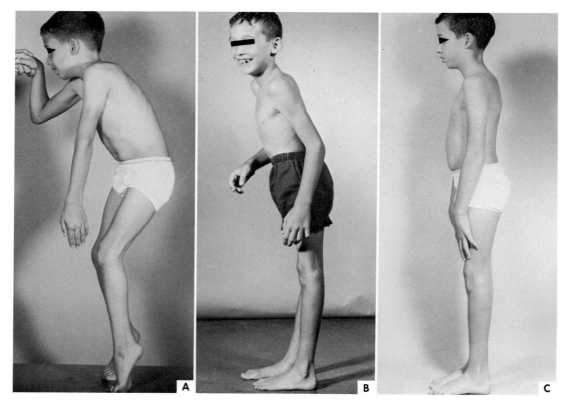

Fig. 3-31. A, A 7-year-old boy with asymmetric spastic diparesis. Contractures at hip, knee, and ankle are more severe on the left. **B,** Nine months after bilateral modified hamstring transfer and left heel cord lengthening. There is bilateral backknee and forward pitch of the trunk. **C,** Two years after surgery the backknee has disappeared and the back is fairly straight. Knee flexion power is only fair. Tendo Achillis lengthening on the right 6 months earlier helped to correct the backknee on that side.

asset. In the moderately affected, it is a handicap.

We readily admit that there are poor results with the modifications of the Eggers procedure. These poor results are really recurrences of deformity, and they may be ascribed as much to a breakdown in postoperative programming as to anything else. The less extensive procedures unquestionably require more carefully planned and executed aftercare than the Eggers procedure.

Whether one tenotomizes, lengthens, or transfers, he is always faced with the dilemma of how much to do to which muscles, whether to operate at more than one level, and when to operate.

We are not arbitrary about the timing of a procedure, but we insist that the patient either be ambulatory or that he have established a reciprocal pattern.

We do not hesitate now to operate at more than one level at a time if there is contracture at more than one level (Fig. 3-32). By doing this rather than operating at one level and waiting to see what spontaneous improvement there will be at the others, we do not increase postoperative morbidity and we do accelerate functional progress in physical therapy. The more conservative practice of doing one level at a time is probably still to be preferred where strict postoperative programming is not available, and there is no question but that in some instances it will be found that surgery at other levels is not needed. Certainly, regarding hamstring surgery, it was a positive dictum of Eggers that the hamstrings only be operated on as an initial measure—with other surgery, if necessary, being reserved for later. Other surgeons, I believe, feel as strongly that the knee should be reserved for the last.

Criteria for surgical procedures in hamstring weakness

For those who would like a formula, Table 3-1 might be a reasonable guide for determining how much surgery to do at the knees.

Table 3-1. Suggested surgery for hamstring weakness

Condition	Suggested surgery
Full active knee extension in recumbency	No hamstring surgery
Active recumbent knee extension to within 5° to 10° of full extension with good quadriceps power	Semitendinosus lengthening or transfer, usually with gracilis tenotomy; occasionally, because of operative testing, aponeurotic lengthening of semimembranosus or biceps
An absolute contracture of greater than 10° but less than 20°	Usually requires gracilis tenotomy, semitendinosus lengthening or transfer, and semimembranosus or biceps lengthening; much depends on quadriceps strength
An absolute contracture of 20° or more and a measurable contracture of 45° or more with the hip at 90°	May require lengthening or transfer of all hamstrings and retinaculum release, again depending on quadriceps strength

Actually, a strict schedule is difficult to follow. All patients do not fit into one of four categories. There is no substitute for repeated observation of the patient while walking, crawling, sitting, and lying. This is the dynamic assessment emphasized by Eggers, who would sooner see a patient walk for 5 minutes than spend an hour testing him on the examining table.

Quadriceps augmentation

One of the features of the original hamstring transfer procedure was the patellar retinacula division to restore the central pull of the quadriceps. We still divide the retinacula when there is a knee flexion contracture in excess of 20° or when active knee extension is significantly less than passive.

In principle, procedures for augmentation of knee extensor strength seem sound enough. The transfer of hamstrings into the patella or quadriceps may be performed occasionally. I have heard the procedure discussed. Advancement of the patella to augment quadriceps strength and to lower a high-riding patella is a more popular procedure. But we question the need for either, since in our experience it has never been necessary to help out the knee extensors. Even those muscles that will take very little resistance prior to surgery will, when allowed to function less opposed by the hamstrings, gain sufficient power for full knee extension without resistance (Fig. 3-30, *B*). If the procedure is to be performed, there is one technical

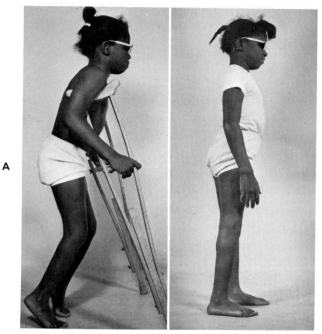

Fig. 3-32. A, A 7-year-old girl with spastic diparesis who had contractures of hip and knee flexors and of the triceps surae. She required crutches for standing and walking. Though she tended to sink into a deeper crouch while upright, she could readily correct the crouch to the limit of her hamstring contracture. She had an excellent walking pattern. **B,** Surgery at all three levels on both sides consisted of recession of the anterior one half of the tensor fasciae latae, division of the anterior fibers of the gluteus medius and minimus, rectus femoris release, gracilis tenotomy, semitendinosus and semimembranosus lengthening, and tendo Achillis lengthening. Thirteen months after surgery she walked without braces or crutches. Lordosis was physiologic, there was no backknee, and there was good knee flexion power.

point worth considering. The advancement in the face of a flexed hip posture will make a tight rectus femoris tighter in spite of straightening the knee, and this muscle may have to be released at its origin.

Rectus femoris and knee function

The functional interrelation of the rectus femoris and the hamstrings is well known, and it is a common practice now for us to release the rectus femoris when we do hamstring surgery. If hip flexion contracture is minimum, we may release the rectus alone, taking out the double tendon of origin down to the muscle belly. This procedure is not carried out basically to increase hip extension but to give a more free knee swing. In spastic patients who have been in a straight-leg paster cast for 2 weeks or more following surgery, active or passive knee motion is often painful, and although total quadriceps shortening may be responsible for much of this restriction, routine rectus femoris release will make it less a problem and will allow better active knee function and hip extension as well. It has been our experience that rectus femoris tightness is difficult to isolate on physical examination. We are not indiscriminate in our selection of cases for its division. But among the moderately to severely involved children, we are of the opinion that the muscle is more often than not offensive regardless of the findings with static testing.

Postoperative programming in knee surgery

Ideally, a spastic child should not be confined to bed after extremity surgery. There is functional hazard even in plaster confinement. In our effort to interrupt a child's functional routine as little as possible, we have adopted a rather active postoperative program. The child is placed on a tilt table 3 days after surgery. He could as easily stand in this manner the first postoperative day were the table available on the ward. While strictly confined to bed, he is begun immediately on stomach-lying and on active trunk and upper extremity exercises as soon as he will cooperate. By the end of the first postoperative week he is standing daily and has resumed all of the therapy and activity that plaster casts will allow (Fig. 3-33). This includes all trunk and upper extremity exercises and even lower extremity exercises within the confines of the cast. We routinely use bilateral long leg plaster casts with the knees in easy extension and with the hips in easy abduction and external rotation. We never force a position. With all tendon or other soft tissue surgery, plaster casts are never used for more than 3 weeks. The patient is then placed in braces and he is kept in these, and often in night splints or night braces as well, until he actively, easily, and efficiently retains the corrected position without them. Knee flexion is restored as soon as possible. Active exercises requiring patient participation are emphasized in all postoperative programming. We involve parents as much as is practical, requiring that they learn the child's routine, participating if necessary.

We have learned that in some children who have walked with a flexed knee posture prior to surgery, walking will be resumed more quickly after surgery if the knees are locked in a few degrees of flexion in the braces. The usual angle for this soft knee posture is 160° to 170°. From this point the knees can be gradually extended as the patient becomes more secure. If the knees are not completely straightened by surgery, they are straightened gradually after surgery by means of calibrated bracing. A softly extended knee is generally preferable to one that slaps into full extension or backknee.

The backknee problem

The backknee gait, if it is not of the abrupt and slapping variety, may be acceptable, particularly if the hyperextension stance is secure for the patient. Occasionally, however, backknee is undesirable, possibly harmful, and to say the least, unsightly. If all of the hamstrings have been sacrificed either by lengthening or transfer, there is little likelihood that adequate support of the back of the knee can be restored by ordinary physical therapeutic means.

In general, the problem is handled in the following ways. If there is hip flexion contracture or gastrosoleus contracture, we correct these surgically since either exaggerates the backknee stance. If the hamstrings have been inserted into the condyles or are simply overlengthened, we may try to restore competency surgically by reinsertion or shortening. This procedure is not, unfortunately, as easy as it sounds, and the results are disappointing. The most important part of the program, whether or not surgery is performed, is the bracing. We place the patient in bilateral long leg braces with a pelvic band. The knee stops are set at 160° and the ankle stops at 85°, or slightly above neutral. The patient is thus forced to return to a slight crouch. It is possible to discard the pelvic band as soon as active hip control is regained, but the knees are restricted indefinitely. Night splinting with the knees in flexion complements this program. It may take months or years to regain a soft knee stance, but there is, to my knowledge, no good alternative to this method. We reject osteotomy.

In those patients who have asymmetric involvement, backknee tendency will likewise be asymmetric (Fig. 3-31). Corrective knee surgery should, accordingly, be asymmetric in extent.

In our enthusiasm we occasionally straighten the knees of patients who would have been better off functionally with their knees in flexion. Such patients are found among the moderately severely involved quadriparetics. It is particularly risky to do knee surgery on a patient who walks independently with slightly flexed knees and whose upper extremities are not good enough to control crutches.

And there are those patients in whom such sufficient improvement can be attained by nonoperative means that surgical correction is unnecessary. Plaster cor-

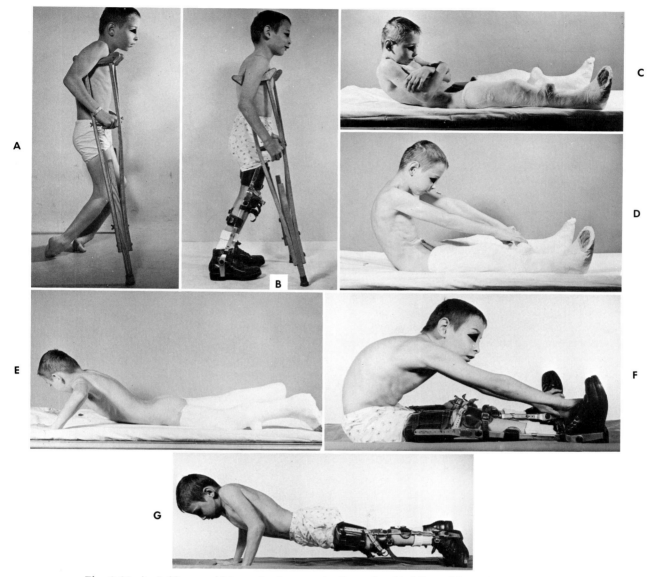

Fig. 3-33. **A,** A 10-year-old boy who has spastic diparesis with bilateral knee flexion and hip adduction contractures and with marked equinovarus deformities of the feet. Hip flexion contracture was minimal. He had a good reciprocal pattern. **B,** Appearance 5 weeks following bilateral adductor tenotomy and medial hamstring and heel cord lengthening. He had been out of the plaster cast and walking for 2 weeks. **C** to **D,** Four days following surgery, he began trunk and upper extremity exercises. Tilt-table standing was begun at the same time. **F** and **G,** Five weeks following surgery, mobility and strength had improved. The only program was therapy at home. He wore his brace with an abduction bar 4 nights a week. He will eventually be able to walk without support.

rection of knee and ankle deformity is particularly rewarding in the mildly to moderately involved children who have good strength, a good reciprocal pattern, and ready voluntary control. Night bracing and a strict physical therapy program may correct the deformity in others.

Surgery is, after all, only a part of the treatment—and a small part at that.

REFERENCE

1. Eggers, G. W. N., and Evans, E. B.: Surgery in cerebral palsy, J. Bone Joint Surg. **45-A:**1275, 1963.

Part IV
Hip deformities in cerebral palsy

EUGENE E. BLECK, M.D.
San Mateo, California

CLASSIFICATION OF HIP DEFORMITIES

The term "hip deformity" is preferred to contracture or contraction since both occur at the same time, making it impossible to differentiate between the two unless the patient is under general anesthesia, thus ensuring complete muscle relaxation. The hip deformities in cerebral palsy can be divided into functional and bony deformities. The functional deformities include those of flexion, adduction, internal rotation, and abduction. The first three of these frequently blend together. As a result of the functional deformities, bony deformities develop, namely, coxa valga and anteversion, subluxation, and finally dislocation. This discussion is concerned with the management of spastic patients. Athetoid patients have entirely different problems, most of which do not appear to be amenable to present physiotherapeutic or orthopaedic surgical methods. The management of these deformities is considered from three aspects: the physiotherapeutic, the orthotic, and the surgical. The sections on physiotherapeutic and orthotic management encompass all functional deformities. Surgical management will be discussed separately for each deformity.

PHYSIOTHERAPEUTIC MANAGEMENT

Stretching. The effectiveness of stretching a spastic muscle to correct a specific deformity must be questioned. As a result of our own experience in the past 10 years and a 16-year follow-up of 550 patients, we have no convincing evidence that hip flexion or hip adduction deformities have been corrected by stretching. Furthermore, recent studies of the gamma system of muscle innervation indicate that the intrafusal fibers of the muscle spindle are stimulated when the muscle is stretched, causing a sensory discharge to the central nervous system. Therefore the more the muscle is stretched, the more muscle contraction occurs.[7]

Exercise. Progressive resistance exercises of hip abductors in order to correct adduction spasticity or strengthen the abductors following surgery have not been effective. Electromyographic studies of the hip abductors in spastic patients with presumably "flaccid zero cerebral muscles" have demonstrated normal motor units. Progressive resistance exercises of the quadriceps in a patient who walks with a flexed knee gait have not effected better extension of the knees when a flexion deformity of the hip is a primary cause of the knee flexion deformity. Hip extension exercises to overcome hip flexion deformities have been unrewarding. Consequently, we have abandoned exercise of individual muscles.

Postural methods. Since 1957 we have used postural or sensory-motor learning methods that have been described in the physical therapy literature.[6,24,34] In essence, these methods are an attempt to develop

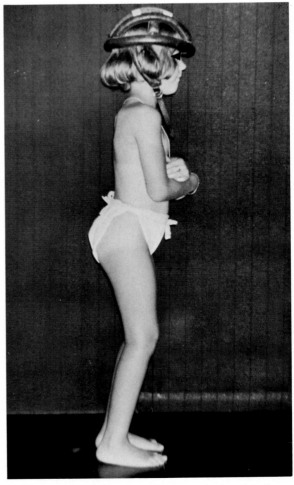

Fig. 3-34. An 8-year-old spastic paraplegic who demonstrates balance between flexor and extensor spasticity. Hamstring spasticity is counteracted by quadriceps spasticity. Hip flexion deformity is compensated by lumbar lordosis.

the best postural control consistent with the neurologic involvement. The most satisfying results are in those patients who strike a balance between spastic flexion and extension patterns (Fig. 3-34). Physiotherapeutic and surgical management can be thought of as a subtraction and addition process in which the correction of one deformity anticipates a compensatory deformity in the opposite direction (Fig. 3-35).

ORTHOTIC MANAGEMENT

Hip flexion deformities have not been controlled with bilateral long leg braces with pelvic bands and hip locks. If the hip joints are locked, the patient either leans forward over the top of the brace or else develops a compensatory lumbar lordosis (Fig. 3-36). Adduction deformities severe enough to cause scissor-

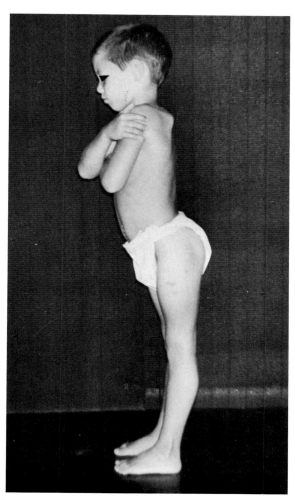

Fig. 3-35. An 8-year-old spastic paraplegic. Hip flexion deformity is compensated only by lumbar lordosis due to spastic knee extension with no hamstring spasticity.

ing have not been controlled with bilateral long leg braces and pelvic bands. Progressive subluxation of the hip has been observed, even with the assiduous application of a restraining brace (Fig. 3-37). If scissoring is severe enough to interfere with either ambulation, sitting, or hygiene, surgical treatment is preferred.

Internal rotation deformities of the hip have not responded to any type of brace. I have used the cable twister brace (Fig. 3-38). If the patient gets an apparent good result from this brace, I have observed the development of external torsion of the tibia with no alteration of the internal rotation deformity of the hip (Fig. 3-39). External torsion of the tibia has been observed even without the application of twister braces in those patients who have good heel contact, probably due to constant torsional stress exerted externally on the tibia as the extremity is carried forward at heel contact.

Crutches are essential for some patients. The dividing line between those patients who use crutches and those who do not is the presence of normal equilibrium reactions. Equilibrium reactions are controlled by the brain. Intermingled with the spastic paralysis, varying degrees of ataxia are present. Crutch use has little to do with muscle imbalance, weakness, or deformity. If the equilibrium reaction loss is severe, no amount of correction of the hip flexion deformity will render the patient crutch free. If the equilibrium reactions are borderline preoperatively, then after hip surgery, crutches may be necessary for a longer time postoperatively until the patient adjusts to the new muscle balance and regains confidence. In evaluating the results of surgery about the hip, crutches mask functional losses after surgery. An accurate assessment of surgery about the hip can be made only in patients who do not use crutches.

SURGICAL MANAGEMENT
Timing of surgery

Based upon long-term clinical examinations and serial motion pictures, I believe that the gait pattern is fixed by the age of 8 years. Physiotherapeutic and surgical methods of treatment after this age yield fewer and fewer good results. Consequently, decisions for surgery should be made before this age, and continuation of physical therapy after this age to produce a better gait pattern can be questioned. Furthermore, early surgery is important if bony deformities, namely, subluxation and dislocation of the hip, are to be avoided. I aim at completing the entire physiotherapeutic and surgical program before the

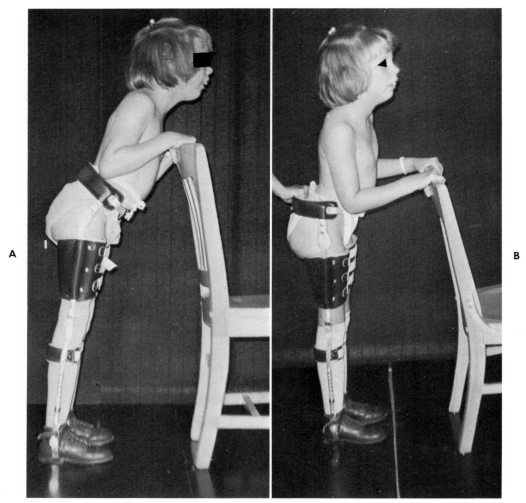

Fig. 3-36. A, A 10-hear-old spastic quadriplegic with severe hip flexion deformity. With the hip joints unlocked, the patient leans forward. **B,** With the hip joints held in extension, the patient still leans forward but must develop lumbar lordosis to keep erect.

age of 9 years; after this age, therapy directed toward the development of the whole child, including activities of daily living, has been more rewarding. In this way the child ceases to be a mere object of "treatment." Any additional surgery as the child becomes older is incidental and not the total program.

How early should surgery be done? Unless subluxation of the hip is developing or fixed hip and knee contractures occur, it is better to wait until the child is ambulatory, either with or without crutches. Preoperative analysis of the locomotor potential of the patient according to the presence or absence of infantile automatisms (for example, persistence of an obligate asymmetric tonic neck reflex and neck-righting reflex or absence of the parachute reaction) has been a reasonably accurate method of predicting

ambulation. There are some children who will never walk because of severe involvement. These nonambulatory children should have surgery of the hip musculature to prevent dislocation of the hip and also to facilitate nursing care and hygiene needs.

Should the surgical procedures be staged? Outmoded adages in cerebral palsy surgery were that the surgeon started at the feet and worked up or started at the hips and worked down. My experience indicates these adages serve no useful purpose; instead, the gait pattern should be analyzed accurately and the surgery accomplished at one stage. Multiple surgical procedures done individually have not been satisfactory because (1) the child becomes more resistant to being "hurt" again and again, (2) the retraining period for gait patterns after surgery rob

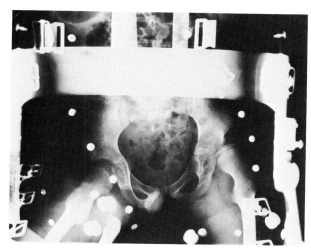

Fig. 3-37. Radiograph of a spastic quadriplegic. Despite application of a full-control brace, subluxation of the right hip has developed. (From Bleck, E. E.: In Adams, J. P., editor: Current practice in orthopaedic surgery, St. Louis, 1966, The C. V. Mosby Co., vol. 3.)

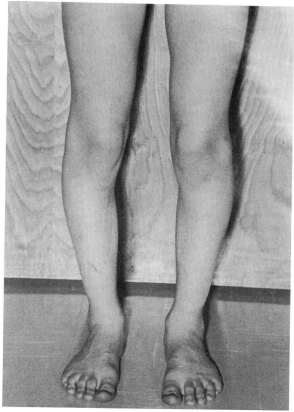

Fig. 3-39. In this spastic paraplegic the patellas point inward due to femoral internal rotation; the feet point straight ahead due to external tibial torsion. (From Bleck, E. E.: In Adams, J. P., editor: Current practice in orthopaedic surgery, St. Louis, 1966, The C. V. Mosby Co., vol. 3.)

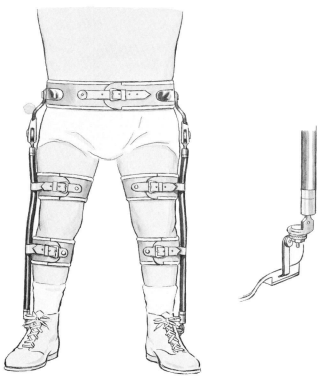

Fig. 3-38. Cable twister brace. (From Bleck, E. E.: In Adams, J. P., editor: Current practice in orthopaedic surgery, St. Louis, 1966, The C. V. Mosby Co., vol. 3.)

the child of development in other areas, for example, speech, education, and self-care, and (3) one deformity corrected does not necessarily lead to correction of all other deformities in the lower extremity; for example, if fixed equinus is present after hip surgery, the result is compromised.

Hip flexion deformity

Measurement. The usual clinical method of hip flexion deformity measurement is to flex the opposite hip on the abdomen to determine the angle the opposite femur makes with the horizontal plane. Varying degrees of hip flexion deformity can be produced by concomitantly flexing the pelvis (Fig. 3-40).

In order to improve the accuracy of measurement of the degree of hip flexion deformity and to analyze its effects on the pelvis and lumbar spine, radiographic studies are helpful. Standing lateral radiographs of the lumbar spine, pelvis, and both hips are made.

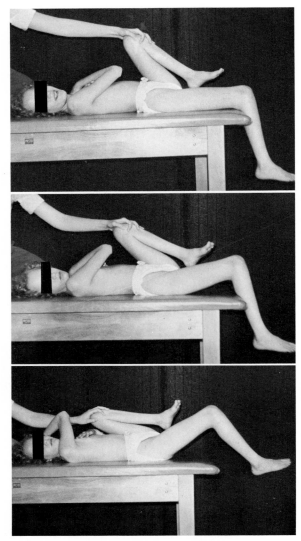

Fig. 3-40. Varying degrees of hip flexion deformity produced by flexing the contralateral hip on the abdomen at varying degrees. (From Bleck, E. E.: In Adams, J. P., editor: Current practice in orthopaedic surgery, St. Louis, 1966, The C. V. Mosby Co., vol. 3.)

The radiographic landmarks used for measurement are the superior aspect of the sacrum and a line drawn along the femoral shaft. I have called this the sacral-femoral angle. The normal angle in the standing patient ranges from 50° to 65° (Fig. 3-41). In patients who have spastic hamstrings and flexed knees the sacral-femoral angle approaches zero, with the femur becoming horizontally parallel with the top of the sacrum (Fig. 3-42). In patients whose knees have been extended either spontaneously due to quadriceps spasticity or surgically due to hamstring

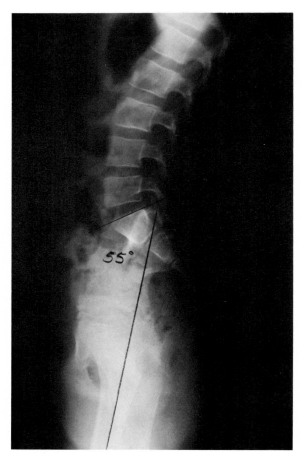

Fig. 3-41. Standing lateral radiograph of the lumbar spine, pelvis, and both hips in a normal 10-year-old child. The sacral-femoral angle is 55°.

lengthening or transfer, the sacral-femoral angle also approaches zero, with the femur becoming vertically parallel with the top of the sacrum (Fig. 3-43). The sacral-femoral angles of patients who have undergone either hamstring lengthening or transfer are less than 30°. Three patients have had low back pain due to excessive lordosis after a hamstring transfer (Fig. 3-44). If the sacral-femoral angle is under 35°, significant hip flexion deformity is present.

Biomechanical analysis. The deforming force of the hip flexor spasm becomes evident as the lumbar spine, pelvis, and knees conform to the hip flexion deformity. Two compensatory mechanisms are noted. One is the development of an anterior inclination of the pelvis in conjunction with spasticity of the quadriceps. The lumbar spine becomes lordotic, but the knees remain straight (Fig. 3-45). A second compensatory mechanism occurs in the presence of spastic hamstrings and causes posterior inclination of the

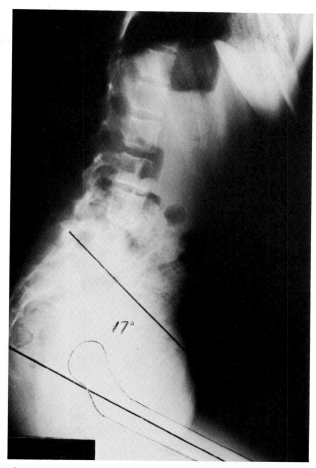

Fig. 3-42. Standing lateral radiograph of the lumbar spine, pelvis, and both hips in an 11-year-old patient with spastic paraplegia. Note flexed hip–flexed knee posture. The femur becomes horizontally parallel with the top of the sacrum. (From Bleck, E. E.: In Adams, J. P., editor: Current practice in orthopaedic surgery, St. Louis, 1966, The C. V. Mosby Co., vol. 3.)

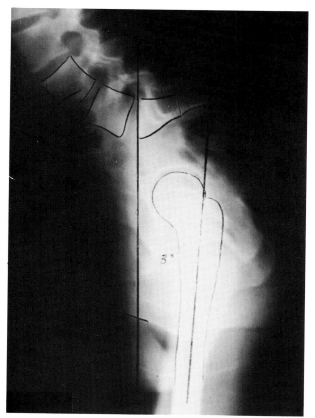

Fig. 3-43. Standing lateral radiograph of a 20-year-old spastic paraplegic who has severe hip flexion deformity with extended knees. The femur becomes vertically parallel with the top of the sacrum. (From Bleck, E. E.: In Adams, J. P., editor: Current practice in orthopaedic surgery, St. Louis, 1966, The C. V. Mosby Co., vol. 3.)

pelvis and flexed knees. These patients are sitting down while standing up (Fig. 3-46). The lack of extension of the lumbar spine and the inability of the pelvis to incline backward due to the tightness of the anterior capsule of the hip joint aggravate the hip flexion deformity so that the knees must flex even more.

In patients with marked hip flexion and knee flexion deformities, methods to extend the knees with braces, hamstring tenotomies and lengthenings or transfers, or patellar advancements increase the amount of functional disability because the balancing effect of the knees in the flexed position is removed. Therefore the patient bends forward at the trunk or else assumes a severe lordotic position and still leans forward (Fig. 3-47).

If spastic equinus is present in a patient with flexed hips and flexed knees, balance becomes precarious. Overlengthening of the Achilles tendon, however, causes a secondary exaggerated flexion deformity of the hips and knees (Fig. 3-48).

As a result of these observations, correction of the hip flexion deformity must be considered.

Function of hip flexors. The iliopsoas is the main flexor of the hip. The rectus femoris and sartorius are flexors, but not beyond 90° flexion. The pectineus, in addition to adduction, flexes in all positions of the joint. The adductors longus, brevis, and magnus act as flexors from the hyperextended to the flexed position, but not beyond 50° to 70°, respectively. The gracilis acts as a flexor up to 20° to 40° flexion.[9] Electromyographic studies of the iliacus have demonstrated that normally there is practically no activity of this muscle during walking.[10] Basmajian[4] found that

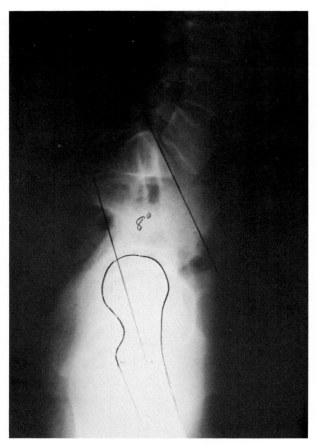

Fig. 3-44. Radiograph of a 17-year-old spastic paraplegic 1 year after modified hamstring transfer. The sacral-femoral angle is 8°. The patient has spondylolisthesis and low back pain. The preoperative sacral-femoral angle was 32°. (From Bleck, E. E.: In Adams, J. P., editor: Current practice in orthopaedic surgery, St. Louis, 1966, The C. V. Mosby Co., vol. 3.)

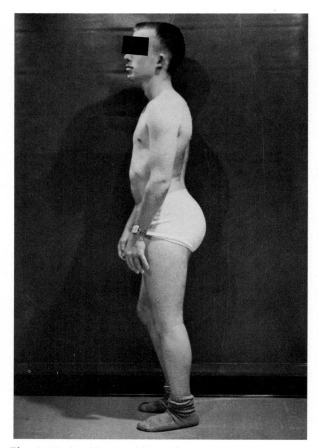

Fig. 3-45. An 18-year-old spastic paraplegic who has bilateral hip flexion deformity with spastic knee extension resulting in compensatory lumbar lordosis. (From Bleck, E. E.: In Adams, J. P., editor: Current practice in orthopaedic surgery, St. Louis, 1966, The C. V. Mosby Co., vol. 3.)

the iliopsoas shows slight to moderate activity during standing. He recorded action potentials in all degrees of flexion and demonstrated that the iliopsoas is neither a medial nor a lateral rotator since both motions produce some slight activity. Keagy et al.[19] demonstrated electrical activity of the psoas major during heel-rise and the initial 40% of the swing phase in level gait (Fig. 3-49).

ILIOPSOAS TENOTOMY

Rationale. Frequent failures of muscle slide operations and fasciotomies in cerebral palsy have been observed. These operations were originally designed to correct hip flexion deformities in poliomyelitis. The pathologic process of a contracture in poliomyelitis is in the fascia layers surrounding the muscle; hence

these operations were fairly successful. However, in cerebral palsy, no contracture in the fascia or, in fact, within the muscle itself has been demonstrated by gross or microscopic analysis. Lamb and Pollock[22] reported a marked recurrence rate in sixty-six patients who had Campbell or Soutter muscle slide operations. Peterson[30] first described iliopsoas tenotomy to relieve hip flexor spasm in ten patients who had spastic paraplegia resulting either from disease or trauma of the spinal cord. Bleck and Holstein[5] performed iliopsoas tenotomy in patients with spastic cerebral palsy. Keats[21] reported a modification of the operative approach for iliopsoas tenotomy in patients with cerebral palsy.

Selection of patients. As the result of my experience with iliopsoas tenotomy, the following criteria are suggested in selecting patients for this procedure.

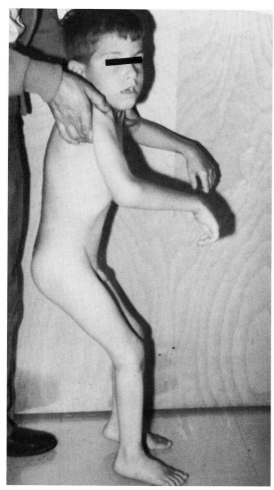

Fig. 3-46. A 7-year-old spastic paraplegic who has severe hip flexion deformity with spastic hamstrings and resultant posterior inclination of the pelvis and a flattened lumbar spine.

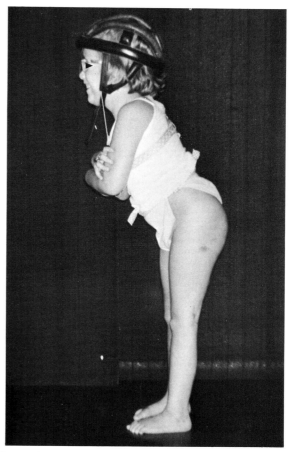

Fig. 3-47. A 7-year-old spastic paraplegic after semitendinosus transfer and semimembranosus and biceps lengthening. The knees formerly were flexed. The patient has a hip flexion deformity and now leans forward in compensation for the extension of the knees.

Spastic paralysis. Tension athetosis can be confused with spasticity, and if iliopsoas tenotomy is done in tension athetosis, a shift of the tension to the extensors may result, precluding even sitting in a wheelchair.

Flexed hip–flexed knee gait. Iliopsoas tenotomy can be combined with hamstring transfer or lengthening to prevent severe lordosis or imbalance of the posture.

Patient who uses crutches. A patient who can walk without external support can be weakened by iliopsoas tenotomy since hip flexion power is diminished considerably in the majority of such patients. Patients who use crutches may compensate for this loss of power.

Patient less than 16 years of age. Patients older than 16 years of age may have too much secondary contracture of the joint capsule and even bony deformity

to expect adequate satisfactory correction by tenotomy alone.

Hip flexion deformity over 45°. A standing lateral radiograph of the lumbar spine, pelvis, and both hips is helpful in the preoperative analysis of the patient. If the sacral-femoral angle is less than 35°, iliopsoas tenotomy may be considered in addition to hamstring or other surgery designed to extend the knees.

Operative technique. Iliopsoas tenotomy was performed using the modified Ludloff approach (Fig. 3-50).[11] A longitudinal incision paralleling the adductor longus muscle was made. The adductor longus was isolated and sectioned, and the anterior branch of the obturator nerve was sectioned if an obturator neurectomy was to be performed at the same time. The adductor brevis was sectioned with a cutting

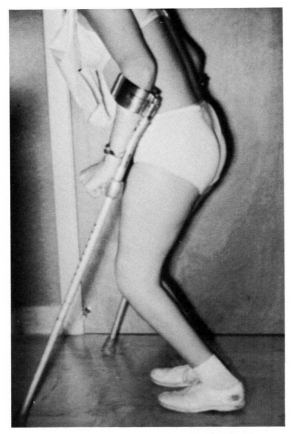

Fig. 3-48. A 14-year-old spastic paraplegic. Achilles tendon lengthening for spastic equinus resulted in exaggerated flexion deformity of the hips and knees. (From Bleck, E. E.: In Adams, J. P., editor: Current practice in orthopaedic surgery, St. Louis, 1966, The C. V. Mosby Co., vol. 3.)

cautery. The hip was externally rotated, flexed, and abducted; and at the depths of the wound, the lesser trochanter was palpated and the iliopsoas tendon isolated and sectioned. Continuous closed suction drainage was used in the wound for 24 hours postoperatively. Postoperative care consisted of long leg plaster casts with an abduction bar for 4 to 6 weeks.

Results. An 8- to 14-year follow-up has been carried out on the first thirteen patients who had iliopsoas tenotomy. Nine patients who were ambulatory continued to maintain the original correction of the hip flexion deformity (Fig. 3-51). The mean anatomic correction obtained was 18° (from a mean preoperative deformity of 60°). Five-year postoperative standing lateral radiographs of the lumbar spine, pelvis, and hips of four patients have shown a sacral-femoral angle of 50°, 48°, 47°, and 45°. One patient who was ambulatory, age 26 years, failed to improve. Three patients who were nonambulatory remained so postoperatively. It should be emphasized that this procedure or any other operative procedure cannot make a nonambulatory patient ambulatory. All patients permanently lost hip flexion power; however, all were able to lift their foot 6 inches from the floor so they could clear curbs.

Because of the permanent weakness after iliopsoas tenotomy, iliopsoas recession was developed to control the lengthening of the iliopsoas and preserve part of its strength.

ILIOPSOAS RECESSION

Selection of patients. Five years' experience with twenty-five patients who had the spastic type of

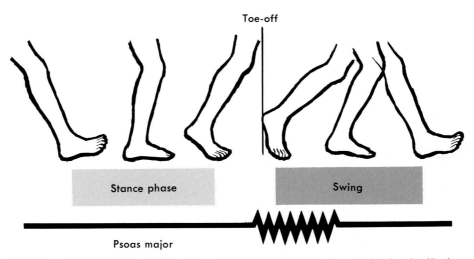

Fig. 3-49. Electromyographic activity of the psoas major muscle during level gait. (Redrawn from Keagy, R. D., Brunlik, J., and Bergan, J. J.: J. Bone Joint Surg. **48-A:** 1377, 1966.)

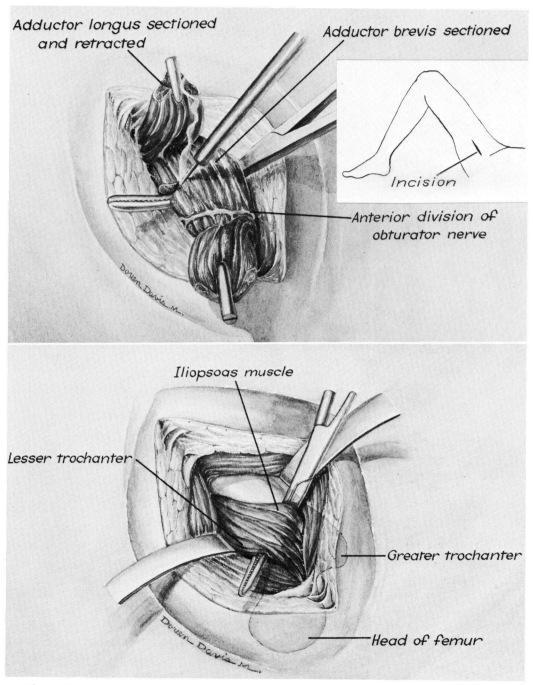

Fig. 3-50. Operative technique for iliopsoas tenotomy. (From Bleck, E. E.: In Adams, J. P., editor: Current practice in orthopaedic surgery, St. Louis, 1966, The C. V. Mosby Co., vol. 3.)

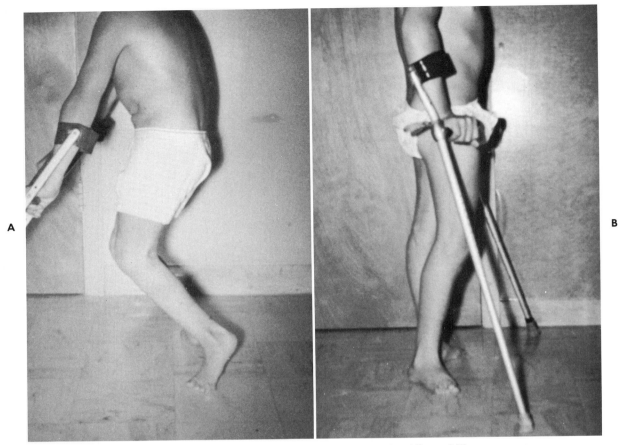

Fig. 3-51. A, A 12-year-old spastic triplegic. **B,** Four years after bilateral iliopsoas tenotomy, hamstring lengthening, patellar advancement, and Achilles tendon lengthening. (From Bleck, E. E.: In Adams, J. P., editor: Current practice in orthopaedic surgery, St. Louis, 1966, The C. V. Mosby Co., vol. 3.)

cerebral palsy was the basis for the development of the following criteria for the selection of patients. These children were categorized according to their gait patterns as follows: (1) flexed hips–internally rotated and flexed knees (spastic hamstrings), (2) flexed hips–internally rotated and hyperextended knees (spastic quadriceps), and (3) flexed hips–internally rotated and normal knee function (Fig. 3-52). The optimum age for the best surgical result was 7 to 9 years. The hip flexion deformity was greater than 15° and the sacrofemoral angle was less than 45°. Twenty-one patients walked without support and four were nonambulatory but had the potential to walk according to the neurologic assessment.

Operative technique. The approach was through an anterior iliofemoral incision that coursed obliquely downward, beginning ½ inch beneath the anterior

superior iliac spine and extending for approximately 4 to 6 inches. The sartorius muscle was retracted laterally. The femoral nerve was defined and separated from the iliacus muscle; the medial and lateral borders of the iliopsoas were defined. It was noted in the dissections that the iliacus muscle fibers overlapped the broad psoas tendon that hugged the anterior medial aspect of the hip joint capsule. The iliacus muscle was then sectioned as far distally as possible and the psoas tendon was cut close to the lesser trochanter. The psoas tendon was sutured to the anterior capsule of the hip near the base of the neck of the femur and the iliacus muscle fibers were sutured into the capsule in this location (Fig. 3-53). Continuous suction drainage was used in all wounds for 24 hours.

In addition to iliopsoas recession, other procedures were performed at the same time, depending upon

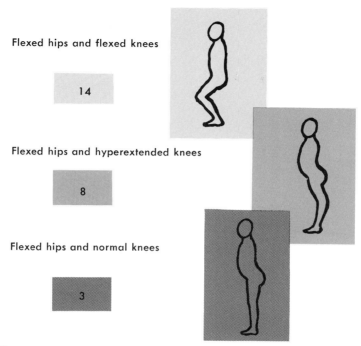

Flexed hips and flexed knees

14

Flexed hips and hyperextended knees

8

Flexed hips and normal knees

3

Fig. 3-52. Diagrammatic representation of the three spastic hip flexion gait patterns in a series of twenty-five patients.

the preoperative analysis of the gait pattern and the examination. In patients who had actual scissoring or limitation of hip abduction to 15° to 20° or less an adductor longus myotomy and anterior branch obturator neurectomy were performed. In those who walked with hyperextended knees a rectus femoris release at its origin was carried out. In those who walked with flexed knee gait patterns, the semi-tendinosus tendon was transferred to the medial femoral condyle and the semimembranosus length-ened. Achilles tendon lengthening was performed on those patients who had a contracture of the gastroc-nemius soleus muscles.

Postoperative care. The hips were not immobilized in plaster. Patients were kept in bed for 3 weeks; no sitting was permitted. All were allowed to lie prone, supine, or on their side. At the end of 3 weeks, gait training was resumed, first of all in parallel bars, then on crutches, and finally independent ambulation for those patients who had good equilibrium reactions.

Results. The mean correction of the hip flexion deformity was 20°, with a range from 0° in one patient to a maximum of 50°. The sacrofemoral angles, measured radiographically, showed decreased lumbar lordosis in the majority of patients and no increased lordosis in those who had the hamstring transfer and lengthening. Muscle testing of the hip flexors demon-

strated grades of good to fair in the majority of patients. An interesting long-term result of iliopsoas recession was a gradual decrease in the passive range of internal rotation of the hips and an increase in the passive range of external rotation. The mean decrease in hip internal rotation was 25° and the mean increase in external rotation was 25°. Subluxation of the hip in all three nonambulatory children was reduced. A 50% improvement in the gait pattern was observed. Physical therapy beyond 12 months postoperatively was not necessary. No deterioration of the gait pattern has been observed. All children are brace free (Fig. 3-54).

Adduction deformities

Biomechanical analysis. Other than that of hip stabilizers, the true role of the adductors has never been established. It has already been pointed out that the adductors can also act as flexors, but after 50° of flexion they become extensors. Regarding the rotary function of the adductors, they appear to be mechan-ically situated as external rotators; however, when the joint is already internally rotated, they may act as internal rotators. Banks and Green's report[3] of eighty-nine patients who had adduction deformities is of interest. Only fifteen of their eighty-nine patients had internal rotation deformities with the adduction

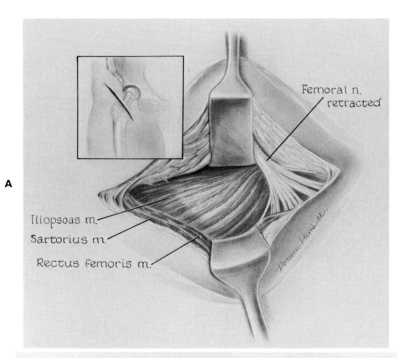

A

Femoral n.
retracted

Iliopsoas m.

Sartorius m.

Rectus femoris m.

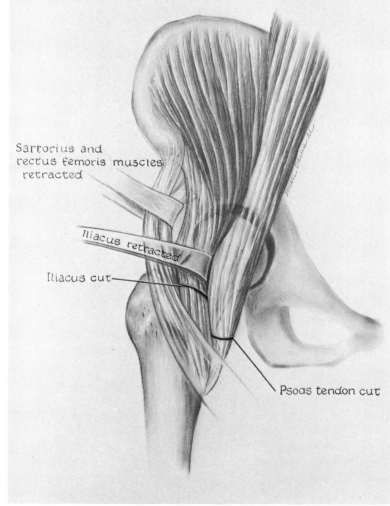

B

Sartorius and
rectus femoris muscles
retracted

Iliacus retracted

Iliacus cut

Psoas tendon cut

Fig. 3-53. For legend see opposite page.

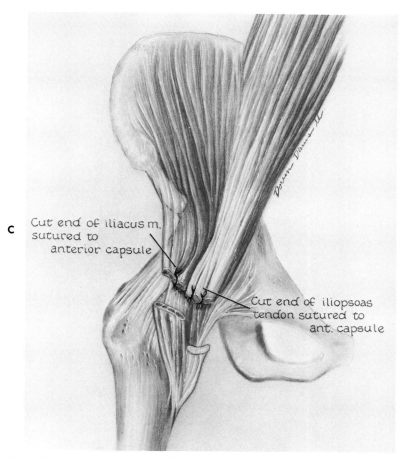

C   Cut end of iliacus m.
     sutured to
     anterior capsule

     Cut end of iliopsoas
     tendon sutured to
     ant. capsule

Fig. 3-53. A, Operative technique for iliopsoas recession. Incision and anatomy of the wound when viewed from the side as it appears to the surgeon. The sartorius and rectus femoris muscles are retracted laterally. The femoral nerve is identified and *gently* retracted. **B,** The tendon of the psoas major is broad medially and hugs the capsule of the hip. The iliacus muscle fibers are sectioned as far distally as possible; the psoas tendon is cut near its insertion on the lesser trochanter. **C,** The psoas tendon is sutured to the anterior capsule of the hip and the iliacus fibers are sutured to the capsule in the same location. (From Bleck, E. E.: J. Bone Joint Surg. [In press.])

deformity. My own observations confirm that internal rotation or flexion deformities are not outstanding features of the posture with pure adduction deformities. Consequently, the surgical treatment of spastic adductors cannot be relied upon to correct internal rotation or flexion deformities of the hip.

Excessive abduction of the hip during gait is not physiologic. The normal base of the gait is from 2 to 4 inches from heel to heel.[13] The hip abductors are stronger when the hip joint is in the neutral position. The data furnished by Murray and Sepic[28] that the mean output of torque of the hip abductor muscles was 82% greater with the hip in the neutral rather than the abducted position should be considered

when contemplating hip adductor surgery as a panacea for gait problems in cerebral palsy.

Surgical procedures. Adductor longus myotomy and anterior branch obturator neurectomy have been established as a satisfactory procedure for ambulatory spastic patients who scissor or nonambulatory patients who may have so much scissoring that hygiene and nursing care become difficult (Fig. 3-55).[3,20] In the ambulatory patient, adductor longus myotomy and anterior branch obturator neurectomy are indicated as the first procedure. If insufficient correction is obtained, an intrapelvic obturator neurectomy is an easier secondary procedure because the posterior branch of the obturator nerve is difficult to find in the

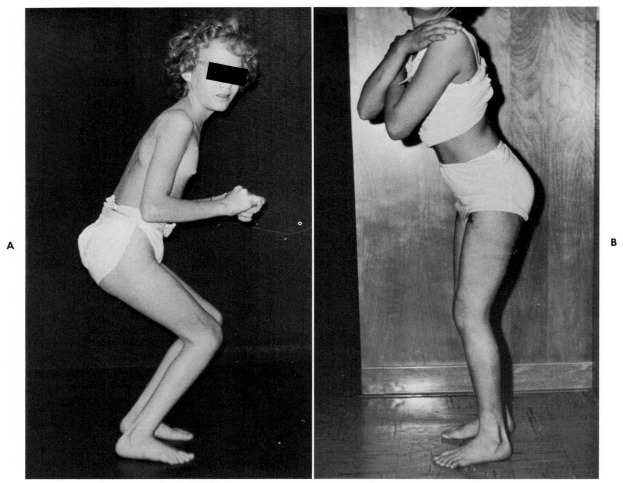

Fig. 3-54. A, A 14-year-old spastic paraplegic. **B,** One year after bilateral iliopsoas recession and modified hamstring transfer. This patient remains balanced and walks without support. Compensatory lumbar lordosis has developed. There is no loss of hip flexion power. It was impossible to correct the hip flexion deformity entirely due to contracture of the joint capsules of the hip and of the knee.

usual postoperative scar. In the nonambulatory patient who scissors severely the first choice is the intrapelvic obturator neurectomy rather than the extrapelvic approach.

Adductor myotomy and anterior branch obturator neurectomy have been combined with iliopsoas tenotomy or iliopsoas recession for the treatment of flexion or internal rotation deformities of the hip. Frequently these deformities blend together and combined operative treatment is required.

Abduction deformity

Abduction deformity of the hip is a rare occurrence. It has been said that this deformity has occurred in spastic patients as a result of weakening of the adductors by obturator neurectomy so that abduction occurs. I have observed postoperative abduction deformities only in those patients whose condition was misdiagnosed as spastic but was, in fact, tension athetosis. In such athetoid patients a shift of the tension from one muscle to another can occur postoperatively (Fig. 3-56).

Two patients without prior surgery had abduction deformities of the hips. Both patients had spastic and hypertrophied tensor fascia femoris muscles. Both had internal torsion of the tibias and equinovarus of the feet. Neither had internal rotation deformities of the hip. Surgical release of the tensor fascia femoris satisfactorily corrected the abduction deformity in both patients.

Internal rotation deformities

Biomechanical analysis. Internal rotation deformities of the hip have been consistently observed in those patients who walk with flexed hips and hyperextended knees. The more the patient walks with the knees flexed, the less the internal rotation deformity becomes (Figs. 3-57 to 3-59). In these patients, excessive medial rotation of the pelvis occurs with internal rotation of the femur (Figs. 3-60 and 3-61). When such a patient is examined in the supine position with the hips extended, the range of external rotation of the femur will be very limited (Fig. 3-62). If the hip, however, is flexed to 90°, external rotation can easily be accomplished due to a combination of two factors: relief of tension on the iliopsoas and abnormal anteversion of the proximal end of the femur (Fig. 3-63). Radiographic studies (Magilligan technique) for femoral anteversion have demonstrated increased femoral anteversion in all patients who had internal rotation deformities of the hip (Figs. 3-64 and 3-65).[26]

Once the hip begins to internally rotate, several muscles contribute to the internal rotation: the medial hamstrings and the gluteus medius and minimus. If the proximal end of the femur is anteverted, with subsequent posterior positioning of the

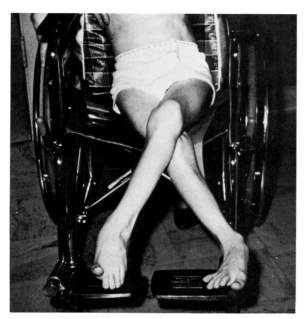

Fig. 3-55. Severe scissoring in a nonambulatory patient.

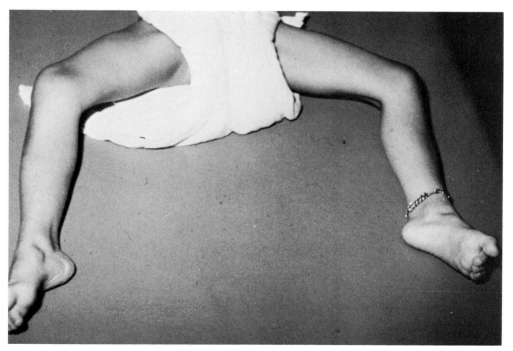

Fig. 3-56. Abduction deformity of the hips after adductor myotomy and anterior branch obturator neurectomy in a patient with tension athetosis. The deformity is not fixed and the extremities can be brought together.

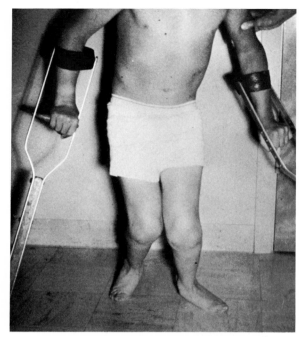

Fig. 3-57

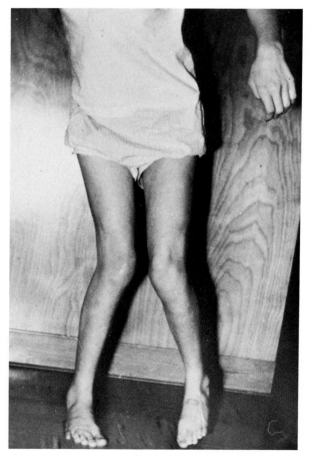

Fig. 3-58

Fig. 3-57. A 13-year-old spastic paraplegic with flexed hip–flexed knee gait. With greater degrees of knee flexion such as this, the rotation deformity is not apparent.

Fig. 3-58. In this 15-year-old spastic paraplegic, as the knees are progressively extended, the internal rotation deformity becomes evident.

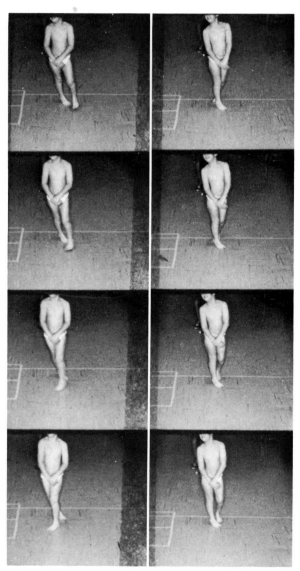

Fig. 3-59. Sixteen-millimeter filmstrip of a spastic paraplegic with internal rotation and flexion deformity of the hip and spastic rectus femoris.

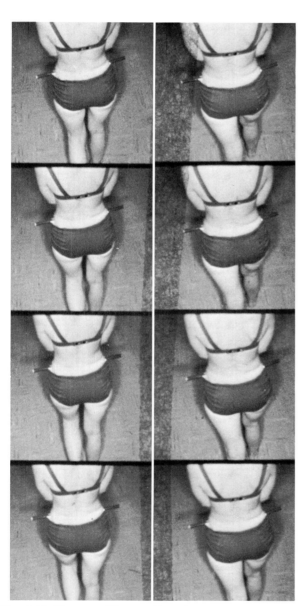

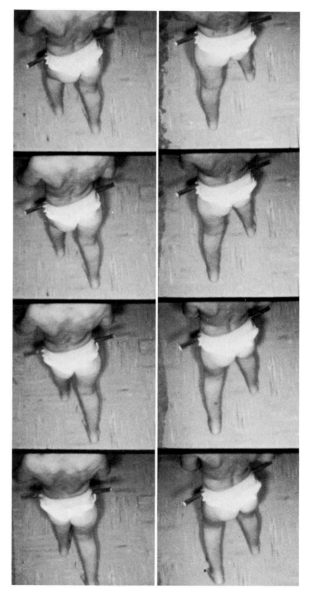

Fig. 3-60. Sixteen-millimeter filmstrip of a normal female; markers on the anterior spine of the ilium demonstrate the degree of medial and lateral rotation of the pelvis during gait.

Fig. 3-61. Sixteen-millimeter filmstrip of an 8-year-old spastic paraplegic; markers on the anterior spine of the ilium demonstrate the excessive medial rotation of the pelvis as the extremity is carried forward.

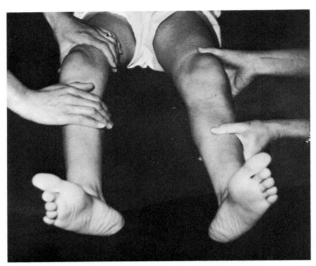

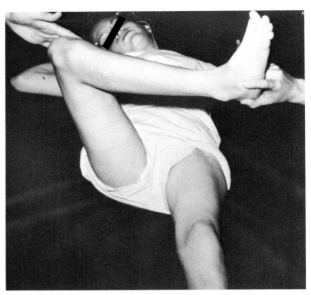

Fig. 3-62. When this spastic paraplegic is supine and the extremities extended, internal rotation deformity of the hip is evident. External rotation of the hip is practically zero.

Fig. 3-63. A spastic paraplegic with internal rotation deformity of the hip. With the hip flexed to 90°, external rotation is possible.

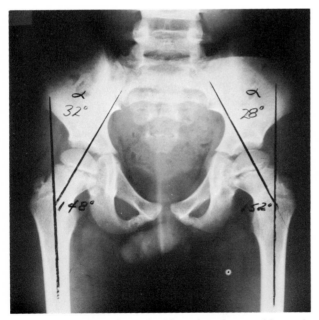

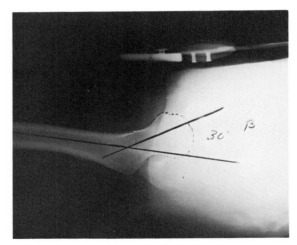

Fig. 3-64. Radiograph of the hips of an 8-year-old spastic paraplegic with internal rotation deformity. The alpha angle is part of the radiographic technique in measuring the degree of anteversion according to Magilligan.

Fig. 3-65. Lateral radiograph of the hip of a spastic paraplegic with internal rotation deformity. The beta angle is measured and the Magilligan chart is used to determine the angle of true anteversion. In this patient the true angle of anteversion of the right hip is 47° and of the left hip 53°. At this age the normal range is between 32° and 7°.

greater trochanter, the greater trochanter must rotate forward to a more neutral position in order for the hip abductors to function most efficiently.[27]

The role of the iliopsoas in the production of the internal rotation deformity has been considered. Because the iliopsoas is inserted lateral to the axis of the femur, this muscle has been considered an internal rotator.[13, 14] However, electromyographic studies of the iliacus show it is neither an internal nor an external rotator. The occurrence and importance of pelvic rotation during gait has been noted.[24, 27] The internal rotation function of the iliopsoas seems to be medial rotation of the pelvis in relation to the femur at the time of push-off in gait so that excessive lateral rotation of the pelvis is prevented.[37]

In the spastic patient the iliopsoas appears to lock the femur to the pelvis, preventing pelvic-femoral freedom during gait as if the hips were ankylosed. Consequently, an alternating internal rotary gait results in a patient who has severe bilateral spasticity.

Surgical procedures. Three procedures for internal rotation deformities can be recommended.

Iliopsoas recession. This procedure has been performed on thirty-five patients under the age of 9 years who have walked with their lower extremities in internal rotation. All have had flexion deformities of the hip and in all the hips have had varying degrees of excessive femoral anteversion (mean 55°) demonstrated by the radiographic techniques of Magilligan.

The operative technique has been described previously. The iliopsoas tendon has been sutured to the anterior capsule of the hip joint. No postoperative immobilization has been used. Three weeks of bed rest without trunk elevation has been sufficient.

The results of iliopsoas recession have been gratifying. However, complete correction of internal rotation has not been observed. Persistence of increased femoral anteversion has explained the failure of complete correction. Poor results have occurred in two patients over 9 years of age who had approximately 60° to 70° of femoral anteversion (Fig. 3-66).

Semitendinosus transfer. The semitendinosus tendon is detached distally and transferred and rerouted through a separate tunnel to the anterior lateral aspect of the femur as described by Baker and Hill[1] and modified by Sutherland et al.[38] The procedure seems to be indicated in those patients who have a mild hip flexion deformity and a passive range of external rotation of the hip to at least 10° with the hip extended. This transfer seems to work mainly

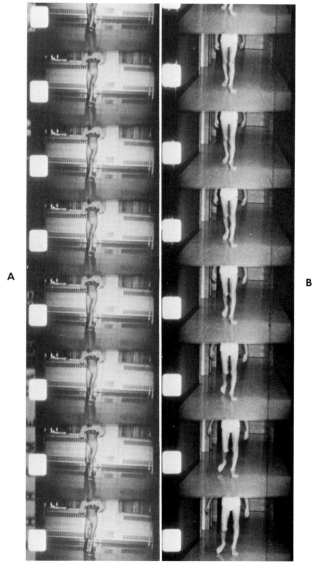

A **B**

Fig. 3-66. A, Filmstrip demonstrates bilateral internal rotation deformities of the hip in an 8-year-old spastic paraplegic. **B,** One year after bilateral iliopsoas recession and modified hamstring transfer.

during the swing phase of gait, removing one additional cause of internal rotation. If a significant hip flexion deformity is present, correction may be disappointing. In my experience, transfer of a semitendinosus to the medial condyle of the femur appears to work as well as rerouting the tendon.

Derotation subtrochanteric osteotomy. The rational of this operation is to correct the internal rotation deformity of the hip by effectively blocking internal

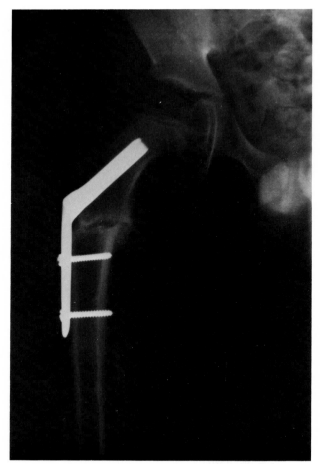

Fig. 3-67. Postoperative x-ray view of derotation subtrochanteric osteotomy fixed with a small Jewett nail.

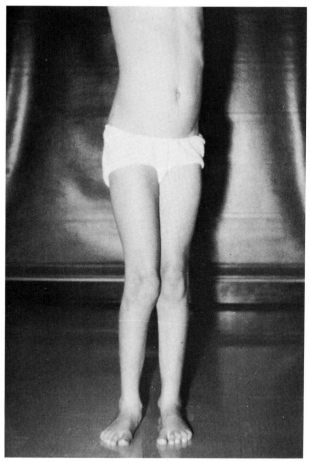

Fig. 3-68. Patient after derotation subtrochanteric osteotomy for internal rotation deformity of the hip. Anterior rotation of the pelvis persisted on the side operated on due to complete elimination of the range of internal rotation of the right hip following osteotomy. If internal rotation of the hip is zero, then external rotation of the pelvis cannot occur.

rotation. Follow-up anteversion radiographs of the hip demonstrate correction of anteversion. The operative technique consists of a subtrochanteric osteotomy using a small-scale Jewett nail for fixation. It is important to insert the nail first into the head and neck of the femur before performing the osteotomy. The assistant holds the hip in internal rotation with the nail and plate in place. The osteotomy is completed and the femur is externally rotated just to the neutral position and then the shaft is fixed to the plate (Fig. 3-67). It is important to avoid overcorrection of the deformity by making sure that the hip is not forced into too much internal rotation. This has been an effective procedure, particularly in unilateral internal rotation deformities of the hip. I have reserved femoral osteotomy for children over the age of 8 years because, with advanced skeletal maturity, spontaneous correction of femoral anteversion after

correction of the hip flexion deformity cannot be anticipated.

Two problems have been noted after subtrochanteric derotation osteotomy: increased lumbar lordosis and persistent anterior rotation of the pelvis on the side on which the osteotomy was performed (Figs. 3-68 and 3-69). Increased lumbar lordosis appears to result from externally rotating the lesser trochanter with the distal fragment, increasing the tension on the iliopsoas. Consequently, iliopsoas recession is now performed in addition to the rotation osteotomy. Persistent forward rotation of the pelvis has been observed only on unilateral derotation osteotomies. It is due to effective blockage of internal rotation of the hip so that the pelvis cannot externally

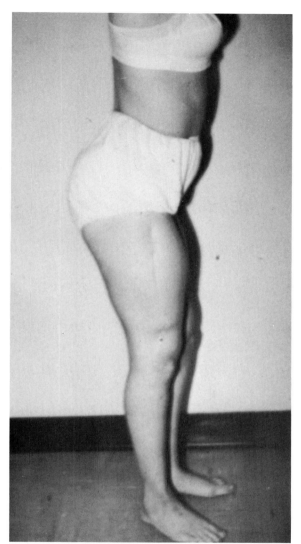

Fig. 3-69. Five years after bilateral derotation subtrochanteric osteotomy. Severe compensatory lordosis developed due to persistence and aggravation of the hip flexion deformity.

rotate on the hip during gait. This secondary deformity can be minimized by avoiding overcorrection and iliopsoas recession.

Bony deformities

The bony deformities of the hip in patients with spastic cerebral palsy are coxa valga, anteversion, subluxation, and dislocation. Complete dislocation of the hip has been observed only in nonambulatory patients. The objective of surgical treatment is to prevent subluxation in the ambulatory patient and dislocation in the nonambulatory patient.

Pathogenesis. Subluxation and dislocation of the hip in cerebral palsy is an acquired and not a congenital deformity (Fig. 3-70). Coxa valga is a radiographic finding indicating that the femoral neck angle is greater than 135°. Lewis and co-workers,[25] after detailed radiographic study, concluded that the true deformity was anteversion rather than coxa valga. My own studies indicate that both deformities are present, but the major deformity accounting for the coxa valga is anteversion of the proximal end of the femur (Fig. 3-71).

The striking correlation between the hip flexion deformity and the presence of excessive femoral anteversion suggests a hypothesis of persistent fetal femoral anteversion. Fetal femoral anteversion has been estimated to be as high as 60°, with a range of 10° to 55° at the eighth month of gestation.[23, 36] The hips are flexed in the fetus, and after birth a rapid decrease in the hip flexion contracture occurs, with full extension completed by 3 months. Children who are born with spastic paralysis of the hip flexors never extend the hips completely. Thus the femoral anteversion persists as in the fetus. In the normal infant, as the hip extends, the pressure of the femoral head against the anterior capsule of the hip results in gradual derotation of the cartilaginous proximal end of the femur. I have observed that patients with postnatal cerebral spastic paralysis and hip flexion deformities (for example, cerebral contusion or laceration at age 2 or 3 years) do not have excessive internal rotation of the femur or abnormal femoral anteversion.

With persistent excessive femoral anteversion, the following can occur: (1) if the spastic child becomes independently ambulatory, internal rotation of the hip during gait occurs, (2) if the child has delayed ambulation and uses crutches, subluxation ensues, and (3) if the child is nonambulatory, dislocation eventually follows subluxation.

Wilkinson[39] consistently produced anteversion of the proximal end of the femur in rabbits by holding the femur in internal rotation. Holding the femur externally rotated produced retroversion. Brookes and Waddle,[8] in attempting to analyze the deformities that would be produced by overpulling of the muscles on the decalcified femur, noted that when the iliopsoas was contracted, a valgus deformity of the neck of the femur resulted. They reported the case of a 4-year-old patient, with flaccid paralysis due to poliomyelitis who had good iliopsoas function on the left and absent iliopsoas function on the right. Seven and a half years later the left side subluxated,

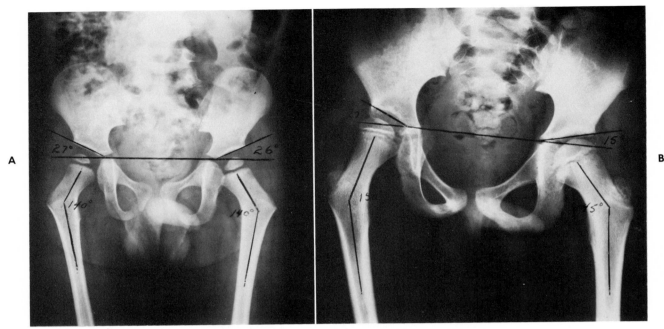

Fig. 3-70. A, Radiograph of the hips of a 3-year-old patient with left spastic hemiplegia. **B,** Radiograph made when the patient was 9 years of age showed development of coxa valga and subluxation of the left hip.

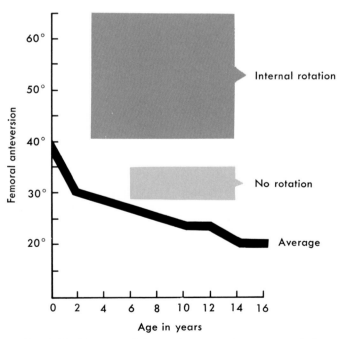

Fig. 3-71. Ranges of femoral anteversion measured in fifty-five spastic paraplegic or diplegic children with internal rotation deformity compared with twenty-two without internal rotation deformity and plotted against the average femoral anteversion in normal children.

but the right side showed no subluxation. In addition to the pull of the iliopsoas, the adductors, and particularly the gracilis, have been incriminated as the cause of progressive coxa valga.[31]

Holstein[16] believed that, in addition to the adductors, the iliopsoas was also responsible for producing the bony deformities leading to subluxation and dislocation. It appeared likely that with the hip already adducted the iliopsoas acted as a powerful adductor. Sharrard[35] has added the concept that the iliopsoas acts as a "nylon cord" suspending the hip in a new center of rotation when the hip is subluxated and thus acts as an effective force levering the hip out of the acetabulum to produce dislocation. Failures of reduction of subluxation of the hip have been observed after adductor myotomy and obturator neurectomy (Fig. 3-72).

Adductor myotomy, anterior branch obturator neurectomy, and iliopsoas tenotomy. Coxa valga without subluxation demands no treatment other than repeated radiographic observation. If subluxation ensues, surgery is indicated. For adduction spasm with minimal hip flexion deformity, adductor myotomy and anterior branch obturator neurectomy are sufficient. If, in addition to adduction spasticity, the medial hamstrings are contracted, medial ham-

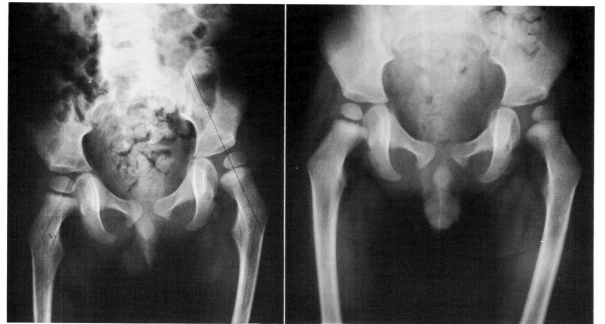

Fig. 3-72. A, A 3-year-old nonambulatory spastic paraplegic with subluxation of the right hip. **B,** Eleven months after adductor myotomy and anterior branch obturator neurectomy. Subluxation of the right hip persisted.

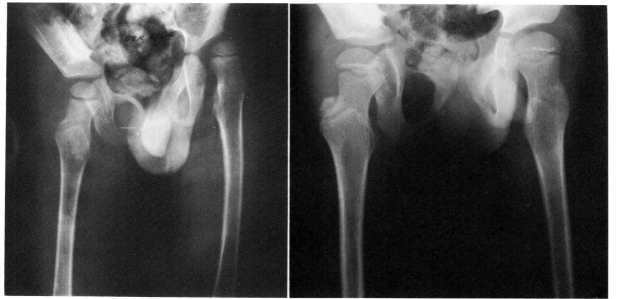

Fig. 3-73. A, A 3-year-old spastic quadriplegic with subluxation of the right hip. **B,** Five years after adductor myotomy, anterior branch obturator neurectomy, and iliopsoas tenotomy. The subluxation of the right hip has been reduced.

string tenotomy or transference is useful. If, however, considerable hip flexion deformity is present, iliopsoas tenotomy is indicated.

Bleck and Holstein[5] performed iliopsoas tenotomy, adductor myotomy, and anterior branch obturator neurectomy in nine patients to correct coxa valga and subluxation of the hip. The results, after a follow-up of 3 to 10 years, showed good restoration of the hip to near normal in all cases, except in one patient who was not spastic but had tension athetosis (Fig. 3-73).

Varus derotation subtrochanteric osteotomy. Varus subtrochanteric osteotomy to correct subluxation of the hip was introduced by Jones.[17,18] The objectives of the osteotomy are to restore the femoral neck angle to normal and to centralize the head of the femur in the acetabulum. A more accurate term for the operation is varus derotation subtrochanteric osteotomy because femoral anteversion frequently must be corrected in order to accomplish the objective of the surgery. Osteotomy is preferable to acetabular shelving procedures because spastic patients who had shelves developed limited hip motion later in life or the shelf melted away. Varus derotation subtrochanteric osteotomy is indicated in patients over the age of 9 years when over half of the femoral head is outside the acetabulum. Lesser degrees of subluxation in patients under the age of 9 years can be treated by muscle release operations alone, as described in the previous section. If acetabular shallowing is present in a patient whose growth is almost completed, an iliac osteotomy can be performed at the same stage.

The operative technique consists of two parts, both done at the same time: (1) adductor myotomy, anterior branch obturator neurectomy, and iliopsoas tenotomy and (2) subtrochanteric osteotomy (Fig. 3-74). This procedure is done on an orthopaedic table so that a spica cast may be applied afterward. After release of the spastic muscles medially the hip is abducted to its maximum. The subtrochanteric region of the femur is approached through a lateral incision. With the hip held in maximum abduction and internal rotation to correct anteversion, two Steinmann pins are inserted, one through the base of the neck of the femur and a second pin just superior to the acetabulum through both walls of the ilium. The pins are crossed externally and held by entwining them with heavy stainless steel wire. A guide pin is introduced through the subtrochanteric region of the femur between the greater and lesser trochanters, and a radiograph is made in order to ascertain the site of osteotomy. After the osteotomy the distal

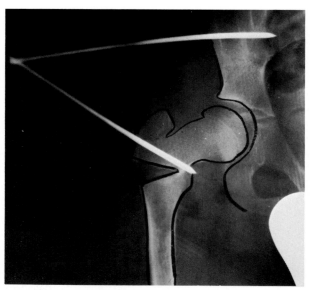

Fig. 3-74. Radiograph made in the operating room shows two-pin fixation and varus derotation subtrochanteric osteotomy in a patient with paralytic subluxation of the hip.

fragment is adducted to restore the femoral neck angle to 125° and externally rotated to place the distal fragment in neutral rotation. The pins are incorporated into a one and a half hip spica plaster cast. Immobilization is necessary for 8 weeks.

The end results of subtrochanteric osteotomy have been satisfactory. The length of follow-up has been 4 to 10 years. The results appear permanent due to the fact that the deforming muscles have been weakened by tenotomy and neurectomy (Fig. 3-75). If acetabular reconstruction is necessary, it can be performed at the same time of the osteotomy.

Dislocation of the hip. Dislocation of the hip in the spastic patient has been seen only in the nonambulatory patient. The dislocated hip frequently becomes painful, precluding even comfortably sitting in a wheelchair. At first the dislocation is usually unilateral. The dislocated hip is in neutral rotation and flexion, with the unaffected hip in marked internal rotation (Fig. 3-76). Reduction of the dislocated hip demands considerable surgical reconstruction in order to centralize and hold the head of the femur in the acetabulum. The most successful procedure has been bilateral adductor myotomy, obturator neurectomy, and iliopsoas tenotomy, followed by varus derotation subtrochanteric osteotomy and an iliac osteotomy (Fig. 3-77).

If one hip is dislocated, it is important to release the spastic adductors and iliopsoas bilaterally in order

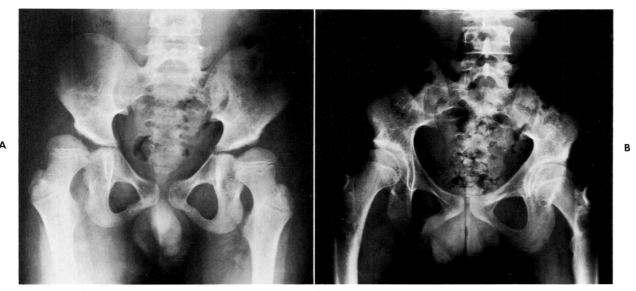

Fig. 3-75. A, A 9-year-old spastic paraplegic with subluxation of both hips. **B,** Five and one-half years after bilateral iliopsoas tenotomy and varus derotation subtrochanteric osteotomy.

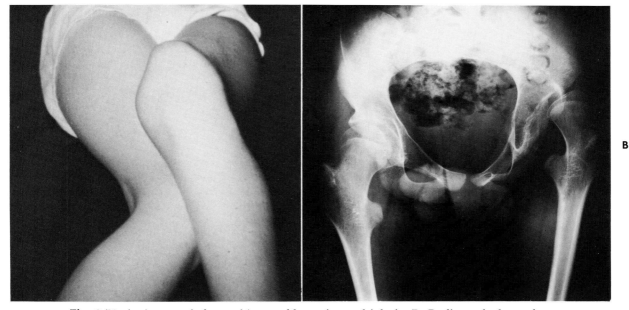

Fig. 3-76. A, A nonambulatory 14-year-old spastic quadriplegic. **B,** Radiograph shows that the left hip is dislocated. The right hip, which is internally rotated, is not dislocated. The pelvis on the dislocated side is rotated posteriorly.

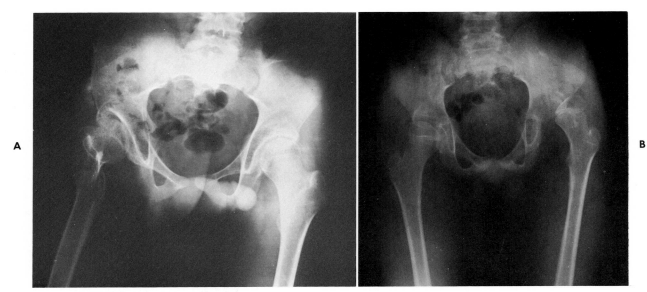

Fig. 3-77. A, An 11-year-old wheelchair-bound spastic quadriplegic who has a dislocated left hip. **B,** Five years after iliopsoas tenotomy, adductor myotomy, anterior branch obturator neurectomy, varus derotation femoral osteotomy, and iliac osteotomy. The hip has remained stable and painless.

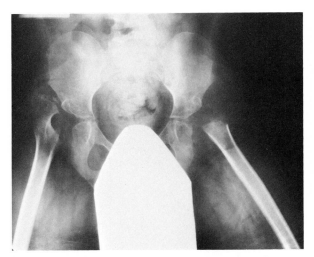

Fig. 3-78. Radiograph of the hips of a nonambulatory 8-year-old spastic quadriplegic shows dislocation of the left hip and the appearance of the right hip after femoral head and neck resection for a painful dislocation. The right hip subsequently became painful and femoral head and neck resection were again performed. The patient could sit comfortably after a short convalescence.

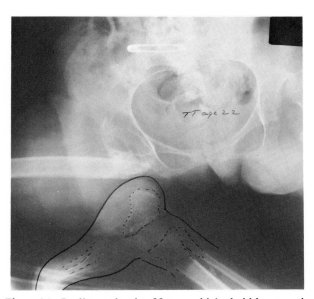

Fig. 3-79. Radiograph of a 22-year-old bed-ridden spastic quadriplegic after femoral head and neck resection of the left hip for painful dislocation. (Courtesy Dr. Jacob Sharp, Porterville State Hospital, Porterville, Calif.)

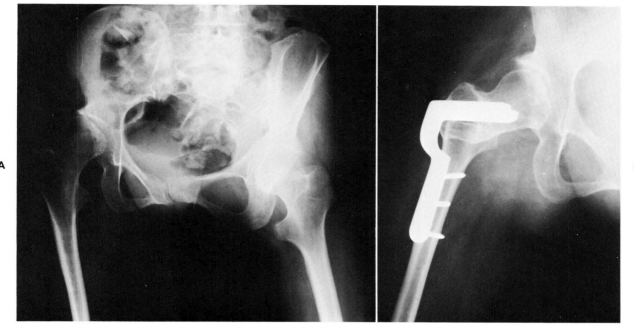

Fig. 3-80. A, Painful subluxation of the hip due to degenerative arthritis in a 40-year-old spastic paraplegic. Bilateral hip flexion deformities of 40° were present. Surgical treatment included bilateral iliopsoas recession and varus displacement osteotomy of the hip. **B,** Radiograph made after varus intertrochanteric osteotomy and iliopsoas recession. There was complete relief of pain. (Courtesy Dr. Leonard Woods, Concord, Calif.)

to obviate the dislocation of the opposite unaffected hip following surgery on one hip alone. In spastic paraplegia, when one hip is dislocated, the pelvis on the side of the dislocation is rotated posteriorly, with anterior rotation of the pelvis on the opposite unaffected side. In addition, the dislocated hip is more adducted than the unaffected hip, holding the opposite hip in abduction. As a result of these two factors, the opposite uninvolved hip is held in a position of abduction and internal rotation, preventing dislocation. Therefore, if the dislocated hip is relieved of the adduction and pelvic rotation deformity by tenotomy, further adduction and external rotation of the opposite hip can be anticipated with a resultant dislocation. Femoral head and neck resection combined with intrapelvic obturator neurectomy, iliopsoas tenotomy, and adductor myotomy has been occasionally successful (Fig. 3-78). However, my experience and that of Samilson[32] is that femoral head and neck resection leaves much to be desired, particularly in the older severely spastic patient (Fig. 3-79). I would now recommend the more difficult and extensive reconstruction by varus derotation subtrochanteric femoral osteotomy, iliac osteotomy, and the soft tissue releases previously referred to.

Painful subluxated hip in the adult with cerebral palsy. Adult patients who have spastic paralysis and a subluxated hip have complained of disabling pain if they are ambulatory. Their hips have gradually succumbed to degenerative arthritis (Fig. 3-80, *A*). Such patients can be surgically treated via hip flexor and adductor release plus the usual reconstructive hip surgery such as a cup arthroplasty or intertrochanteric femoral varus displacement osteotomy (Fig. 3-80, *B*).

REFERENCES

1. Baker, L. D., and Hill, L. M.: Foot alignment in the cerebral palsy patient, J. Bone Joint Surg. **46-A:**1, 1964.
2. Baker, L. D., Dodelin, N. D., and Bassett, F. H.: Pathological changes in the hip in cerebral palsy: incidence, pathogenesis, and treatment, J. Bone Joint Surg. **44-A:**1331, 1962.
3. Banks, H. H., and Green, W. T.: Adductor myotomy and obturator neurectomy for the correction of adduction contracture of the hip in cerebral palsy, J. Bone Joint Surg. **42-A:**111, 1960.
4. Basmajian, J. V.: Muscles alive, Baltimore, 1962, The Williams & Wilkins Co.
5. Bleck, E. E., and Holstein, A.: Iliopsoas tenotomy for spastic paralytic deformities of the hip, Presented at the annual meeting of The American Academy of Orthopaedic Surgeons, Chicago, 1963.
6. Bobath, K., and Bobath, B.: Control of motor function

in the treatment of cerebral palsy, Physiotherapy **43:** 295, 1957.

7. Boyd, I. A., Eyzaguirre, C., Matthews, P. B. C., and Rushworth, G.: The role of the gamma system in movement and posture, New York, 1964, Association for the Aid of Crippled Children.

8. Brookes, M., and Waddle, E. N.: Muscle action and the shape of the femur, J. Bone Joint Surg. **44-B:**398, 1962.

9. Brunnstrom, S.: Clinical kinesiology, Philadelphia, 1962, F. A. Davis Co.

10. Close, J. R.: Motor function in the lower extremity, Springfield, Ill., 1964, Charles C Thomas, Publisher.

11. Crenshaw, A. H., editor: Campbell's operative orthopaedics, ed. 5, St. Louis, 1971, The C. V. Mosby Co., vol. 2.

12. Dunlap, K., Shand, A. R., Jr., Hollister, L. C., Gual, S., Jr., and Streit, H. A.: A new method for determination of torsion of the femur, J. Bone Joint Surg. **35-A:** 289, 1953.

13. Frankel, V. H.: Fundamentals of biomechanics, Instructional Course Lectures, The American Academy of Orthopaedic Surgeons, Chicago, 1968.

14. Grant, J. C. B.: A method of anatomy, ed. 5, Baltimore, 1952, The Williams & Wilkins Co.

15. Hollinshead, W. H.: Functional anatomy of the limbs and back, Philadelphia, 1951, W. B. Saunders Co.

16. Holstein, A.: Personal communication, 1958.

17. Jones, G. B.: Paralytic dislocation of the hip, J. Bone Joint Surg. **36-B:**375, 1954.

18. Jones, G. B.: Paralytic dislocation of the hip, J. Bone Joint Surg. **44-B:**573, 1963.

19. Keagy, R. D., Brunlik, J., and Bergan, J. J.: Direct electromyography of the psoas major muscle in man, J. Bone Joint Surg. **48-A:**1377, 1966.

20. Keats, S.: Combined adductor-gracilis tenotomy and selective obturator-nerve resection for correction of adduction deformity of the hip in children with cerebral palsy, J. Bone Joint Surg. **33-A:**698, 1951.

21. Keats, S.: A simple anteromedial approach to the lesser trochanter of the femur for the release of the iliopsoas tendon, J. Bone Joint Surg. **49-A:**632, 1967.

22. Lamb, D. W., and Pollock, G. A.: Hip deformities in cerebral palsy and their treatment, Develop. Med. Child Neurol. **4:**488, 1962.

23. Lanz, T., and Mayet, A.: Zeitschrift fur Anatomie, Berlin, 1953, Julius Springer.

24. Levitt, S.: Physiotherapy in cerebral palsy, Springfield, Ill., 1962, Charles C Thomas, Publisher.

25. Lewis, F. R., Samilson, R. L., and Lucas, D. B.: Femoral torsion and coxa valga in cerebral palsy, Presented at the annual meeting of The Western Orthopaedic Association, Seattle, 1963.

26. Magilligan, D. J.: Calculation of the angle of anteversion by means of horizontal lateral roentgenography, J. Bone Joint Surg. **38-A:**1231, 1956.

27. Merchant, A. C.: Hip abductor muscle force, J. Bone Joint Surg. **47-A:**462, 1965.

28. Murray, M. P., and Sepic, S. B.: Maximum isometric torque of hip abductor and adductor muscles, Phys. Ther. **48:**1327, 1968.

29. Murray, M. P., Drought, A. B., and Kory, R. C.: Walking patterns of normal men, J. Bone Joint Surg. **46-A:**335, 1964.

30. Peterson, L. T.: Tenotomy in the treatment of spastic paraplegia with special reference to the iliopsoas, J. Bone Joint Surg. **32-A:**875, 1950.

31. Phelps, W. M.: Prevention of acquired dislocation of the hip in cerebral palsy, J. Bone Joint Surg. **41-A:**440, 1959.

32. Samilson, R.: Dislocation of the hip in cerebral palsy, Instructional Course, Lectures, The American Academy for Cerebral Palsy, Houston, 1970.

33. Saunders, J. B., Dec, M., Inman, V. T., and Eberhart, H. D.: The major determinants in normal and pathological gait, J. Bone Joint Surg. **35-A:**543, 1953.

34. Semans, S.: Physical therapy for motor disorders resulting from brain damage, Rehabilitation Literature of National Society for Crippled Children and Adults **20:**99, 1959.

35. Sharrard, J.: Discussion on surgery of the hip in cerebral palsy, Instructional Course Lectures, The American Academy for Cerebral Palsy, Houston, 1970.

36. Sommerville, E. W.: Persistent foetal alignment of hip, J. Bone Joint Surg. **51-A:**1070, 1957.

37. Strange, F. G. St. Clair: The hip, Baltimore, 1965, The Williams & Wilkins Co.

38. Sutherland, D. H., Schottstaedt, E. R., Larsen, L. J., Ashley, R. K., Callander, J. N., and James, P. M.: Clinical and electromyographic study of seven spastic children with internal rotation gait, J. Bone Joint Surg. **51-A:**1070, 1969.

39. Wilkinson, S. A.: Femoral anteversion in the rabbit, J. Bone Joint Surg. **44-B:**386, 1962.

Chapter 4

The painful shoulder

GEORGE HAMMOND, M.D., WILLIAM R. TORGERSON, JR., M.D.,
WILLARD E. DOTTER, M.D., and ROBERT E. LEACH, M.D.
Boston, Massachusetts

Next to backache, pain in the shoulder is the most frequent complaint of orthopaedic patients at the Lahey Clinic Foundation. Despite the frequency and importance of shoulder lesions in producing disability, it is surprising that physicians have allowed so much confusion to exist as to terminology, diagnosis, and treatment. This confusion is rampant in our formal and informal discussions, in the medical literature, and in textbooks.

Supraspinatus tendinitis, supraspinatus syndrome, painful arc syndrome, subdeltoid and subacromial bursitis, calcific or calcified bursitis, calcific or calcified tendinitis, and tendinitis calcarea are terms that refer to the same syndrome. Adhesive capsulitis, periarthritis, frozen shoulder, adhesive bursitis, periarticular adhesions, and check-rein shoulder are all terms referring to the same syndrome.

Subdeltoid bursitis to one physician may be diagnosed as frozen shoulder by another. Painful arc syndrome to one is bicipital tenosynovitis to another, and so on. It seems that some physicians have given up and diagnose bursitis in all instances of shoulder pain and treat all patients the same whatever the pathologic findings.

Confusion is even greater concerning treatment as one reads of rest in a sling versus exercise, use the arm versus do not use the arm, manipulate the shoulder versus never manipulate, diathermy, x-ray therapy, ultrasound, phenylbutazone (Butazolidin), cortisone, indomethacin (Indocin), needling, irrigation and injection of hydrocortisone, sympathetic blocks, and open operations. At present the standard treatment seems to be repeated injections of a steroid preparation in and about the shoulder without regard to diagnosis or results.

This confusion seems to be directly related to our lack of understanding of shoulder pain. A proper diagnosis can be made and proper treatment instituted without much difficulty in the great majority of patients.

Emphasis will be on the diagnosis and treatment of the two conditions that account for the vast majority of cases of shoulder pain—supraspinatus tendinitis and adhesive capsulitis. Certain other shoulder lesions will be reviewed briefly since clinically they closely resemble and must be differentiated from the two most common lesions.

It is helpful to divide the discussion into two groups of conditions:

I. Conditions associated with normal range of motion
  A. Supraspinatus tendinitis (acute, subacute, chronic; with or without calcific deposit)
    1. Primary degeneration (majority)
    2. Degeneration associated with chronic tears of musculotendinous cuff
    3. Degeneration secondary to any lesion encroaching on coracoacromial space
      a. Malunion fracture of greater tuberosity
      b. Malunion or nonunion fracture of acromion
      c. Adduction fracture of neck of humerus
      d. Exostoses or spurs of tuberosity, acromion, or acromioclavicular joint
      e. Tumors
  B. Bicipital tenosynovitis
II. Conditions associated with limited range of motion
  A. Adhesive capsulitis (majority)
  B. Chronic, unrecognized posterior dislocation
  C. Degenerative arthritis

Since the diagnosis of degenerative arthritis of the acromioclavicular joint is frequently missed and treated as a shoulder condition, we wish to mention this disease.

ANATOMIC AND PATHOLOGIC CONSIDERATIONS

The unique anatomy of the shoulder joint contributes to the physiologic degeneration that gradually develops in the musculotendinous cuff after the age of 40 years. The coracoacromial arch, consisting of the acromion, the coracoacromial ligament, and the coracoid process, lies directly over and in close relationship with the superior portion of the musculotendinous cuff (Fig. 4-1). The subacromial bursa is interposed between the coracoacromial arch and the musculotendinous cuff to provide a gliding mechanism. The musculotendinous cuff provides joint stability by holding the humeral head against the glenoid and helps initiate abduction. With the arm at the side, the capsule of the shoulder is very loose and lies in a fold inferiorly.

When the arm is abducted, the supraspinatus portion of the musculotendinous cuff is impinged between the humeral tuberosity and the overlying coracoacromial arch. This repeated trauma accelerates and intensifies the normal degeneration so that the tendinous fibers become frayed, fibrillated, avascular, and even necrotic. A tear of the cuff may occur in the deteriorated area. Degenerative changes also occur in the tendon of the long head of the biceps. Since this tendon is surrounded by synovium, it shares any inflammatory reaction that may occur in the joint.

The musculotendinous cuff is often the site of a calcific deposit. The mechanism by which calcium is deposited is not understood. It may be similar to calcification in collagenous tissue in which local tissue necrosis and low oxygen tension exist together. A Ghon tubercle surrounding a necrotic tubercular focus and endochondral bone formation in which calcium is laid down on a necrotic matrix after the death of the chondrocyte are two examples of such calcification.

If degeneration in the rotator cuff occurs with such frequency, why do some shoulders become painful? Simmonds[2] proposed a theory of "focal necrosis in the musculotendinous cuff" to account for the painful shoulder. This theory states that when cuff

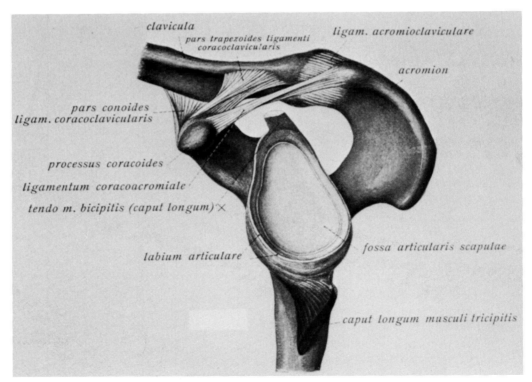

Fig. 4-1. Socket of the left shoulder. The coracoacromial arch, consisting of the coracoid process, the coracoacromial ligament, and the acromion, is shown to good advantage. (From Sobotta and Becher: Atlas of descriptive anatomy of the human being, ed. 16, Munich, 1967, Urban and Schwarzenberg, part I.)

degeneration develops without actual tissue necrosis there is no inflammation and no pain in the shoulder. Conversely, when local or "focal" necrosis occurs with or without a calcific deposit, an inflammatory reaction to the degenerated area develops, producing a painful shoulder. In some cases this inflammation may spread to involve the capsule and synovium of the shoulder joint, producing a capsulitis.

CONDITIONS ASSOCIATED WITH NORMAL RANGE OF MOTION
Acute calcific tendinitis

Of the conditions under discussion, acute calcific tendinitis is the easiest to delineate. It is an extremely painful, self-limiting process with a natural history lasting 6 to 14 days. The pathologic finding is usually in the supraspinatus portion of the rotator cuff, where a zone of degeneration becomes infiltrated with calcium salts. The calcium salts plus the degenerated area cause an acute inflammatory reaction in the surrounding viable tendinous fibers and the overlying subdeltoid bursa, producing swelling and tension. Any shoulder motion will cause impingement of the acutely inflamed area upon the coracoacromial arch, resulting in pain.

The patient has a sudden onset of acute disabling pain in the shoulder, usually without any preceding significant trauma. He may or may not have had a previous attack. When seen, the patient often guards and splints his arm against his body. Generally, there is exquisite tenderness directly over the calcific deposit and loss of active motion because of severe pain. Radiographs, which must include three views (neutral, internal, and external rotation), usually show a fluffy calcific deposit (Fig. 4-2). Often these patients have so much pain that the patient rather than the shoulder must be rotated to obtain these views.

There are several options for treatment, depending upon the patient's desires and the stage of the disease when the patient is seen. Some patients are seen when the acute pain is subsiding, indicating spontaneous rupture of the calcium deposit (Fig. 4-3). In such a case, symptomatic treatment with pain medication, resting the arm in a sling for a few days, and progressive exercises are indicated. Recovery is usually prompt.

In most instances, rupture will not have occurred by the time of consultation, and the pain remains severe. The patient may help to decide the treatment after discussion of the self-limiting nature of the process. Some may elect symptomatic treatment consisting of pain medication, ice packs, and a sling and

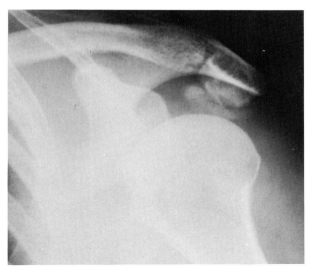

Fig. 4-2. This patient has had acute pain for 3 days. The large calcium deposit appears soft and flocculent.

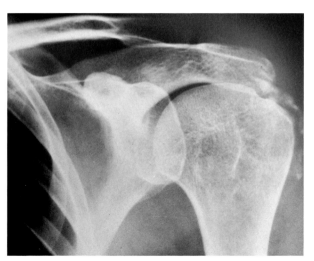

Fig. 4-3. This patient has had acute pain for 5 days. The pain has now started to decrease. The calcific deposit has spontaneously ruptured from the tendon into the bursa, where it will be absorbed. The process is subsiding spontaneously.

wait for spontaneous rupture of the calcific deposit, which usually occurs 4 to 10 days from the onset of symptoms. A course of phenylbutazone treatment may be helpful. Other patients choose more aggressive treatment to shorten the duration of severe pain.

Decompression of the acute calcium furuncle by needle punctures may be effective. Two needles are inserted into the zone of maximum tenderness and into the calcific deposit using strict aseptic technique and local anesthesia. Aspiration of calcific material is evidence of rupture of the deposit. Irrigation of the bursa with saline solution may then be carried out. The injection of a steroid that reduces the local inflammatory reaction is often performed before withdrawal of the needles, but it should be realized that the essential part of this procedure is rupture of the acute deposit. The local anesthetic relieves the pain immediately, but the patient must be aware that some pain of a milder nature will return after the anesthesia has worn off. After needling, conservative treatment, as already mentioned, is carried out. The patient should be reexamined in 24 to 48 hours. If the original severe pain has not disappeared and the needling has failed, either a second needling procedure or other mode of treatment may be instituted. As soon as possible, progressive exercises and use of the arm should be insisted upon to avoid adhesive capsulitis. There is a definite danger of introducing infection by the needling operation, and again a strict aseptic technique must be emphasized (Fig. 4-4).

Evacuation of the calcium by open operation is occasionally performed, particularly if the patient refuses needling, if there are multiple deposits, or if the deposit is inaccessible to a needle. A short, anterolateral, deltoid-splitting incision is used, the bursa opened, and the rotator cuff exposed. By rotating the shoulder, the deposit is found and incised longitudinal to the tendon fibers. The tense calcific material, frequently having the consistency of milk or toothpaste,

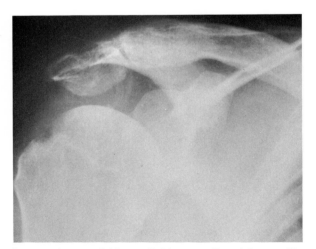

Fig. 4-4. Acute calcific tendinitis was relieved by needling in this patient, but in 10 days severe shoulder pain recurred. Osteomyelitis of the humeral head is present.

is evacuated and the wound closed. The postoperative care is identical to that after needling.

Chronic tendinitis

Chronic tendinitis of the shoulder is much more common than acute calcific tendinitis. It is caused by chronic inflammation of the viable tendinous tissue surrounding a degenerated zone in the rotator cuff with mild secondary inflammation of the overlying subdeltoid bursa. There may or may not be a calcific deposit in the deteriorated area of the tendon. The mild inflammatory swelling of chronic tendinitis, often increased by a calcific deposit, encroaches upon the small space between the tuberosity and the acromion and coracoacromial ligament, resulting in increased impingement and pain.

Chronic, dull, aching pain of considerable duration is the usual complaint. There may be a history of previous acute attacks of "bursitis." The pain is usually in the deltoid area of the shoulder and may extend down the arm. It is increased by motions of the shoulder, particularly above 60° of abduction or flexion. Night pain is very common.

On physical examination, shoulder motion, actively or passively, is normal, with a painful arc occurring in the ranges of flexion and abduction beyond 60°. Establishing the presence of a full range of motion, actively or passively, is very important since *normal motion distinguishes this condition from adhesive capsulitis.* Mild local tenderness of the cuff is common. Roentgenograms taken in three different projections may or may not demonstrate a calcific deposit. At times calcium may be present in such small amounts that it cannot be seen, or it may be hidden by superimposed bone.

It is thought that if calcium is deposited rapidly and superficially in a zone of focal necrosis of the cuff, an acute calcific tendinitis may ensue, but if the calcium is deposited slowly and more deeply in the tendinous tissue, a chronic calcific tendinitis is more likely. Finally, if there is no calcium deposited in the zone of attrition and focal necrosis, inflammation of the cuff may still occur and cause a chronic noncalcific tendinitis.

Spontaneous recovery of patients with chronic tendinitis is common. Conservative treatment is often helpful in relieving symptoms and preventing complications. Avoiding activities in the painful arc of motion is of help. Pendulum exercises that avoid impingement of the rotator cuff against the coracoacromial arch and range of motion exercises will prevent adhesive capsulitis. Aspirin and heat may be beneficial in relieving pain. Anti-inflammatory drugs such as phenylbutazone may help to decrease pain in subacute tendinitis. In the majority of patients with chronic tendinitis, needling procedures are ineffective and often aggravate the pain. Many patients have had multiple steroid injections without any lasting effect. More than 90% of patients with chronic tendinitis recover spontaneously without heroic measures.

In a small group of patients, despite good conservative treatment, there is persistent *disabling* shoulder pain that may be benefited by operative treatment. Simple removal of the inspissated calcific deposit that is infiltrated in the tendinous tissues has not been successful in our hands, and a symptomatic tendinitis remains. An acromionectomy, which relieves the impingement and friction upon the chronically inflamed zone of the cuff, has proved very beneficial. The calcific deposit is not touched, as it is gradually absorbed after operation (Fig. 4-5).

Although primary degeneration in the cuff is the most important cause of tendinitis, certain other conditions can intensify the degenerative process and bring about a symptomatic tendinitis. Any lesion encroaching upon the space between the acromion and tuberosity increases impingement upon the cuff and may precipitate a painful tendinitis. Examples of such lesions are a nonunited or malunited fracture of either the acromion or the greater tuberosity; healed adduction fracture of the neck of the humerus; exostoses or spurs of the tuberosity, acromion, or acromioclavicular joint; and tumors. Tendinitis in such instances

can be relieved promptly by acromionectomy if the pain is disabling and does not respond to a conservative program.

In summary, chronic tendinitis, a common cause of shoulder pain, can be controlled in the majority of patients by good conservative treatment, and spontaneous cure is the rule. In a small group of patients who have persistent disabling symptoms of long duration, an acromionectomy will relieve the symptoms and yield a high percentage of good and excellent results.

Differential diagnosis of tendinitis of shoulder

Acute calcific tendinitis should not present any problem in differential diagnosis.

In the differential diagnosis of chronic tendinitis of the shoulder the three conditions that should be considered are degenerative arthritis of the acromioclavicular joint, chronic tears of the musculotendinous cuff, and bicipital tenosynovitis.

In *degenerative arthritis of the acromioclavicular joint* the patient complains of pain in the shoulder that may extend down the arm. There may or may not be a history of remote injury. When asked where the worst pain is located, the patient will usually point to the acromioclavicular joint. The range of motion is normal on examination, and there is frequently a painful arc of motion. Tenderness is localized to the acromioclavicular joint and not over the cuff or deltoid area. Roentgenographic examination shows degenerative changes in the acromioclavicular joint. The

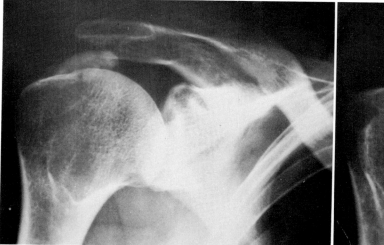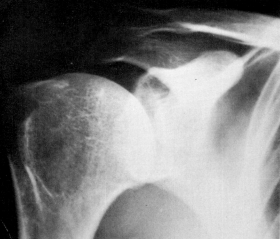

A **B**

Fig. 4-5. A, This patient has had chronic disabling pain for 3 years. A large calcific deposit is obvious. **B,** Three and one-half months after acromionectomy, the calcium has been absorbed spontaneously.

combination of pain and tenderness localized to the joint and the roentgenographic findings are usually sufficient to establish the diagnosis. If there is doubt that the acromioclavicular joint is causing the pain, the diagnosis can be verified by the temporary complete relief of symptoms on injection of a local anesthetic into the joint.

Chronic tears of the cuff may or may not produce symptoms. These tears usually occur through degenerated tendinous tissue. A chronic inflammatory reaction in the viable tissues around the degenerated and torn tendon fibers may occur. The bursa is often swollen. These patients often complain of pain, not weakness, and on cursory examination a normal range of motion with a painful arc leads to the diagnosis of tendinitis alone. We often fail to examine these patients for a torn cuff and thereby miss this diagnosis. A history of trauma is frequently absent, which speaks for the tear occurring spontaneously in the course of ordinary activities. Results of the roentgenographic examination are frequently negative. In our experience, patients who have a disabling painful arc syndrome and have negative findings on roentgenograms have a high incidence of cuff tears. The examination of chronic painful shoulders should include the strength of initiation of abduction and the strength of maintaining the abducted arm against gravity and mild resistance. An arthrogram is diagnostic and may be helpful in certain instances.

Bicipital tenosynovitis was not a frequent diagnosis in our series of patients with painful shoulders. Inflammation of the biceps tendon and its sheath may be the cause of a painful arc syndrome in a shoulder with normal motion. The pain is usually located anteriorly, and tenderness is localized to the bicipital groove. Flexion of the shoulder against resistance with the elbow extended may cause pain in the groove. Supination of the forearm against resistance with the elbow flexed may cause pain in the groove. Displacing the tendon with the fingers 3 inches below the shoulder and suddenly releasing it may cause pain in the same area. The roentgenographic findings are usually negative. Bicipital tenosynovitis can be an isolated lesion, but much more commonly it is associated with and is involved in a diffuse capsulitis—an adhesive capsulitis.

CONDITIONS ASSOCIATED WITH LIMITED RANGE OF MOTION
Adhesive capsulitis

Adhesive capsulitis is a distinct clinical entity characterized by a chronic inflammatory process of the articular and periarticular tissues of the shoulder joint accompanied by pain and loss of active and passive motion. This syndrome is usually self-limiting and runs a long and protracted course lasting from 1 to 2 years. Gradual, spontaneous recovery of a full and painless range of motion may or may not be complete. The cause is unknown, but inactivity of the arm, for various reasons, is a causative factor in one half of the patients.

When the disease is established, a low-grade inflammatory process involving the capsule, synovium, and musculotendinous cuff results in adhesions between the folds of the capsule and between the capsule and the humeral head. There are no adhesions in the subacromial bursa, nor are there adhesions between the humeral head and the glenoid.

History and examination. Adhesive capsulitis is twice as common in women as in men. Its occurrence is rare in patients less than 40 years of age and it seldom occurs in patients more than 70 years of age. There is usually a gradual onset of increasing pain in the involved shoulder, which has existed several weeks or months before the patient seeks medical attention. The patient locates the pain in the deltoid area with extension down the arm and forearm as far as the hand. The pain is moderately disabling, aggravated by certain motions and positions of the arm, and often interferes with sleep. On rare occasions the chief complaint is stiffness and not pain. Often the history includes a factor that encouraged lack of use of the arm.

The examination must include the range of passive motion in all patients with shoulder pain. *A definite limitation of passive shoulder motion is essential to the diagnosis of adhesive capsulitis.* Progressive pain is obvious as the shoulder is manipulated into the restricted zone. It is important to compare the range of motion of both shoulders. The rotator cuff is usually not tender. Wasting of the deltoid and scapular muscles is evident if the capsulitis has existed any length of time. Because of restriction of true shoulder motion, the shoulder and shoulder girdle elevate on abduction, indicating abnormal scapulothoracic motion. The patient may have the so-called periarthritic personality and appear to be an apprehensive and depressed person with a low threshold of pain.

Roentgenograms of the shoulder usually appear normal or show demineralization. If a calcific deposit is present, it is considered incidental and not the primary cause of symptoms.

Prevention and treatment. Prevention is a most important feature in adhesive capsulitis as no mode of treatment promotes an early cure of the established disease. The disease is often iatrogenic and can be prevented in many patients by simple exercises through a full range of motion of the shoulder in all those conditions that promote inactivity of the arm.

The aims of treatment are to shorten the period of disability and to ensure a more complete recovery. Most patients respond to a conservative treatment program that includes instruction in the nature of adhesive capsulitis and an active stretching exercise program. The patient is urged to use the shoulder as normally as possible rather than protect and splint the extremity. Muscular activity is beneficial in overcoming the stiffness. Cooperation of the patient is essential. Both the physician and physical therapist should instruct the patient in three or four simple stretching exercises that carry the shoulder joint into the painful zone of flexion, abduction, and the rotations. Each of these exercises should be persistently performed slowly, five times every waking hour. When performed properly, the exercises are painful, and the patients are benefited by adequate analgesics during the first few weeks of treatment as well as sedation for sleep at night. Adequate medication for relief of pain is very important as it encourages use of the arm and allows the patient to perform stretching exercises more vigorously. An anti-inflammatory drug such as

prednisone may also be helpful during the first 4 weeks of treatment. The physician must see the patient at regular intervals to follow up his progress, to encourage him, and to add more difficult exercises as motion increases. For best results the doctor must assume this responsibility and should not relegate these duties to the therapist. With this program, 95% of the patients gradually recover in 4 to 6 months.

Some patients have difficulty making any improvement. If the patient will not cooperate in carrying out the program of use and stretching exercises, there is little hope of improvement from any form of therapy. They may benefit from daily visits to a physical therapist for active stretching exercises using the hold-relax technique. These visits may provide motivation and encouragement. A few patients may benefit from hospitalization with intensive physical therapy, close supervision, and adequate analgesia.

Other types of treatment have been advocated. These include manipulation, forceful intracapsular injection of saline solution, and operation. These methods should never be considered unless the patient has demonstrated his cooperation in an intensive exercise program that has failed to bring improvement. The only method of aggressive treatment that has been utilized infrequently at the Lahey Clinic

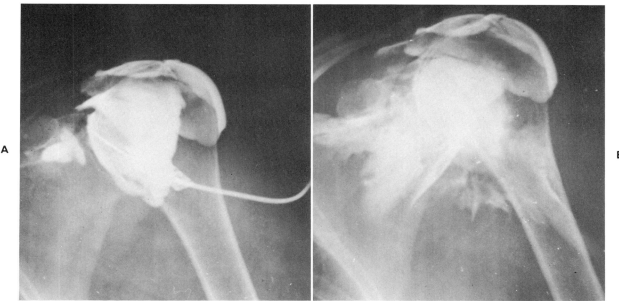

Fig. 4-6. A, Arthrogram of shoulder of a patient with severe adhesive capsulitis before manipulation. Conservative treatment had failed. Note that the subacromial bursa is filled with contrast media, indicating a cuff tear. **B,** Following manipulation. The dye has escaped from the joint anteroinferiorly, indicating tears of the inferior capsule and subscapularis tendon.

Foundation has been manipulation. Only three or four manipulation procedures per year are performed in the treatment of 150 to 200 patients with adhesive capsulitis. A few patients who have truly cooperated in conservative therapy but have failed to make any progress may benefit from manipulation. The patient should be informed that considerable pain will follow the procedure and that the exercise program must be carried out promptly and just as meticulously as before the manipulation. A physical therapist will help ensure the success of this procedure. One must be cautious when carrying out manipulation of the shoulder because this procedure has its dangers. The joint capsule is always torn, and the subscapularis and the biceps tendons may also be ruptured (Fig. 4-6). Other possible complications are compression fracture of the humeral head, fracture of the shaft of the humerus, and dislocation of the shoulder. The contra-indications to this procedure include recent fractures of the humerus, osteoporosis, hemiplegia, severe parkinsonism, and a history of blood dyscrasia. The manipulation should always be gentle. It is better to do a second manipulation after 7 to 10 days than to traumatize the joint too severely at the first procedure. Because of the possibility of dislocation, the arm is not fixed in wide abduction and external rotation after manipulation but is placed in approximately 60° of abduction and neutral rotation.

Arthrotomy of the shoulder joint with lysis of adhesions under direct visualization, as advocated by Neviaser,[1] may be considered for the individual who has not improved on a program of conservative treatment or who has some contraindication to manipulation. This operation may also be considered for those patients in whom manipulation has failed to improve the situation.

Differential diagnosis. In the differential diagnosis of adhesive capsulitis of the shoulder we must consider two conditions: chronic, unrecognized posterior dislocation and degenerative arthritis of the shoulder.

Chronic posterior dislocation is a rare condition that is seldom thought of and therefore remains undiagnosed for long periods. After the acute onset the shoulder becomes stiff and painful and is often treated unsuccessfully as an adhesive capsulitis. A history of trauma to the adducted, internally rotated arm followed by acute pain at the onset would be suggestive. About 30% follow a convulsive seizure. The diagnosis is quite evident if we are on the alert for this lesion. The important physical signs are a fixed internal rotation deformity, prominence of the coracoid process, diminished anterior bulge of the humeral head, and the palpable and often visible prominence of the head posteriorly. Otherwise the findings are identical with those in adhesive capsulitis. In the acute dislocation the usual anteroposterior roentgenogram with the shoulder internally rotated may not reveal the condition. A lateral view of the scapula will show the dislocation. In the chronic dislocation the anteroposterior film will reveal (1) an incongruity of the articular surfaces of the head and glenoid cavity; (2) a double line representing two apparent articular surfaces of the head, one of which overlaps the glenoid margin; and (3) interruption of the smooth line along the inferior border of the neck and head of the humerus to the lateral border of the scapula. An axillary view is usually diagnostic. This view shows the head displaced posteriorly and jammed and compressed against the posterior glenoid margin. The most important points in the diagnosis are a history of acute injury, a fixed internal rotation deformity, and an adequate roentgenographic examination and interpretation. Above all, keep this lesion in mind in the painful, stiff shoulder.

The findings in *degenerative arthritis of the shoulder* are identical with those in adhesive capsulitis. There may or may not be a history of previous major trauma to the shoulder. The diagnosis is not made until roentgenograms are taken and degenerative joint changes are seen.

REFERENCES

1. Neviaser, J. S.: Adhesive capsulitis of the shoulder (the frozen shoulder), Med. Times **90:**783, 1962.
2. Simmonds, F. A.: Shoulder pain, with particular reference to "frozen" shoulder, J. Bone Joint Surg. **31-B:** 426, 1949.

Chapter 5

Fractures of the shafts and distal ends of the radius and ulna

FRED P. SAGE, M.D.
Memphis, Tennessee

Fractures of the shaft of the bones of the forearm allow one to show his expertise as a fracture surgeon. The decision to do a closed reduction or an open reduction depends on the knowledge of the anatomy of the forearm and dynamics of the forearm muscles and on the ability to neutralize those forces that act on the bones. It also depends, to a great degree, on the level of the fracture and whether one or both bones are broken. To achieve a satisfactory closed reduction itself can be trying or impossible. Open reduction may require a combination of several techniques of fixation. Furthermore, one must decide whether to do a primary bone graft or not. In addition, rehabilitation of a well-united forearm may not be as simple as one would be inclined to believe.

Finally, overcoming the complications inherent in treating fractures of the forearm in adults can test one's expertise in reconstructive surgery. Reconstructive procedures may run the gamut from soft tissue loss to diaphyseal loss from trauma or infection, from delayed union to malunion or refracture, and from arterial injury to Volkmann's contracture.

ANATOMIC CONSIDERATIONS

Some fractures in the shaft of the forearm bones can be treated by closed reduction. Closed reductions are difficult to obtain because of several factors. First, the muscles that arise on one bone and insert on the other, the supinator and pronator quadratus, cause angulation at the fracture site as well as rotary displacement. Second, the extrinsic muscles of the forearm, the flexor-pronator group and the extensor-supinator group, run diagonally across the forearm and cross the interosseous space obliquely and tend to cause

angulation, compression of the bones, or overlapping of the fractured ends and rotational malalignment. The biceps brachii has a strong rotary influence on the radius as well as a flexor force at the elbow. The tension of the biceps on the proximal fragment of a radius determines the amount of pronation or supination present in the proximal fragment. Third, an adequate interosseous space must be maintained. The ulna is locked in the olecranon notch and cannot rotate; it merely abducts and adducts slightly in pronation and supination. The radius rotates around the ulna, and if the interosseous space is not kept clear of bony projections (Fig. 5-1), pronation and supination may be lost. The normal dorsal and lateral curves (Fig. 5-2) in the radius must be restored as well, for if they are lost, the relative width of the interosseous space is decreased.

Another obstacle to closed reduction is failure to secure accurate rotational alignment of the fragments of the radius. It is easy to see if one has not restored length or linear alignment to the fracture, but alignment in rotation is difficult to assess. Correct rotational alignment is a must in the radius. If a pronated distal fragment is placed on a supinated proximal fragment, supination is limited. Conversely, if a supinated distal fragment is placed on a pronated proximal fragment, pronation is limited. In 1949 Knight and Purvis[7] reviewed forty-one adult patients with fresh fractures in the shaft of both bones of the forearm treated by closed reduction at the Campbell Clinic in Memphis and found rotary malalignment to be the greatest cause for unsatisfactory results. There was rotary malalignment in 65% of the cases. Evans[5] in 1945 advocated the use of a tuberosity view

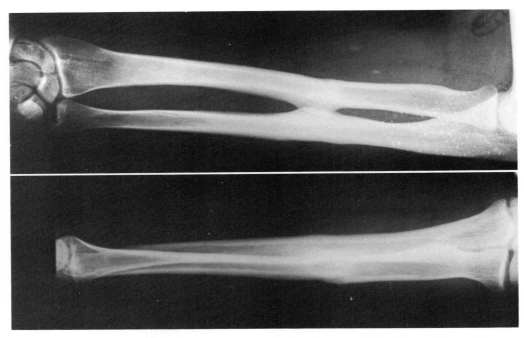

Fig. 5-1. Incomplete synostosis after healing of a fracture in the middle of the radius and ulna.

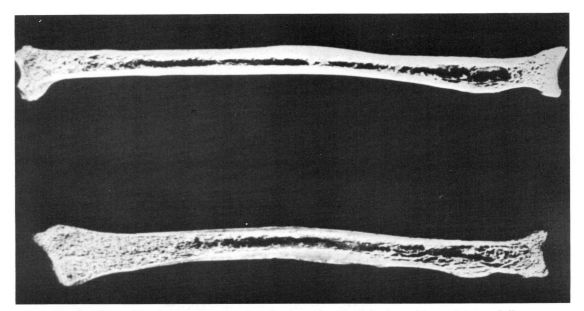

Fig. 5-2. Bisected cadaver radius showing the dorsal bow and the lateral bow of the medullary canal.

of the upper end of the radius to ascertain the degree of pronation or supination in the proximal fragment of the radius (Fig. 5-3). The bicipital tubercle appears in full profile toward the ulna with the proximal radius in full supination, and in full pronation it appears in full profile on the lateral side of the radius.

This change in position of the bicipital tuberosity is a guide to the degree of pronation or supination present in the proximal fragment. Since the fracture surgeon has no control over the degree of rotation of the proximal fragment of the radius, he must determine its position relative to pronation and supination.

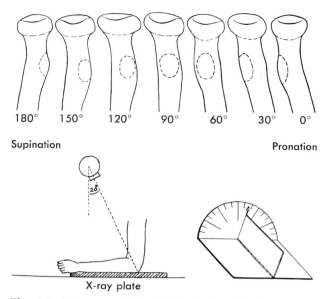

Fig. 5-3. Diagram of the bicipital tuberosity in various stages of pronation and supination. The technique for obtaining the tuberosity view is shown. (From Evans, E. M.: J. Bone Joint Surg. 27:373, 1945.)

He must then accurately place the distal fragment in the proper plane of rotation to correspond with the proximal fragment. Restoration of rotational alignment to the radius and the use of sling suspension of the cast near the elbow will produce a greater number of satisfactory results by closed reduction.

A long arm cast from the upper arm to the proximal palmar crease is a necessity until all fractures are healed. The weight of the cast against the forearm can cause the bones to angulate (Fig. 5-4). The proximal one half of the forearm bones are covered by tendons and thick muscles. The heavier muscles in the upper half of the forearm will atrophy when the arm is immobilized. The cast can then sag down against the radius, causing either the radius or the radius and ulna to angulate toward the ulnar side of the arm.[8] One has only to review a few roentgenograms of forearm fractures that have angulated to see this is the direction of angulation, almost without exception (Fig. 5-5).

The constant use of a sling through a wire loop incorporated in the cast near the elbow will prevent the

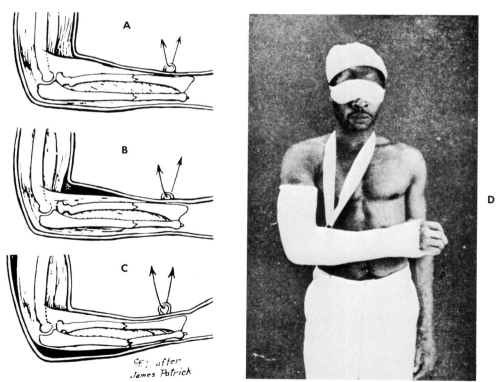

Fig. 5-4. Mechanism of ulnar angulation of fracture fragments when the cast is suspended from a loop distal to the fracture site. **A,** Immediately following cast immobilization. **B,** Atrophy of upper forearm musculature. **C,** Effect of gravity on the loosened cast causing angulation of the fracture fragments. **D,** Proper method of suspending cast through a loop proximal to the forearm fracture (From Knight, R. A., and Purvis, G. D.: J. Bone Joint Surg. **31-A:**735, 1949.)

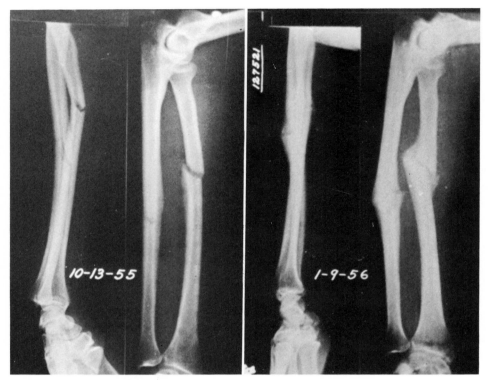

Fig. 5-5. Preoperative and postoperative roentgenograms showing ulnarward angulation after closed treatment of a minimally displaced fracture.

cast from sagging against the forearm. We have seen a strategically placed wire loop and sling suspension effect a satisfactory reduction of fractures that had angulated toward the ulnar side of the forearm. The use of this method of cast suspension is equally as applicable to the child as to the adult.

The same muscular forces that oppose reduction also tend to cause displacement during the healing period.

TECHNIQUES OF CLOSED REDUCTIONS

Those fractures most suited to closed reductions are fractures in the upper fifth of the radius, solitary fractures in the middle and distal thirds of the ulna, and two bone fractures in the distal third of the radius and ulna (Fig. 5-6). Transverse fractures in the midshaft of the radius or in the ulna (Fig. 5-7) can be manipulated, but nothing short of an anatomic restoration should be accepted. Any loss of alignment will result in a loss of function in almost every instance.

A satisfactory closed reduction in adults is predicated first on satisfactory anesthesia, which relaxes the muscles. This is best obtained by a general anesthetic, but an axillary block may be adequate. With the patient supine, the thumb and one or two of the fingers

are suspended from an overhead frame, with the elbow flexed at 90°. Chinese finger traps, Spanish hitches of muslin, or any other suitable device may be used to suspend the fingers. A sling of silence cloth muslin is placed across the anterior surface of the upper arm just above the elbow. A 5-pound sandbag is suspended in this loop for traction. At this point the Evans tuberosity view is obtained (Fig. 5-3) by placing the x-ray film posterior to the elbow in line with the forearm and tilting the x-ray tube 20° cephalad. The tube bisects the antecubital space at a 70° angle with the forearm. Again, it must be emphasized that the operator has no control over the degree of rotation of the proximal radial fragment. He must rotate the distal fragment of the radius properly on the proximal fragment of the radius to obtain satisfactory rotational alignment. While the roentgenograms of the tuberosity view are processed, the 5-pound sandbag is allowed to exert traction on the fragments, and the ulna is manipulated by palpating its subcutaneous border. After the ulna is clinically aligned and the rotation of the proximal radius is determined, the distal fragment of the radius is reduced by rotating the wrist to correspond with the rotation of the proximal fragment. As an assistant holds the forearm in the

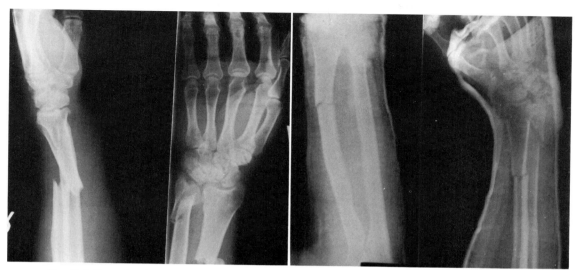

Fig. 5-6. Prereduction and postreduction roentgenograms of fractures in the distal third of the radius and the ulna treated satisfactorily by closed reduction.

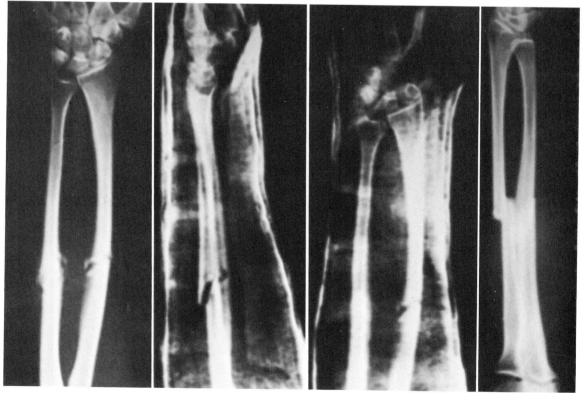

Fig. 5-7. Preoperative and postreduction roentgenograms of fractures in the middle third of the radius and the ulna treated by closed reduction. An excellent position was maintained by cast fixation alone until solid union occurred. (From Sage, F. P.: In Adams, J. P., editor: Current practice in orthopaedic surgery, St. Louis, 1963, The C. V. Mosby Co., vol. 1.)

proper position and with traction continuously maintained, a sugar-tongs cast is applied over cotton padding. After the cast is hardened, the sandbag is removed from the silence cloth sling, and while the arm is still suspended from overhead by gravity, roentgenograms in the anteroposterior and medial to lateral planes are made. If an unsatisfactory reduction is present, the sugar-tongs cast can be removed and these steps repeated to correct the malalignment. If reduction is satisfactory, the sugar-tongs cast can be incorporated in a long arm cast and a wire loop placed near the elbow from which to constantly suspend the cast during the period of healing. This period of healing averages 20 weeks. Nonunion from closed reductions occurred in 12% of the cases reviewed by Knight and Purvis.[7]

In the immediate postoperative period there is a tendency of the hand to swell. It should be suspended uppermost for 48 hours, with the hand higher than the elbow and the elbow higher than the shoulder. Ice packs should be placed about the cast at the level of the fracture for the first 24 hours. The patient is encouraged to exercise the fingers in full flexion and extension 5 minutes of each waking hour. In the ensuing weeks during healing the sling must be maintained and the shoulder adequately exercised to prevent adhesive capsulitis. The position of the frag-

ments should be checked by roentgenograms each 2 weeks, for until adequate healing has occurred, malposition is always a possibility. If there is any loss in position, the fragments should be either remanipulated or subjected to open reduction. Function is primarily predicated on union, but union in good position, not malunion.

TECHNIQUES OF OPEN REDUCTIONS
Indications

Fractures not suited to closed reduction are comminuted fractures, segmental fractures, Monteggia's fractures, and the solitary fractures of the distal third of the radius or at the junction of the middle and distal third of the radius (Fig. 5-8). This latter fracture has been called the reverse Monteggia fracture or the Piedmont fracture, as it was thoroughly studied by the Piedmont Orthopaedic Society. It was also termed by the late Dr. Willis Campbell as a fracture of necessity, necessitating open reduction to ensure adequate fixation in good position and a competent distal radioulnar joint.

Complications

An open reduction carries with it some inherent danger to the patient and certain obligations to the patient on the part of the surgeon. The foremost dan-

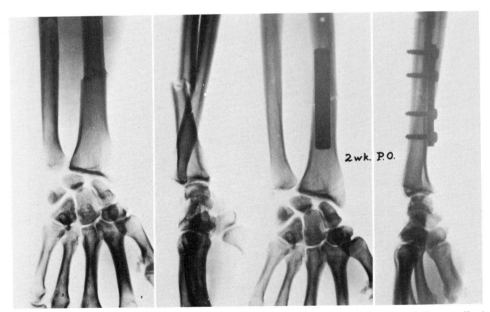

Fig. 5-8. Wide canal in the distal fragment prevented secure fixation by a medullary nail. A Mueller compression plate is shown 2 weeks postoperatively. Note the screw hole in the radius proximal to the plate to which the compression device had been secured. (From Sage, F. P.: In Adams, J. P., editor: Current practice in orthopaedic surgery, St. Louis, 1963, The C. V. Mosby Co., vol. 1.)

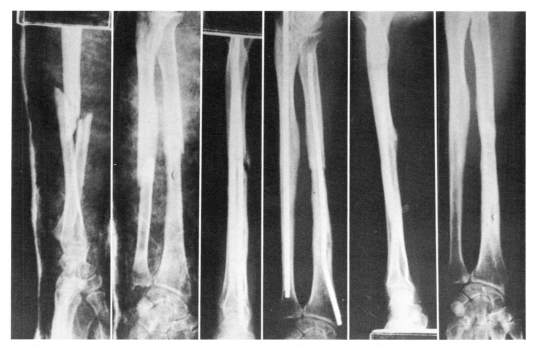

Fig. 5-9. Moderate infection following medullary nailing. In spite of infection, union occurred and drainage ceased. The nail was removed following union. (From Sage, F. P.: J. Bone Joint Surg. **41-A:**1489, 1959.)

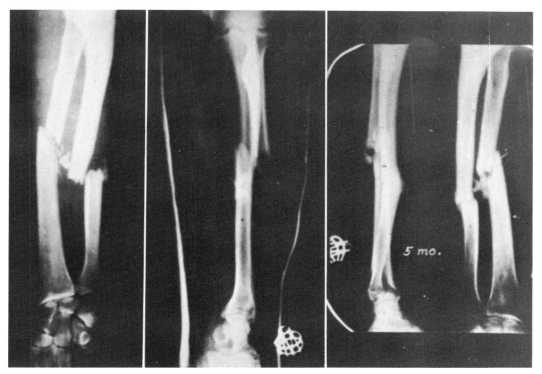

Fig. 5-10. Preoperative and postoperative roentgenograms showing loss in position from thin wire fixation.

ger, of course, is the hazard of infection (Fig. 5-9); meticulous aseptic technique is mandatory. To convert a clean forearm with an excellent chance for healing into an infected forearm may be a tragedy. Another hazard of open reduction is nonunion. It is more common after open reduction than after closed reduction. Knight and Purvis[7] reviewed fifty-nine patients in whom two bone fractures of the forearm were treated by the staff at the Campbell Clinic using a variety of open reduction techniques; nonunion occurred in more than 20% of the cases. In another series of 555 forearm fractures subjected to open reduction in eighteen orthopaedic centers in the United States and reviewed by Smith and Sage,[10] nonunion occurred in 20% of the fractures. Because of the high incidence of nonunion following open reduction, a primary bone graft must be considered. Since it has a greater likelihood of success than homologous bone, autogenous bone should be used. This, of course, affords another possible site for infection or some other complication.

If open reduction is done, internal fixation should be used. To lose position in the healing stage after one has already done an open reduction without internal fixation would be embarrassing. This, of course, does not include compound fractures that are reduced openly but no internal fixation used because of potential infection.

The fixation device should be adequate to hold the fracture and not homeopathic (Fig. 5-10). To have the fracture slip from inadequate internal fixation is likewise embarrassing.

Medullary fixation

The type of fixation device to use depends on the level of the fracture, the bone fractured, the comminution of the fracture, and the choice of the particular surgeon. For intramedullary fixation to be adequate the medullary nail should firmly engage the inner cortices of the bone above and below the fracture site. Fractures at the junction of the middle and distal thirds of the radius are not suited to medullary fixation, for here the canal in the distal fragment is too wide and the nail will not control rotation or alignment (Fig. 5-11). It may allow motion at the fracture site and increased absorption of bone. In the upper third of the ulna where the canal is wide a medullary nail can be used, but a transfixation wire loop across

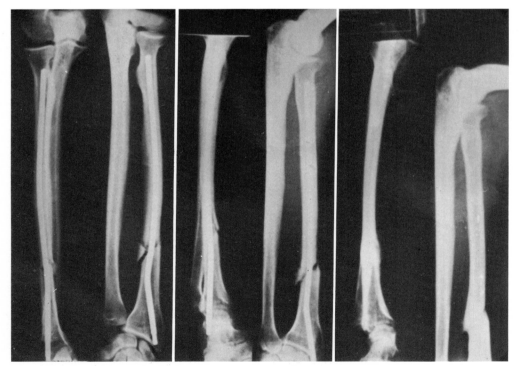

Fig. 5-11. Derangement of the distal radioulnar joint from shortening of the radius and relative lengthening of the ulna. Note proximal migration of the distal fragment of the radius on the nail. (From Sage, F. P.: J. Bone Joint Surg. **41-A:**1489, 1959.)

the fracture site may be necessary to avoid rotary displacement. In these two locations, rigid plate fixation is better. There is no doubt, as Anderson[1] has pointed out, that the presence of an indwelling medullary nail retards endosteal bone healing, which accounts for the healing of the inner two thirds of the cortex (Fig. 5-12). This endosteal healing may not occur until after the medullary nail is removed (Fig. 5-13). Medullary nails require less soft tissue exposure than plate and screw fixation and considerably less than when a com-

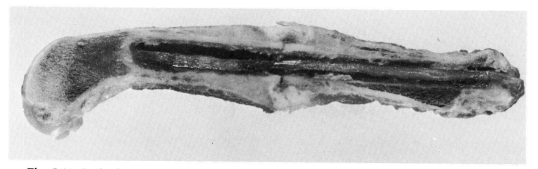

Fig. 5-12. Sagittal section of an experimental fracture in the femur of a dog; the femur was immobilized with a tightly fitting medullary nail. Note the lack of bone along the inner border of the medullary canal and between the cortical fragments. (Courtesy Dr. L. D. Anderson; from Sage, F. P.: In Adams, J. P., editor: Current practice in orthopaedic surgery, St. Louis, 1963, The C. V. Mosby Co., vol. 1.)

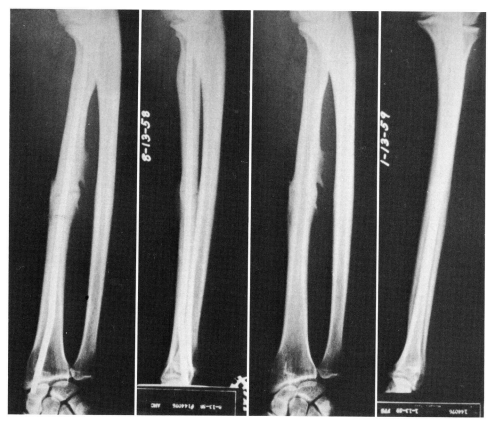

Fig. 5-13. Excellent fixation of a fracture in the middle third of the radius by a prebent triangular medullary nail. Interstitial bone formation was delayed until the medullary nail was removed. (From Sage, F. P.: J. Bone Joint Surg. **41-A:**1489, 1959.)

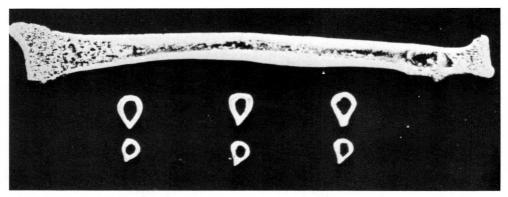

Fig. 5-14. Cross-sectional cuts at three levels in two radii showing the oblong cross section of the medullary canal. (From Sage, F. P.: J. Bone Joint Surg. **41-A**:1489, 1959.)

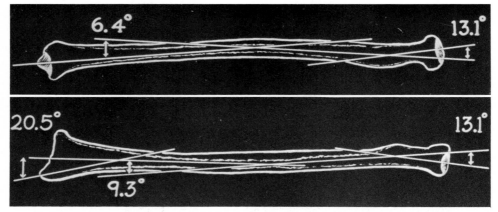

Fig. 5-15. Average angles in the medullary canal of the radius and ulna in the anteroposterior and medial to lateral projections and the angle of insertion from the radial styloid. (From Sage, F. P.: J. Bone Joint Surg. **41-A**:1489, 1959.)

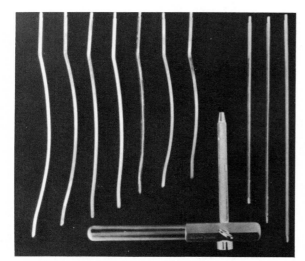

Fig. 5-16. Full complement of 4 mm. medullary nails for the radius and ulna and a combination driver-extractor. (From Sage, F. P.: J. Bone Joint Surg. **41-A**:1489, 1959.)

pression device is used. The cosmetic effect of scarring should likewise be considered.

If medullary fixation is used, the device should not be round in cross section. Since the medullary canal is oval in contour (Fig. 5-14), a square-, triangular-, or diamond-shaped pin may be used. A nail for the radius should have a bow in it to correspond to the bows in the medullary canals. In a series of 100 cadaver radii, the average radial bow measured 9.3° and a dorsal bow averaging 6.4° was also present (Fig. 5-15).[9] The prebent triangular pins that we devised for medullary fixation of the radius have the radial bow placed in the pins; a second angle of 20° is prebent in the distal portion of the pin to accommodate an angle of insertion from the radial styloid (Fig. 5-16). The nails measure either 4 or 5 mm. on each side. Street[11] inserts a square medullary nail, which he designed (Fig. 5-17), just proximal to Lister's tubercle on the dorsum of the distal radius; from this

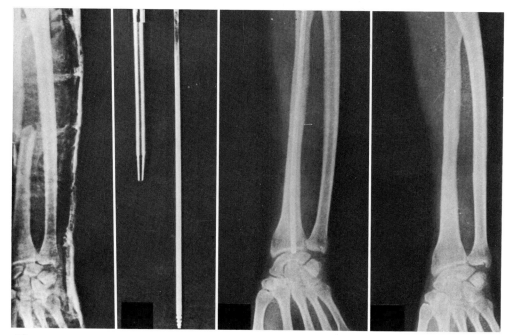

Fig. 5-17. Street's square nail for the forearm. Note the broached end. (From Street, D. M.: Spectator Club Letter, Nov. 18, 1955.)

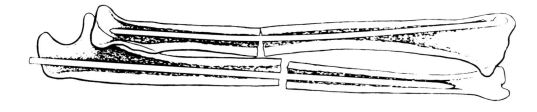

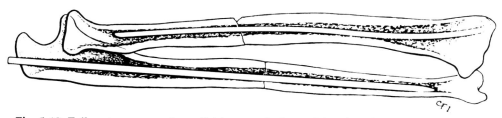

Fig. 5-18. Failure to preserve the radial bow results in straightening of the radius and distraction of the ulnar fragments. (From Smith, H., and Sage, F. P.: J. Bone Joint Surg. **39-A**:91, 1957.)

insertion it does not need an angle of insertion. He recommends that the square medullary nail be bent in its middle third prior to insertion to accommodate the normal radial bow. There are others who contend that the curves in the radius are not significant and that a straight nail will be adequate. Such a nail can cause a relative lengthening of the radius with loss in the width of the interosseous space and distraction of the ulnar fracture, with malunion in the radius and nonunion in the ulna (Fig. 5-18). A medullary nail should be springy but resilient so that it might snake its way up the medullary canal from an eccentric in-

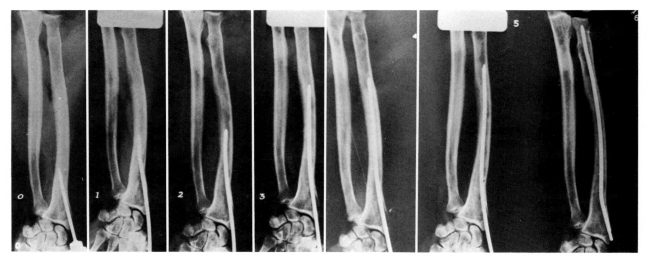

Fig. 5-19. Nail being driven up the radius of an amputated specimen. The nail must bend as it traverses the canal and then finally spring back to its prebent shape. (From Stewart, M. J.: In American Academy of Orthopaedic Surgeons, Instructional Course Lectures, Ann Arbor, 1958, J. W. Edwards, vol. 15.)

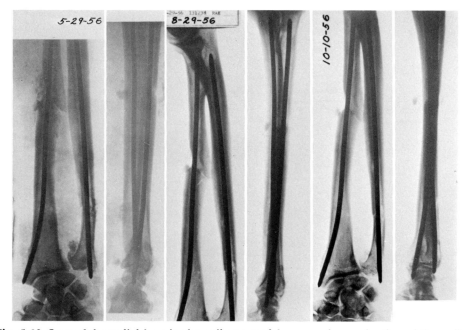

Fig. 5-20. Loss of the radial bow in the nail occurred because of comminution of the radius. (From Sage, F. P.: J. Bone Joint Surg. **41-A:**1489, 1959.)

sertion and spring back to its prebent shape once it has been finally seated (Fig. 5-19).

The ulna has two curves in its medullary canal. In the proximal third the canal bows toward the radius and in the distal third it bows convexly away from the radius. These two curves are slight and are offsetting in their deviation from a straight line; accordingly, a straight nail in the ulna can be used.

Fractures better suited to medullary fixation are those in the distal three fourths of the ulna and in the proximal two thirds of the radius, whether they are comminuted or not. Comminuted fractures may need

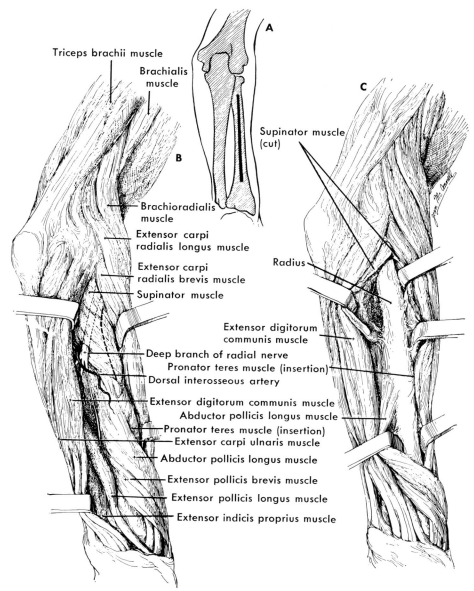

Triceps brachii muscle

Brachialis muscle

Supinator muscle (cut)

Brachioradialis muscle

Extensor carpi radialis longus muscle

Extensor carpi radialis brevis muscle

Supinator muscle

Radius

Extensor digitorum communis muscle

Deep branch of radial nerve

Pronator teres muscle (insertion)

Dorsal interosseous artery

Extensor digitorum communis muscle

Abductor pollicis longus muscle

Pronator teres muscle (insertion)

Extensor carpi ulnaris muscle

Abductor pollicis longus muscle

Extensor pollicis brevis muscle

Extensor pollicis longus muscle

Extensor indicis proprius muscle

Fig. 5-21. Thompson's approach to the upper one half of the forearm (From Crenshaw, A. H., editor: Campbell's operative orthopaedics, ed. 5, St. Louis, 1971, The C. V. Mosby Co.; modified from Anson and Maddock.)

accessory fixation in addition to the medullary nails. This may be in the form of accessory wire loops or extra screw fixation to hold the fragmented segments in position. If the comminuted fragments are small and particularly if the comminution is on the lateral side of the radius, the bow in the prebent pin should be accentuated. If it is not increased, the fracture fragments will telescope (Fig. 5-20) and allow a loss in the bow of the nail, with some loss in the width of the interosseous space.

Union failed to occur in 6% of the first fifty prebent medullary nails placed in the radius. This led us to recommend primary autogenous iliac cancellous grafts about each fracture. With such treatment, no nonunions have occurred in the last twenty-five cases of fractures in the radius.

OPERATIVE TECHNIQUE

Radius. The technique of insertion of the triangular prebent nail is exacting and should be meticulously

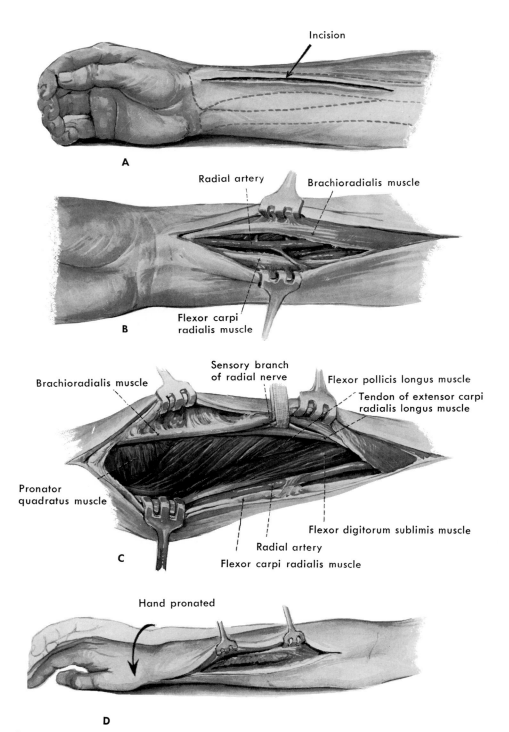

Fig. 5-22. Henry's anterior approach to the distal half of the forearm. (From Crenshaw, A. H., editor: Campbell's operative orthopaedics, ed. 5, St. Louis, 1971, The C. V. Mosby Co.; modified from Banks and Laufman.)

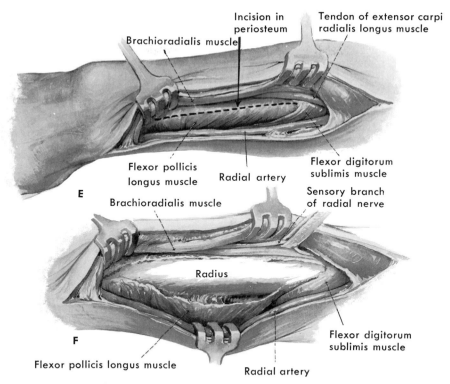

Fig. 5-22, cont'd. For legend see opposite page.

followed. It has been described in detail elsewhere,[7] but some points need to be emphasized. The fractures in both bones should be exposed and the canals found to be adequate to accommodate the nails proximally and distally or made so by reaming before either bone is fixed. It is important not to greatly enlarge a canal that is unusually small as this may thin the cortex so that it fragments during seating of the nail. The posterolateral Thompson approach (Fig. 5-21) is used to expose the proximal half of the radius. Either the Thompson or the Henry approach (Fig. 5-22) is used in the distal half. A straight subcutaneous incision along the posterior border of the ulna is usually all that is needed to expose the fracture here. The radial nails should be inserted on the styloid process directly into an unnamed ridge on the bone that separates the abductor pollicis longus and the extensor pollicis brevis tendons from the extensor carpi radialis longus and brevis. We previously tried inserting the nail at Lister's tubercle; it resulted in rupture of the extensor pollicis longus tendons in four patients during the postoperative period. Lister's tubercle as a point of insertion for the prebent triangular nail has been abandoned. A hole into the bone should be reamed in an oblique direction from the radial styloid toward the lateral epicondyle (Fig. 5-19). The nail for the radius then should be inserted 2½ inches by hand up the medullary canal. After the nail has been inserted 2½ inches by hand, it is driven up the proximal fragment and into the distal fragment. During the driving of the nail the ends of the fractured bones should be tightly clamped with small bone-holding forceps to prevent any butterfly fragments from becoming dislodged. The same precaution should be observed when reaming the medullary canals. If advancement of the nail becomes impeded, efforts to seat the nail should cease until roentgenograms show there is no obstruction to the passage of the nail.

Ulna. The ulnar nail is placed in the canal last, for it lies subcutaneously and the bone ends are not as difficult to deliver from the wound. The nail is inserted into the ulna from the fracture site. It may be driven in a retrograde fashion up the proximal fragment and out the olecranon or driven distally out the ulnar styloid prior to reducing the fracture and the final seating of the ulnar nail. Autogenous iliac cancellous grafts speed union and enhance the success of the procedure. They should not encroach on the interosseous space. Their use on the upper third of the radius is particularly prone to cause synostosis.

The tourniquet used during the operation should be released prior to skin closure and all deep bleeding stopped. The deep fascia should not be closed as a further prophylaxis against Volkmann's contracture. On the contrary, it is advisable to open the fascia to prevent ischemic pressure from occurring as a result of swelling. A simple skin closure is adequate. Immediately after the operation the arm is immobilized in a sugar-tongs splint so that any pressure from swelling can easily be relieved. When wound healing is complete, the arm is immobilized in a routine long arm cast until union is secure. Roentgenograms need to be repeated only at each cast change. The average time required for union is about 20 weeks.

Compression plate fixation

Indications. Those fractures not suited to medullary fixation are best treated by compression plate insertions. Some of the proponents of this type of fixation actually recommend it for all fractures of the forearm that are subjected to open reduction, while others recommend compression plates for the radius and medullary nails for the ulna. Compression plate fixation is the best method of fixation in the cases of nonunion in either forearm bone. Fresh forearm fractures that unequivocally are best suited to compression plate fixation are those in the proximal ulna, as in Monteggia's fractures[2] (Fig. 5-23), and those in the distal third of the radius, exclusive of the distal end (Fig. 5-8). In fresh fractures treated by compression plate fixation, primary bone grafting is not needed, except in cases of comminution where compression cannot actually be applied. Here it is used simply as an excellent holding device, and bone grafting will be beneficial.

Technique. The technique for applying the ASIF compression plate with which we are familiar is well detailed elsewhere.[3] A few points learned from personal experience may be of help. First, the plates are bulky and should be well covered by muscles. In the distal third they should be placed on the volar surface of the radius and ulna; in the upper and middle thirds they should be placed on the dorsal surface of the bones so as not to block pronation. The plates should be placed on the bone over the periosteum, leaving the periosteum intervening between the plates and the bone. Plating in this manner leaves the periosteum on the remaining uncovered bone intact and enhances earlier union. A full complement of tools in good condition (Fig. 5-24) should be available and a thorough knowledge of their use is a prerequisite. If a four-hole plate is used (it is most often used in the forearm unless there is an area of nonunion or comminution to bridge), full compression should not be

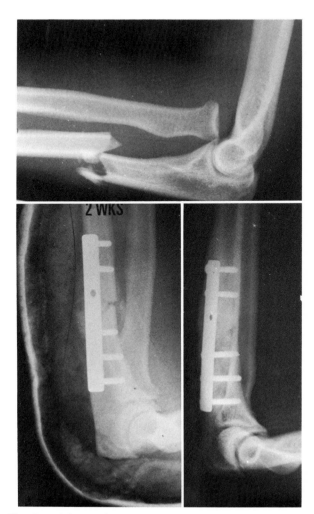

Fig. 5-23. Monteggia's fracture treated with an ASIF plate. (From Anderson, L. D.: Orthop. Clin. N. Amer. **1:**151, 1970.)

attempted, for this may cause the bone to split in line with the four screw holes. In the six-hole plate the screw holes are offset from one another and splitting in line with the holes in the bone is not as likely to occur. Anderson[1] found that excessive compression did not necessarily stimulate osteogenesis, but compression did aid in securing good bone contact and immobilization and thus aid in securing union. As compression is applied, the plate should be kept aligned with the unsecured fragments by forceps to prevent angulation at the fracture site rather than compression. If the screw securing the compression device to the unsecured bone fragment is off-center, angulation at the fracture site is prone to occur or the screw in the compression device may shear out of the bone. At times it is difficult to be sure how well united

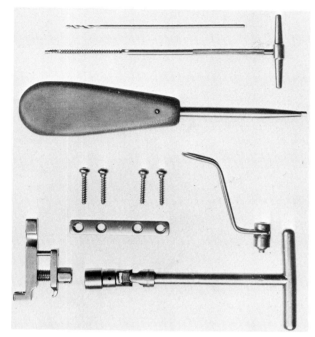

Fig. 5-24. Photograph of ASIF equipment used in plating of forearm fractures. (Courtesy AO-Instrumente, Synthes AG Chur, Biel, Switzerland; from Crenshaw, A. H., editor: Campbell's operative orthopaedics, ed. 5, St. Louis, 1971, The C. V. Mosby Co.)

the fracture has become, as it is usually stable and may be completely obliterated roentgenographically at the time of open reduction and fixation by compression plates. For this reason the plates and screws should remain on the bone for at least 12 months before they are removed. Even then, because the plate has taken much of the stress off the bone, there may be such a disuse osteopenia present that a few weeks in the protective cast is indicated to ensure against refracture.

All bones that have open reduction and internal fixation should be immobilized in a long arm cast until union is assured. To fail to do so has resulted in delayed union and malunion in some patients.

Open fractures

Open or compound fractures are best treated without internal fixation until soft tissue healing has occurred; then the surgeon may treat the fracture as a fresh wound. To initially load the compound fracture with metal could be disastrous. The exception to this rule is when there are large soft tissue losses to be grafted that do not allow use of external support. In such instances (Fig. 5-25), or in cases of vascular repair in which immediate immobilization is needed, a

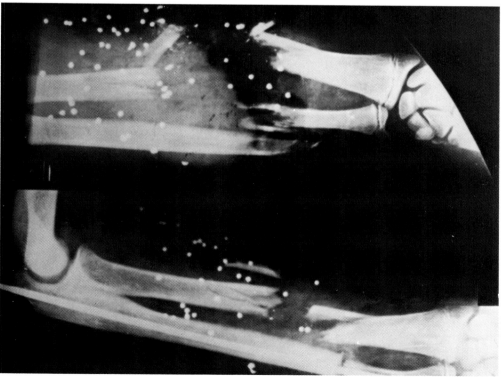

Fig. 5-25. Shotgun wound to forearm. Medullary nail placed down ulna for stability until soft tissue healing has occurred.

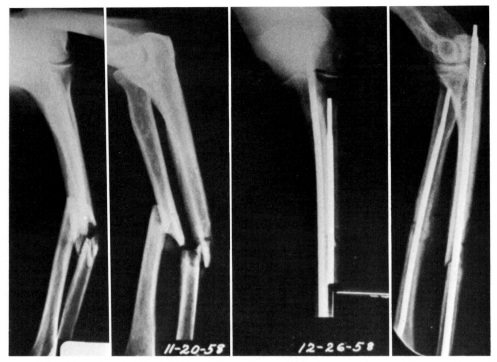

Fig. 5-26. Nonunion in the middle of the radius and ulna treated by medullary nails and iliac grafts.

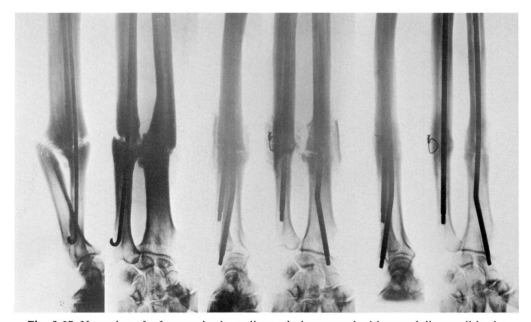

Fig. 5-27. Nonunion of a fracture in the radius and ulna treated with a medullary nail in the ulna and a wire loop in the radius. The immediate postoperative films show the medullary fixation in the radius and ulna, the wire loop in the ulna to prevent distraction, and iliac grafts about the fracture. One year following the initial injury, union occurred in excellent position. (From Boyd, H. B., Lipinski, S. W., and Wiley, J. H.: In Proceedings of the Société Internationale de Chirurgie Orthopedique et de Traumatologie, Brussels, 1960, Imprimerie des Sciences, pp. 29-52.)

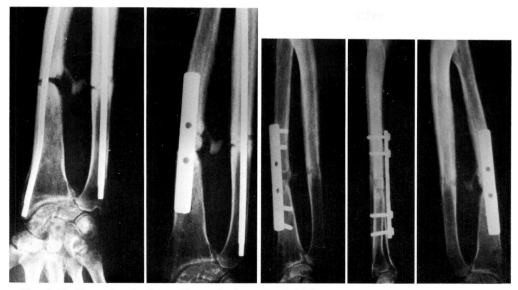

Fig. 5-28. Nonunion in the radius and ulna after initial treatment with medullary nails. A Nicoll graft was inserted in the defect in the radius and fixed with a compression plate. Note that the middle two screw holes in the plate were not used.

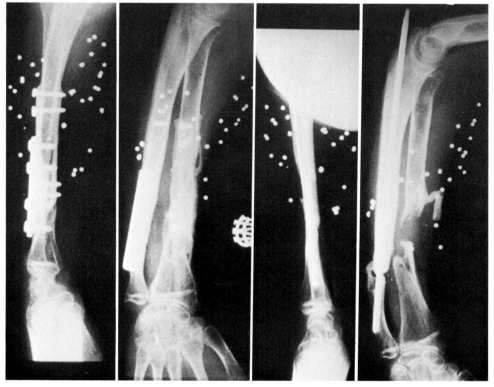

Fig. 5-29. Same patient as in Fig. 5-25. The defect in the radius was treated with a dual onlay bone graft.

medullary nail may preserve length and give enough stability to the forearm to permit extensive soft tissue reconstruction.

Nonunion

Nonunion in the forearm in most instances is best treated by compression plate fixation and autogenous bone grafting. In cases where the bone is overlapped a medullary nail and autogenous bone may be used (Fig. 5-26), for as length is regained from the overlapped bone, the ends will be compressed and afford compression fixation. In nonunion in the ulna when a medullary nail is used it is best to add a wire loop about both fragments to secure better stability (Fig. 5-27). When there is a defect to be bridged, a plug of iliac bone, as advocated by Nicoll, placed between the bone ends and compressed by a six-hole compression plate is excellent (Fig. 5-28). The two innermost holes are unused since this part of the plate bridges the graft. It has been our experience that nonunited fractures in the distal third of the radius with distal radioulnar joint derangement are best treated by securing union in the radius first before resecting the distal ulna. The nonunited radius that has become osteopenic does not hold metallic fixation too well and the distal end of the ulna adds stability. Once union has occurred, then the distal ulna can be resected, obliterating the distal radioulnar joint derangement.

If the gaps in the bone are large and must be

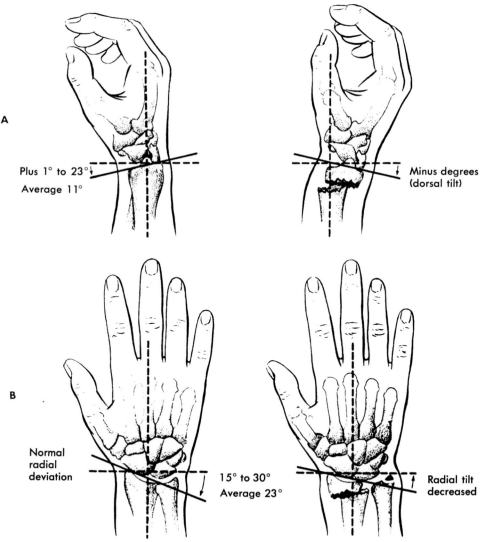

Fig. 5-30. Line drawings showing the deformities in a typical Colles fracture. (From DePalma, A. F.: J. Bone Joint Surg. **34-A**:651, 1952.)

bridged, there is no better source of fixation to osteopenic bone fragments than the use of the classic Boyd dual onlay graft (Fig. 5-29). This affords fixation, clamping the osteopenic fragments between the good bone used in the dual onlay graft. The defect thus bridged is filled with cancellous bone fragments.

FRACTURES OF THE DISTAL RADIUS

There are three fractures in the distal end of the radius, near the articulation between the radius and carpal bones, that are worthy of discussion. The first and the most frequent, of course, is the Colles fracture, the second is the reverse Colles or Smith fracture, and the third is the Barton fracture. In the Barton fracture a part of the articular surface of the radius is broken and dislocated either dorsally or volarly with the carpal bones.

Colles' fracture

Colles' fracture is produced by falling on the outstretched hand. The distal fragment of the radius rotates into supination and the proximal fragment pronates. The Smith fracture is produced by falling on the flexed wrist. The distal fragment of the radius is pronated on the proximal fragment. The mech-

anism of injury in Barton's fracture is also a fall on the outstretched hand with the wrist dorsiflexed. The direction of the displacement or dislocation of the fractured articular surface with the carpal bone depends on that portion of the articular surface that receives the greatest strain. If the strain to the articular surface is greater to the volar half, then an anterior Barton fracture occurs; if the strain is greater to the posterior half, then the bone is fractured in the posterior half and dislocates dorsally.

The classic Colles fracture is one in which there is dorsal dislocation of the distal fragment (Fig. 5-30, *A*). The angulated distal fragment causes a dorsal tilt of the distal articular surface of the radius. The distal fragment may be radially deviated (Fig. 5-30, *B*), as is the hand, and there is usually radial shortening. As mentioned, these deformities occur when the hand and the wrist supinate off of a pronated proximal fragment. In order to reduce the displacement the distal fragment must be pronated on the relatively pronated proximal fragment. The pronation must be maintained in order to prevent recurrence of the displacement. To maintain the arm in a pronated position, the cast must extend around the elbow and block supination. This is adequately accomplished

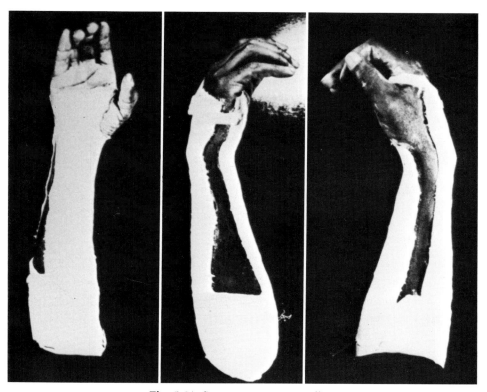

Fig. 5-31. Sugar-tongs cast or splint.

using a sugar-tongs cast (Fig. 5-31) extending from the proximal palmar crease around the volar surface of the forearm, posteriorly about the elbow, and then over the dorsal aspect of the forearm and over the dorsum of the hand to the neck of the metacarpals. This is applied over cotton padding or directly to the skin except for a minimal amount of padding over the bony prominences at the wrist and hand and elbow. This immobilization should be used even if the fracture is undisplaced, for as the fracture line undergoes absorption, during the first 2 weeks after the injury the fracture may become displaced if the patient supinates the forearm. A simple short arm cast that does not include immobilization of the elbow will allow the distal fragment to supinate off of the pronated proximal fragment. The sugar-tongs cast has an added advantage in that it is readily split down to the skin on both sides. If there is any doubt about adequate vascular supply to the hand, one is more prone to simply take the scissors and split the gauze that binds the plaster slabs to the front and back of the forearm down to the skin. This cast is adequate to immobilize these fractures until they unite.

The mechanism of reduction of the Colles fracture is simple. It is preferable that there be good muscle relaxation, which is best obtained with a general anesthetic or an axillary block. We do not recommend local infiltration of the fracture, for the fracture hematoma is already present under pressure, and to add more fluid into the area may cause more pressure, resulting in a Volkmann's contracture. The hematoma is a nutrient broth and will allow propagation of any bacteria that might be introduced locally. Once anesthesia is accomplished, the fractured hand is taken by the same hand of the surgeon, as if the surgeon were merely shaking hands with the patient. As an assistant maintains pressure over the front of the arm just above the antecubital space, the elbow is flexed at 90°. The fracture site is palpated, and the opposite thumb is placed on the proximal end of the distal fragment. As traction is exerted, angulation at the fracture site is increased and pressure by the surgeon's opposite thumb is made on the proximal end of the distal fragment. The forearm is carried into pronation, flexion, and ulnar deviation. This maneuver will effect reduction in practically every instance. The arm can then be encased in a sugar-tongs cast. After the cast is dried, a satisfactory position should be ascertained with two plane roentgenograms. It is our policy to hospitalize the patient for 24 hours following the reduction. With the hand elevated from an overhead frame, ice caps are placed

about the wrist and the patient is advised to exercise the fingers in full flexion and extension 5 minutes out of each hour while awake.

The routine Colles fracture should be immobilized in a sugar-tongs cast for a period of approximately 6 weeks. Then the cast is removed, but the wrist is still protected for 4 weeks in a metal volar splint that can be removed for exercise, eating, and normal hygiene purposes.

The comminuted Colles fracture (Fig. 5-32) requires different treatment. Unless the fracture is stabilized in some way it will collapse and cause radial deviation of the hand, thickening of the wrist, shortening of the radius, and distal radioulnar joint derangement, with prominence of the ulna and limited supination in the forearm. This fracture can be immobilized using continuous traction that is incorporated in the cast (Fig. 5-33). A small Kirschner wire can be inserted in the thumb transversely from the lateral to the medial side and through the proximal phalanx at 90° to the longitudinal axis of the

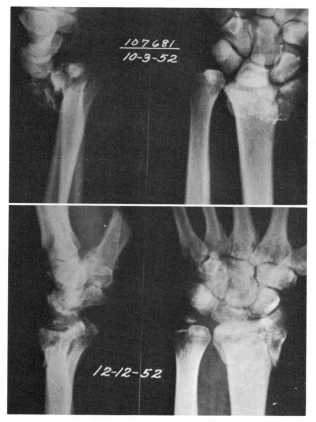

Fig. 5-32. Comminuted Colles' fracture treated by skeletal traction through the thumb. There was early union at 9 weeks.

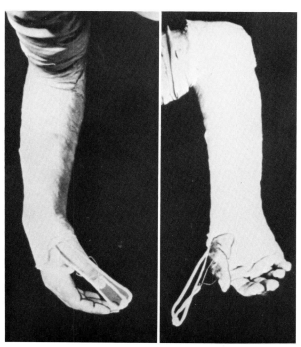

Fig. 5-33. Skeletal traction through the thumb for comminuted Colles' fractures.

thumb. To the wire, rubber band traction is attached and stretched to a wire loop outrigger incorporated in the sugar-tongs cast. The pin should go through the proximal phalanx and not penetrate either the nail bed or the pulp of the thumb. It is now my preference to use a modification of the DePalma method (Fig. 5-34) of immobilization for this fracture.[4] Two small unthreaded Kirschner wires are inserted from the radial styloid across the comminuted fracture site into the medial cortex of the proximal fragment. I believe that two pins inserted across this area, parallel to one another, prevent the fracture from slipping. It is not necessary to carry the pins or Kirschner wires across into the ulna. There is almost always a styloid process that has a fragment big enough to hold two small Kirschner wires, and as an assistant holds the fracture in reduction, the styloid process is usually easily palpated. The Kirschner wires are usually very easily inserted. After the wires have been seated in the bone and their position ascertained by x-ray examination, a small bend is placed in them. The wires then do not migrate further up into the bone. The ends of the wires should be buried beneath the skin, but easily felt, so that they can be removed under local anesthesia when the fracture is united. The postoperative management is the same as it was for the uncomminuted Colles fracture.

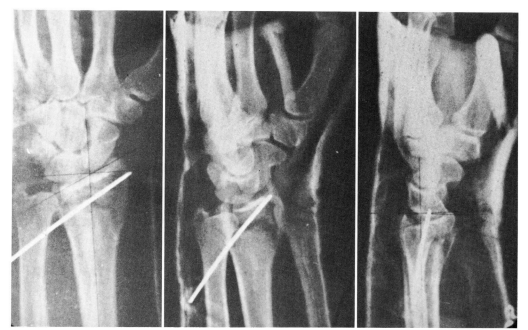

Fig. 5-34. DePalma method of pinning the distal radius. (From DePalma, A. F.: J. Bone Joint Surg. **34-A**:651, 1952.)

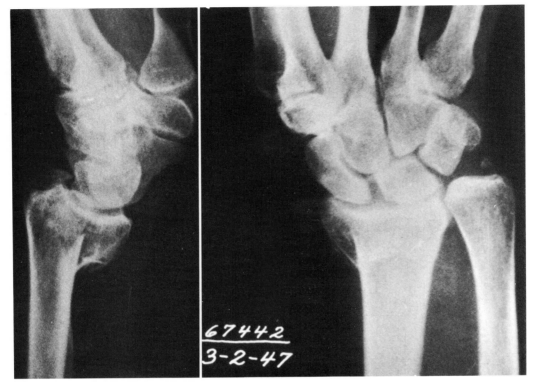

Fig. 5-35. Smith's fracture.

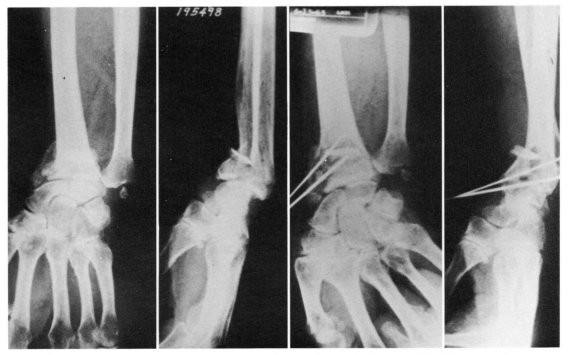

Fig. 5-36. Anterior Barton's fracture treated by Kirschner wire fixation. The Kirschner wires should have penetrated the opposite cortex of the proximal fragment at the radius.

Smith's fracture

Smith's fracture (Fig. 5-35) is exactly the reverse of Colles' fracture. The displacement is volarward. The fracture occurs in pronation; so in order to reduce the fracture it should be in dorsiflexion and supination and maintained in this position with a sugar-tongs cast. The mechanics of reduction are not difficult. The postoperative management in the sugar-tongs cast and following its removal should be the same as for the uncomplicated Colles fracture.

Barton's fracture

Barton's fractures themselves are not difficult to reduce but are difficult to hold with plaster immobilization. For this reason I use the fixation method employing two parallel Kirschner wires, the same as for the comminuted Colles fracture (Fig. 5-36). This ensures a stable fracture in the postreduction period. When simple cast immobilization alone is used, this fracture is prone to redislocate until good solid union has occurred.

• • •

The fracture surgeon's primary responsibility to the patient is to restore the function of the patient's extremity to as near normal as possible. The primary function in the upper extremity is that given by the hand, and for this reason the hand is of primary importance in any injury to the upper extremity. If at any time a question arises as to the adequacy of the blood supply of the hand, all efforts should be made to restore the blood supply to the hand without too much concern about loss of reduction of the fracture. A fracture can always be remanipulated, but an avascular hand is not easy to restore.

REFERENCES

1. Anderson, L. D.: Compression plate fixation and the effect of different types of internal fixation on fracture healing, J. Bone Joint Surg. **47-A:**191, 1965.
2. Anderson, L. D.: The use of plates in the patient with multiple injuries, Orthop. Clin. N. Amer. **1:**151, 1970.
3. Crenshaw, A. H., editor: Campbell's operative orthopaedics, ed. 5, St. Louis, 1971, The C. V. Mosby Co., pp. 669-675.
4. DePalma, A.: Comminuted fractures of the distal end of the radius treated by ulnar pinning, J. Bone Joint Surg. **34-A:**651, 1952.
5. Evans, E. M.: Rotational deformity in the treatment of fractures of both bones of the forearm, J. Bone Joint Surg. **27:**373, 1945.
6. Hughston, J. C.: Fracture of the distal radial shaft. Mistakes in management, J. Bone Joint Surg. **39-A:**249, 1957.
7. Knight, R. A., and Purvis, G. D.: Fractures of both bones of the forearm in adults, J. Bone Joint Surg. **31-A:**755, 1949.
8. Patrick, J.: A study of supination and pronation with especial reference to the treatment of forearm fractures, J. Bone Joint Surg. **28:**737, 1946.
9. Sage, F. P.: Medullary fixation of fractures of the forearm. A study of the medullary canal of the radius and a report of 50 fractures of the radius treated with a prebent triangular nail, J. Bone Joint Surg. **41-A:**1489, 1959.
10. Smith, H., and Sage, F. P.: Medullary fixation of forearm fractures, J. Bone Joint Surg. **39-A:**91, 1957.
11. Street, D. M.: Spectator Club Letter, Nov. 18, 1955.

Chapter 6

Lower extremity bracing

Part I

Introduction to lower extremity orthotics

NEWTON C. McCOLLOUGH, III, M.D.
Miami, Florida

There is little question that until very recently the field of orthotics has lagged significantly behind its sister field of prosthetics in terms of development. The needs of the amputee are more immediate and obvious, and the wars of the past 30 years have resulted in large numbers of young men with extremity loss, thus stimulating interest and research in prosthetics. Medical, engineering, and the prosthetic professions have responded to the needs of the amputee through extensive research and development, improved fabrication and fitting techniques, widespread educational programs, and better delivery of services. The field of orthotics has developed more slowly, with more limited, though no less sophisticated research activities, few educational endeavors, and little improvement upon local fabrication and delivery services over the past 50 years.

On the other hand, the comparative need for further research, development, and education in orthotics is much greater than in prosthetics when measured in terms of sheer patient volume. According to a recent estimate,[1] patients with orthotic needs in the United States number 3,370,000, and 54% of these have lower extremity bracing problems. The total number of amputees in this country is approximately 311,000, so that there are roughly ten times as many patients in need of orthotic service as there are patients with prosthetic requirements.

A number of centers in the United States and Canada engaged in orthotic research for the past few years have produced stimulating and encouraging results. The traditional concept of bracing in the static sense is being revolutionized to a more dynamic approach to control of body or extremity motion. As an example, control of ankle position or movement by bracing techniques is being used to influence control at the knee, either by producing an extension or a flexion moment about the knee axis. In addition, it has been recognized that traditional bracing may often limit to some degree the normal functions that coexist in an impaired extremity, and efforts are being made to develop orthotic systems that more accurately substitute for lost functions, yet preserve those normal functions which remain in the same extremity. As an example, the University of California Biomechanics Laboratory has developed a dual-axis ankle control system that, while controlling ankle motion, will still allow normal subtalar motion.[2]

There are three major factors that should be identified as being influential upon modern concepts of lower extremity bracing.

1. New materials such as plastics, plastic laminates, and thermoplastics have been introduced into the orthotic field, permitting more varied design and altering time-honored fabrication techniques.
2. Principles of biomechanics and human locomotion, which have been the basis for improved prosthetic design over the years, are being recognized as having great relevance to the design of braces for the lower extremity.
3. A method for systematically identifying the biomechanical losses present in a given extremity as a basis for accurate orthotic prescription has been developed.

With regard to the latter, it is obvious that the physician's prescription for a brace has often in the past been somewhat less than exact, calling frequently for a "short leg brace" or a "long leg brace." All too frequently little thought is given to analyzing specific biomechanical defects present in an extremity with

Text continued on p. 124.

116

DIAGNOSIS _____ NAME _____

_____ NO. _____ SEX _____

_____ AGE _____ HEIGHT _____ WEIGHT _____

MAJOR IMPAIRMENTS: DATE _____

A. Musculoskeletal:
  1. Bone & Joint: Normal ☐ Abnormal _____
  2. Muscle: Normal ☐ Flaccid ☐ Spastic ☐
    Other _____
  3. Ligament: Normal ☐ Abnormal ☐: Knee: AC ☐ PC ☐ MC ☐ LC ☐
    Ankle: MC ☐ LC ☐
    Other _____

B. Sensation: Normal ☐ Abnormal ☐
  1. Anaesthesia ☐ Location _____
    Protective Sensation: Lost ☐ Retained ☐
  2. Proprioceptive Loss ☐
    Location _____ Degree: Mild ☐ Moderate ☐ Severe ☐
  3. Pain ☐ Location _____

C. Skin: Normal ☐ Abnormal _____

D. Vascular: Normal ☐ Abnormal ☐ RT ☐ LT ☐
  1. Arterial ☐ 2. Venous ☐ 3. Coagulation Defect ☐

E. Balance: Normal ☐ Impaired: Mild ☐ Moderate ☐ Severe ☐

F. Extremity Shortening: None ☐ LT ☐ RT ☐
  Amount of Discrepancy:

    I.T. — Heel _____
    I.T. — M.T.P. _____
    M.T.P. — Heel _____

    X-ray _____

———————————— LEGEND ————————————

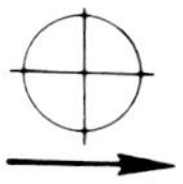

⊕ ↑ = Direction of Translatory Motion

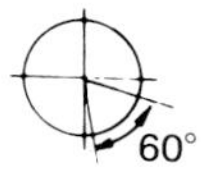

= Abnormal Degree of Rotary Motion (60°)

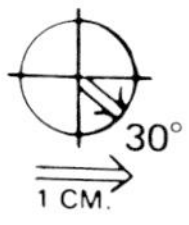

= Fixed Position (30°, 1 CM.)

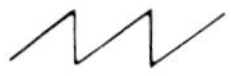

= Fracture

Volitional Force
G = Good
F = Fair
P = Poor
T = Trace
Z = Zero

Spastic Muscle (SP)
SP$_M$ = Mild
SP$_{MO}$ = Moderate
SP$_S$ = Severe

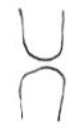

= Pseudarthrosis

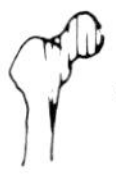

= Absence of Segment

E = Edema

D = Local Distension or Enlargement

Continued.

Fig. 6-1. A, Front sheet of lower extremity patient analysis form, including legend. **B** and **C,** Skeletal outlines of the right and left lower extremities for diagramming abnormalities of bone, joint, and muscle. **D,** Final page includes space for summarizing the functional disability and making orthotic recommendations based on this summary. (From McCollough, N. C., III, Fryer, C. M., and Glancy, J.: Artif. Limbs **14**:68, 1970.)

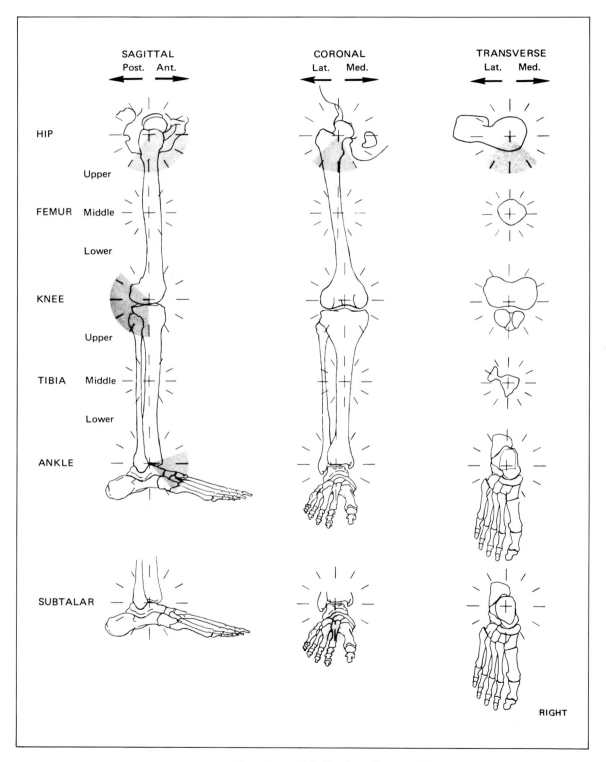

Fig. 6-1, cont'd. For legend see p. 117.

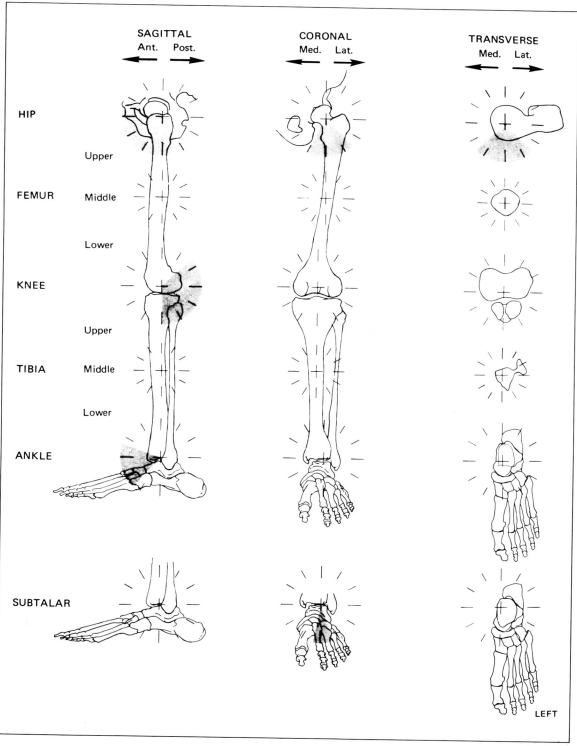

Fig. 6-1, cont'd. For legend see p. 117.

Continued.

Summary of Functional Disability _____

_____

_____

_____

_____

Orthotic Recommendation _____

_____

Fig. 6-1, cont'd. For legend see p. 117.

INSTRUCTIONS FOR USE OF THE LOWER EXTREMITY ANALYSIS FORM

Major impairments

Most of this portion of the form is self-explanatory. Abnormal *bone and joint* conditions may include such entities as osteoporosis, Paget's disease, coxa vara, etc. *Muscle* may be normal, flaccid, or spastic, but a space is provided for description of rarer disorders such as muscular dystrophy, fibrosis of muscle, etc. Under the heading of *ligament*, check boxes are provided for the major ligaments of the knee and ankle to indicate abnormal laxity. The sections on *sensation*, *skin*, and *vascular* impairments cover considerations that may influence orthotic design and are self-explanatory.

Balance is either normal or impaired, and if impaired, the following definitions are applicable:

1. *Mild impairment* is compatible with independent ambulation.
2. *Moderate impairment* is compatible with ambulation utilizing external support.
3. *Severe impairment* indicates the need for maximal support or personal assistance in ambulation.

Extremity shortening is recorded as follows: (1) ischial tuberosity to sole of heel; (2) ischial tuberosity to medial tibial plateau; and (3) medial tibial plateau to sole of heel.

In leg-length discrepancies exceeding ½ inch, x-ray studies of leg length may be indicated and an appropriate space is provided for this measurement.

Legend and extremity diagrams

Two terms must first be defined:

1. *Translatory motion* is motion in which all points of the distal segment move in the same direction, with the paths of all points being exactly alike in shape and distance traversed (Fig. 6-2).
2. *Rotary motion* is motion of a distal segment in which one point in the distal segment or in its (imaginary) extension always remains fixed (Fig. 6-3).

The symbols described in the legend are used in conjunction with the right and left extremity diagrams according to the following rules:

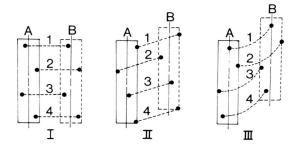

Fig. 6-2. Diagram illustrating translatory motion. (From McCollough, N. C., III, Fryer, C. M., and Glancy, J.: Artif. Limbs **14**:68, 1970.)

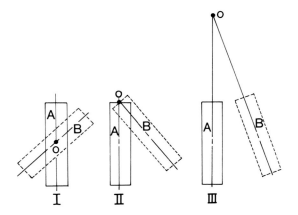

Fig. 6-3. Diagram illustrating rotary motion. (From McCollough, N. C., III, Fryer, C. M., and Glancy, J.: Artif. Limbs **14**:68, 1970.)

INSTRUCTIONS FOR USE OF THE LOWER EXTREMITY ANALYSIS FORM—cont'd

1. Rules pertaining to recording motion:
   a. The degrees of rotary motion or centimeters of translatory motion are to be obtained from passive manipulation and are to reflect passive, not active motion at the site being examined. In the lower extremity, joints are to be observed during weight bearing, and if the degree of joint excursion is greater under conditions of loading than by passive manipulation, this figure is diagrammed rather than the smaller figure (for example, recurvatum of the knee).

   Translatory motion
   b. Linear arrows horizontally placed below the circle indicate the presence of (abnormal) translatory motion at one or more of the six designated levels of the lower extremity listed on the left side of the form. The head of the arrow always points in the direction of displacement of the distal segment relative to the proximal segment. Linear arrows vertically placed on the right side of the circle indicate (abnormal) translatory motion along the vertical axis at the site indicated.

   Rotary motion
   c. Normal ranges of rotary motion about joints are preshaded on the diagram. Abnormal rotary motion, either as limited or as excess motion, is indicated by double-headed arrows placed outside and concentric to the circle to indicate the extent of available motion present in the affected joint. In certain instances, it may be more meaningful to use two double-headed arrows in order to describe the range of motion to either side of the neutral joint axis rather than a single arrow which describes the total range of motion present. If one head of an arrow fails to reach the preshaded margin, limitation of joint motion is denoted. Conversely, if one head of an arrow projects beyond the preshaded margin, excess motion is designated. Numbers in degrees are placed adjacent to the arrows to indicate the arc described. In addition, radial lines drawn from the center of the circle and passing through its perimeter at the tips of the double-headed arrow are to be used for more graphic representation of the arc of available motion. At sites where rotary motion does not occur (for example, fracture site or knee joint in the coronal plane) the presence of abnormal rotary motion is similarly designated by a double-headed arrow with an adjacent numerical value in degrees.

   Fixed position
   d. Double radial arrows indicate a fixed joint position and describe in degrees the deviation from the neutral joint position. Horizontal or vertical double arrows indicate a fixed joint position in a translatory sense, and the extent of abnormal translation is indicated in centimeters adjacent to the arrow (for example, subluxated tibia in a hemophiliac knee).

2. Rules pertaining to muscle dysfunction:
   Flaccid muscle
   a. Flaccid muscle is designated as such under the section on major impairments. Muscle group strength, not individual muscle strength, is determined by conventional means on the examining table, and the letter grade corresponding to volitional force is recorded adjacent to the skeletel outline at the proper location for each muscle group. The letter grades correspond to the standard muscle grading system used in poliomyelitis. No symbol is used if muscle strength is normal.

   Spastic muscle
   b. Spastic muscle is designated as such under the section on major impairments. It is further identified in the legend as "SP." The letter grade (for example, SP$_{MO}$) for muscle group tone, not individual muscles, is to be placed adjacent to the skeletel outline at the proper location for each muscle group. Spastic muscle estimates are to be made with the patient in the functional position for the lower extremity, that is, observation during standing and walking. The subletter grades for spastic muscles are as follows:

   M   mild degree of spasticity
   MO moderate degree of spasticity sufficient for useful holding quality
   S   severe spasticity, obstructive in terms of function

   In certain instances, muscle groups in a patient with spastic paralysis may be more appropriately graded according to volitional force, for example, dorsiflexors of the foot in a hemiplegic.

3. Rules pertaining to fracture or bone deformity: All translatory or rotary motions at the fracture on the shaft of a long bone are diagrammed on the circle located at the midshaft of each bone. The actual fracture site is indicated by the fracture symbol. All bony deformities such as valgus angulation of the shaft are likewise diagrammed on the circle located at the center of the shaft, regardless of the position of the angular deformity. The location of the angular deformity is designated by circling the appropriate level on the left-hand side of the chart.

DIAGNOSIS *Poliomyelitis*

NAME *W. S.*
NO. *89416*   SEX *Male*
AGE *22*   HEIGHT *5' 11"* WEIGHT *195*
DATE *3/9/70*

MAJOR IMPAIRMENTS:

A. Musculoskeletal:

Triple Arthrodesis Ⓛ foot

1. Bone & Joint: Normal ☐   Abnormal *Old supracondylar fracture Ⓛ fem*
2. Muscle: Normal ☐   Flaccid ☑   Spastic ☐
    Other _____
3. Ligament: Normal ☐ Abnormal ☑:   Knee: AC ☐ PC ☑ MC ☑ LC ☐
    Ankle: MC ☐ LC ☐
    Other _____

B. Sensation: Normal ☑   Abnormal ☐

1. Anaesthesia ☐   Location _____
    Protective Sensation: Lost ☐   Retained ☐
2. Proprioceptive Loss ☐
    Location _____ Degree: Mild ☐ Moderate ☐   Severe ☐
3. Pain ☑   Location *Anterior distal thigh*

C. Skin: Normal ☑   Abnormal _____

D. Vascular: Normal ☑   Abnormal ☐   RT ☐   LT ☐
1. Arterial ☐   2. Venous ☐   3. Coagulation Defect ☐

E. Balance: Normal ☑   Impaired: Mild ☐   Moderate ☐   Severe ☐

F. Extremity Shortening: None ☐   LT ☑   RT ☐
    Amount of Discrepancy:

    I.T. — Heel *1 3/4 "*
    I.T. — M.T.P. *1/2 "*
    M.T.P. — Heel *1 1/4 "*

    X-ray _____

─────────── LEGEND ───────────

⊕ ↑ = Direction of Translatory Motion

⊕ 60° = Abnormal Degree of Rotary Motion

⊕ 30° = Fixed Position
1 CM.

∧∧∧ = Fracture

Volitional Force

G   = Good
F   = Fair
P   = Poor
T   = Trace
Z   = Zero

Spastic Muscle (SP)

SP$_M$ = Mild
SP$_{MO}$ = Moderate
SP$_S$ = Severe

⊔ = Pseudarthrosis

= Absence of Segment

E   = Edema

D   = Local Distension or Enlargement

Fig. 6-4. A, Front sheet of lower extremity analysis form completed for patient with poliomyelitis. **B,** Skeletal outline shows loss of full extension at the hip, 20° of hyperextension at the knee, and loss of dorsiflexion above 90° at the ankle. There is a valgus deformity of 10° in the lower one third of the femur, 15° of valgus instability at the knee, and abnormal inversion and eversion at the ankle joint secondary to a triple arthrodesis and a fixed subtalar joint. External tibial torsion of 15° is also found. Muscle group strength is depicted throughout the extremity; for example, hip flexors are good and hip extensors are fair.

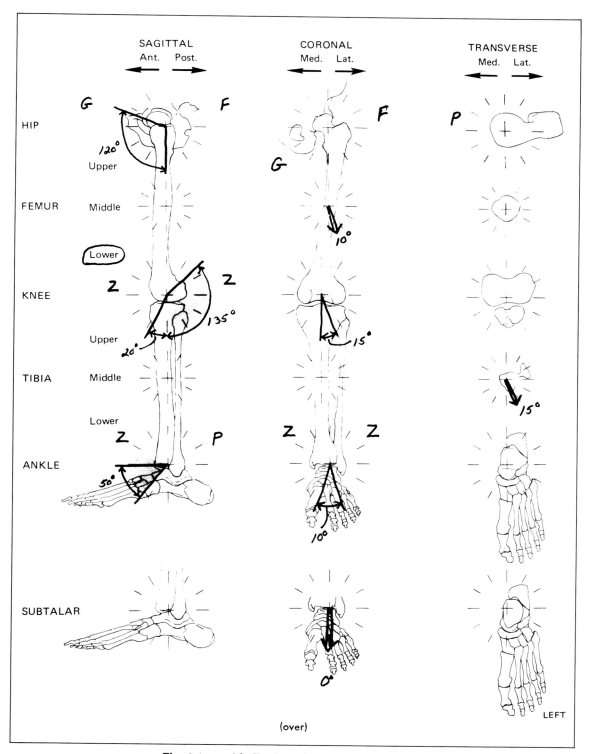

	SAGITTAL Ant. Post.	CORONAL Med. Lat.	TRANSVERSE Med. Lat.

HIP

FEMUR — Middle — Lower

KNEE — Upper

TIBIA — Middle — Lower

ANKLE

SUBTALAR

(over)

Fig. 6-4, cont'd. For legend see opposite page.

the aim of translating them into an appropriate mechanical substitute.

Recognizing the need for a more organized and systematic approach to orthotic prescription, the Committee on Orthotics and Prosthetics of the American Academy of Orthopaedic Surgeons has developed a lower extremity analysis form whereby one can diagramatically plot the biomechanical defects in a given extremity.[3] Once properly identified, these losses can then be matched against specific components or component systems to substitute for the functions lost. In this manner, a more rational and scientific approach to brace prescription can be achieved. The use of such a form may also serve to identify areas or functions for which satisfactory components are not presently available and thus become the basis for future design.

Inherent in this new approach to orthotic prescription is elimination of the old concept of "disease bracing." The basis for prescription should be a careful appraisal of the defects present, regardless of etiology, followed by a selection of components to control these defects, and finally the creation of an orthotic system incorporating the appropriate components selected.

LOWER EXTREMITY ANALYSIS FORM

The lower extremity analysis form consists of four pages of appropriate size for insertion into the hospital chart. The first page (Fig. 6-1, *A*) contains spaces for patient data, including diagnosis and a summary of major impairments existing in one or both extremities. At the bottom of the first page there is a legend for symbols to be used on the extremity diagrams. The second and third pages (Fig. 6-1, *B* and *C*) contain skeletal outlines of the right and left lower extremities, respectively, in the sagittal, coronal, and transverse planes. Overlaying the major joints are shaded areas representing the normal ranges of joint motion within a circle divided into 30° segments. Similar smaller circles overlay the midshafts of the long bones for diagramming angular, rotational, or translational deformities of the femur and tibia. The fourth page (Fig. 6-1, *D*) includes spaces for summarizing the functional disability and for making orthotic recommendations based upon this summary.

The technique of completing the lower extremity analysis form is shown in Fig. 6-4. It is hoped that such a form will lead to a closer working relationship between the physician and the orthotist by providing a common ground upon which to make rational decisions for orthotic design.

REFERENCES

1. Committee on Prosthetics Research and Development, National Academy of Sciences, National Research Council: Unpublished data, 1970.
2. Inman, V. T.: UC-BL dual axis ankle control system and UC-BL shoe insert: biomechanical considerations, Bull. Prosth. Res. Spring, 1969.
3. McCollough, N. C., III, Fryer, C. M., and Glancy, J.: A new approach to patient analysis for orthotic prescription, Artif. Limbs **14:**68, 1970.

Part II

Biomechanics of the lower extremity

CHARLES M. FRYER, M.A.
Chicago, Illinois

Any study of normal or pathologic gait must, of necessity, include information related to body motion and to the forces acting on the body to produce those motions.

Considerable data have been collected regarding motion of the body as a whole, motion of individual body segments, and the angular changes that occur at the major joints of the lower extremity during gait.

Collectively, these data constitute what may be referred to as the kinematics of gait.

During normal and pathologic gait the forces acting on the body and its segments are those produced by gravity and by muscle contraction. Information on the forces acting on the body during gait deals with the subdivision of mechanics called kinetics.

In this discussion an attempt will be made to correlate the salient kinematic and kinetic features of normal gait.

KINEMATICS

For ease of identification and reference the cycle of gait has been arbitrarily divided into various components that are visually discernible without recourse to special equipment or techniques.

A cycle of gait consists of all the activity that occurs between *heel-strike* on one side and the following heel-

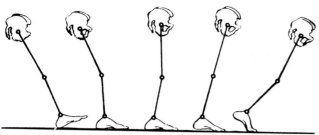

Heel-strike Foot-flat Midstance Heel-off Toe-off

Fig. 6-5. Stance phase and its subdivisions. (From Peizer, E., Wright, D. W., and Mason, C.: Bull. Prosth. Res. **10**:48, 1969.)

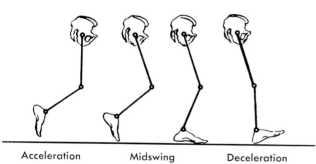

Acceleration   Midswing   Deceleration

Fig. 6-6. Swing phase and its subdivisions. (From Peizer, E., Wright, D. W., and Mason, C.: Bull. Prosth. Res. **10**:48, 1969.)

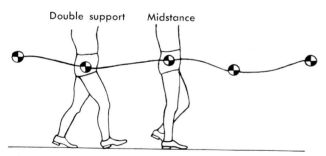

Double support   Midstance

Fig. 6-7. Vertical excursion of the center of gravity. (From Peizer, E., Wright, D. W., and Mason, C.: Bull. Prosth. Res. **10**:48, 1969.)

strike on the same side. It should be noted that during a single cycle there is a period of time when the extremity is supporting the body weight, the *stance phase*, and a period of time when the extremity is swinging freely, the *swing phase*. When walking at a rate of around 95 steps per minute, the stance phase occupies approximately 60% of the time spent in the cycle and the swing phase 40%. Both the stance phase and the swing phase are further subdivided. The stance phase (Fig. 6-5) begins at the instant the heel of the shoe contacts the ground. Simultaneously with heel-

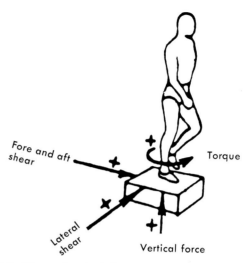

Fore and aft shear   Torque

Lateral shear   Vertical force

Fig. 6-8. Illustrating the information gained from the use of a force plate.

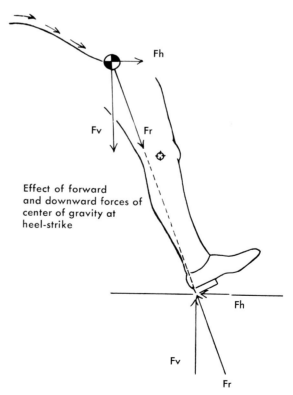

Fh

Fv   Fr

Effect of forward and downward forces of center of gravity at heel-strike

Fh

Fv

Fr

Fig. 6-9. Floor-reaction force is the resultant of horizontal and vertical forces acting through the foot during stance phase.

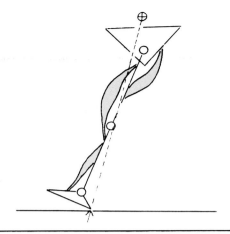

Heel-strike

Joint	Angular attitude	Mechanical force	Muscular activity
Ankle	90° Neutral position	2 ft.-lb. Plantar flexion moment	Dorsiflexors
Knee	180° Complete extension	10 ft.-lb. Flexion moment	Extensors
Hip	25° Flexion	20 ft.-lb. Flexion moment	Extensors

Fig. 6-10. Mechanical forces and muscular activity at heel-strike.

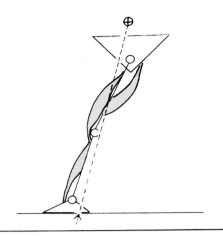

Foot-flat

Joint	Angular attitude	Mechanical force	Muscular activity
Ankle	15° Plantar flexion	10 ft.-lb. Plantar flexion moment	Dorsiflexors
Knee	20° Flexion	50 ft.-lb. Flexion moment	Extensors
Hip	23° Flexion	30 ft.-lb. Flexion moment	Extensors

Fig. 6-11. Mechanical forces and muscular activity at foot-flat.

strike, the foot begins to move in the direction of plantar flexion and continues to so do until the sole of the shoe is in firm contact with the ground; this is the period of *foot-flat*.

With the foot firmly fixed on the floor, the leg and the rest of the body begin to move forward over the foot. When the body reaches a point where the weight is directly over the ankle joint, the *midstance phase* is reached. As the body and leg continue to rotate forward over the foot, the heel of the shoe on the supporting side loses contact with the ground at *heel-off*. The final instant of the stance phase occurs when the shoe of the supporting foot loses contact with the ground: *toe-off*.

Next, the extremity enters the swing phase of gait (Fig. 6-6). Since at this point in the cycle the swinging extremity is behind the body, it must be accel-

erated in a forward direction to be in position for the following heel-strike. Thus the early part of the swing phase is referred to as a period of *acceleration*. During the next part of the cycle, *midswing*, the primary requirement is that the extremity be shortened sufficiently to clear the ground. During this period of midswing we may expect to see maximum flexion angled at the hip, knee, and ankle joints. In order to be in position for the next heel-strike it is necessary that the forward acceleration of the swinging limb be controlled. The last portion of the swing phase is therefore referred to as the period of *deceleration*.

A *step*, or *stride*, is simply the distance covered from toe-off to heel-strike on the same side and is measured in centimeters or inches.

The period of *double support* consists of that portion of the walking cycle when both feet, the heel of one

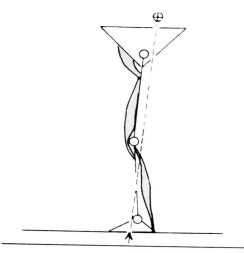

Midstance

Joint	Angular attitude	Mechanical force	Muscular activity
Ankle	2° to 3° Dorsiflexion	25 ft.-lb. Dorsiflexion moment	Plantar flexors
Knee	10° Flexion	20 ft.-lb. Flexion	Extensors
Hip	10° Flexion	30 ft.-lb. Extension moment	Flexors

Fig. 6-12. Mechanical forces and muscular activity at midstance.

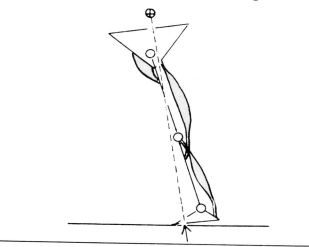

Heel-off

Joint	Angular attitude	Mechanical force	Muscular activity
Ankle	15° Dorsiflexion	80 ft.-lb. Dorsiflexion moment	Plantar flexors
Knee	2° Flexion	20 ft.-lb. Extension moment	Flexors
Hip	−10° Hyperextension	40 ft.-lb. Extension moment	Flexors

Fig. 6-13. Mechanical forces and muscular activity at heel-off.

foot and the toe of the other foot, are both in contact with the ground at the same time. During normal walking speed, approximately 95 steps per minute, the period of double support occupies some 20% to 25% of the entire cycle.

Cadence is measured in steps, not cycles, per minute. The data referred to in this discussion were recorded with the assistance of adult male subjects whose average walking cadence was 96 steps per minute. It should be noted that there is a direct relationship between cadence and stride length; as the walking cadence increases, so too does the length of the stride. Cadence and the period of double support are, on the other hand, inversely related; as cadence increases, the length of time spent in double support decreases.

Angular changes occur at the hip, knee, and ankle joints during the various parts of the walking cycle.

The amplitude of the angular changes at the major joints of the extremity will change with variations in cadence or walking speed. For example, between heel-strike and foot-flat the ankle joint moves from a neutral position to approximately 15° of plantar flexion (Figs. 6-10 and 6-11). At slower cadences the ankle motion required to place the sole of the shoe flat on the floor would be less than 15°. Similar changes at the hip and knee joints occur during different parts of the walking cycle.

KINETICS

During normal walking the center of gravity of the body deviates vertically through an excursion of approximately 2 inches. During double support the center of gravity is at its lowest point. During midstance the center of gravity is at its highest point

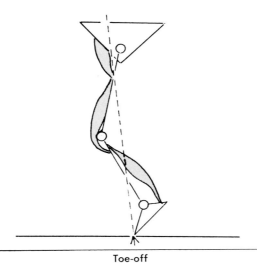

Toe-off

Joint	Angular attitude	Mechanical force	Muscular activity
Ankle	20° Plantar flexion	5 ft.-lb. Dorsiflexion moment	Plantar flexors
Knee	40° Flexion	20 ft.-lb. Flexion moment	Extensors
Hip	10° Flexion	10 ft.-lb. Flexion moment	Flexors

Fig. 6-14. Mechanical forces and muscular activity at toe-off.

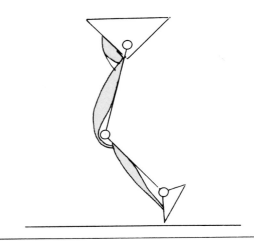

Acceleration

Joint	Angular attitude	Mechanical force	Muscular activity
Ankle	22° Plantar flexion	Plantar flexion moment	Dorsiflexors
Knee	65° Flexion	5 ft.-lb. Flexion moment	Extensors
Hip	5° Flexion	Extension moment	Flexors

Fig. 6-15. Mechanical forces and muscular activity during acceleration.

(Fig. 6-7). Consequently, at the time of heel-strike the center of gravity is moving forward and downward.

Through the use of force plates (Fig. 6-8) it has been possible to determine the magnitude of both the vertical and horizontal forces acting at the center of gravity throughout the stance phase of gait. With these values known, the resultant of these two forces was computed and the mechanical moments about the hip, knee, and ankle joints determined (Fig. 6-9).

The resultant force, or floor-reaction force, may be thought of as a line passing from the center of gravity to the point of maximal pressure of the foot on the floor.

At *heel-strike* (Fig. 6-10) it may be seen that the resultant force passes anterior to the hip joint, posterior to the knee joint, and posterior to the ankle joint. The mechanical moment created by the force of gravity is flexion at the hip joint, flexion at the knee joint, and plantar flexion at the ankle joint. In order to counteract or control the tendency for rotation about the respective joints, the hip extensors, knee extensors, and ankle dorsiflexors must act.

At *foot-flat* (Fig. 6-11) a similar situation exists, and the same muscles are active in controlling joint motion.

During the period of *midstance* (Fig. 6-12) the floor-reaction force passes slightly behind the hip and knee joints, producing an extension moment at the hip and a flexion moment at the knee. It now passes anterior to the ankle joint, creating a dorsiflexion moment. Muscular activity in this phase includes the hip

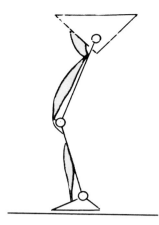

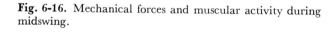

Joint	Angular attitude	Mechanical force	Muscular activity
Ankle	90° Neutral position	Plantar flexion moment	Dorsiflexors
Knee	65° Flexion	1 ft.-lb. Extension moment	Extensors
Hip	25° Flexion	Extension moment	Flexors

Fig. 6-16. Mechanical forces and muscular activity during midswing.

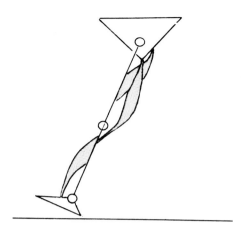

Joint	Angular attitude	Mechanical force	Muscular activity
Ankle	90° Neutral position	Plantar flexion moment	Dorsiflexors
Knee	180° Extension	10 ft.-lb. Extension moment	Flexors
Hip	25° Flexion	Flexion moment	Extensors

Fig. 6-17. Mechanical forces and muscular activity during deceleration.

flexors, knee extensors, and plantar flexors of the ankle joint.

At *heel-off* (Fig. 6-13) the resultant force continues to pass slightly behind the hip joint, requiring hip flexor activity to control the extension moment, but now passes anterior to the knee joint, creating an extension moment, and anterior to the ankle joint, creating a further dorsiflexion moment. The knee flexors now become active, and the plantar flexors of the ankle are strongly active.

Finally, during the period of *toe-off* (Fig. 6-14) the floor-reaction force passes anterior to the hip joint, creating a flexion moment; however, the hip flexors remain active to initiate swing phase activity. It again passes posterior to the knee joint, creating a flexion moment controlled by the knee extensors, and it con-

tinues to remain anterior to the ankle joint as the ankle plantar flexors contract strongly.

The angular attitudes for the hip, knee, and ankle, with the corresponding mechanical forces and muscular activity for the subdivision of swing phase, are shown in Figs. 6-15 to 6-17.

The path of the floor-reaction force at *midstance* when viewed in the frontal plane is illustrated in Fig. 6-18. It may be seen that it passes medial to the hip joint, tending to cause downward rotation of the pelvis on the femoral head and requiring activity of the hip abductors to control this moment of rotation. It likewise passes medial to the knee joint, creating a varus moment counteracted by the lateral collateral ligament and ileotibial band. At the same time it passes lateral to the subtalar joint, causing a valgus

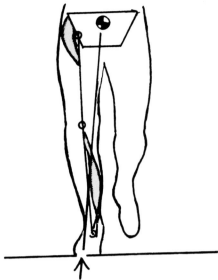

Joint	Mechanical force	Muscular activity
Subtalar	Varus: Maximum 3 to 5 ft.-lb. between heel-strike and foot-slap and between heel-off and toe-off Valgus: Maximum 15 ft.-lb. between foot-flat and heel-off	Peroneus longus, peroneus brevis Posterior tibial, flexor digitorum longus, flexor hallucis longus
Knee	Varus: Maximum 30 ft.-lb. at heel-off Valgus: Maximum 0 ft.-lb.	Lateral collateral knee structures
Hip	Varus: Maximum 60 ft.-lb. Valgus: Maximum 0 ft.-lb.	Gluteus minimus, gluteus medius, tensor fascia lata

Fig. 6-18. Mechanical forces and muscular activity at midstance in the frontal plane.

moment that is controlled by the invertors of the foot.

• • •

In summary, it may be said that knowledge of the kinematics and kinetics of normal human locomotion is necessary to making a rational decision regarding the appropriate mechanical substitute for replacement of a missing function or biomechanical loss.

Part III
Principles of orthotic alignment in the lower extremity*

HANS RICHARD LEHNEIS, C.P.O.
New York, New York

The construction and alignment of a brace cannot be based solely on the condition of the disabled limb for which the brace is intended. Rather, a functionally or structurally deficient extremity must be considered as part of the body as a whole. Special attention must be given to the normal static and dynamic relationships of the hip, knee, ankle, and subtalar joints. If these normal relationships are not taken into account during alignment procedures, the brace may hinder the performance of the wearer and may tend to increase further any existing deformities.

Orthotic alignment deals with the angular relationship of the orthotic components to each other and to a reference line relating the orthosis to the body as a whole. The objectives of proper alignment are as follows:

1. Flat heel and sole contact of the brace shoe with the ground
2. Anatomic-mechanical joint congruency
3. Horizontal orientation of joint axes
4. Conformity to anatomic contours and landmarks

Before proceeding to analyze how these objectives are achieved, it will be helpful to briefly review pertinent characteristics of the joints of the lower extremity.

JOINT CHARACTERISTICS RELATED TO ORTHOTIC ALIGNMENT

Hip joint. The hip joint is a ball-and-socket joint that permits universal motion of the lower extremity, that is, abduction-adduction, flexion-extension, and transverse rotation.

Knee joint. In normal standing the axes of the knee joints lie in the same plane and are perpendicular to the line of progression (Fig. 6-19). The knee is considered a polycentric joint. During the normal range of motion in walking the knee not only exhibits a rotary but also a translatory component; that is, the femur not only flexes with respect to the

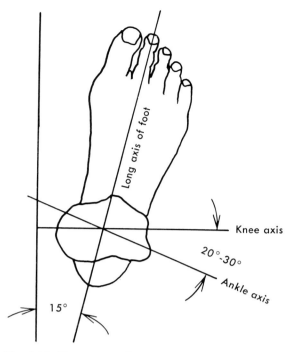

Fig. 6-19. Transverse plane alignment. The knee axis is perpendicular to the line of progression, toe-out is 15°, and the ankle axis is rotated externally 20° to 30° with respect to the knee axis. (From Lehneis, H. R.: Orthop. Prosth. Appl. J. **18**:110, 1964.)

tibia but also translates forward from an extended to a flexed position. In addition, the femur also has a transverse rotation of approximately 10° with respect to the tibia, with the femur rotating externally as the knee joint moves from flexion to extension.

Ankle joint. Because of the natural torsion of the tibia, the axis of the ankle joint is rotated externally 20° to 30° with respect to the knee axis (Fig. 6-19). Tibial torsion is a developmental phenomenon that increases from a minimal amount of about 2° in the newborn infant to a permanent value of 20° to 30° by the age of 7 years. This developmental adaptation places the ankle joint in the best position for upright walking.

The line of progression is a term used to denote the direction in which we walk. Though it is a straight line, we know that the center of gravity oscillates from side to side as it moves forward (Fig. 6-20). Hence the line of progression actually represents a summation of the excursions of the center of gravity during locomotion. The externally rotated ankle joint axis is *not* perpendicular to the line of progres-

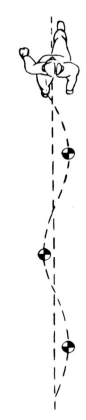

Fig. 6-20. Oscillation of the center of gravity in walking. (From Lehneis, H. R.: Orthop. Prosth. Appl. J. **18**:110, 1964.)

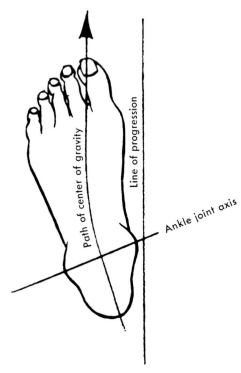

Fig. 6-21. Relationship of external rotation of the ankle joint axis to path of center of gravity over foot. (From Lehneis, H. R.: Orthop. Prosth. Appl. J. **18**:110, 1964.)

sion during the first half of the stance phase (Fig. 6-21). Rather, it is approximately perpendicular to a tangent of the path of the center of gravity from heel-strike to the midstance phase of walking.

Subtalar joint. The subtalar joint performs three especially important functions:

1. In standing it permits mediolateral shifting of the center of gravity while the foot retains flat heel and sole contact with the floor.
2. It permits the feet to adapt to uneven ground.
3. During flexion of the knee, as in squatting, it helps to compensate for the difference in alignment of the ankle joint and the knee joint, as projected in the transverse plane.

In the discussion that follows it must be borne in mind that anatomic joints rarely exhibit a single axis of rotation. Rather, they are more or less polycentric throughout their normal range of motion, whereas the conventional orthotic components are single-axis joints. It is therefore not possible to achieve absolute congruency between mechanical and anatomic joint

axes. Nevertheless, close approximation can be achieved by the application of alignment criteria.

CRITERIA FOR ALIGNMENT
Alignment in the frontal plane

As mentioned earlier, a reference line is needed to relate the orthosis and the disabled limb to the body as a whole. In normal standing with a base of 2 to 4 inches between the centers of the heels, a vertical line dividing the body into equal right and left halves passes through the nose, the umbilicus, the center of gravity, and the symphysis pubis. This line is referred to as the midsagittal line. It is important to note that the midsagittal line bisects the space between the knee and ankle joints (Fig. 6-22).

In the same standing position a line through the center of the hip, the knee, and ankle joints, projected on the frontal plane, will be parallel to the midsagittal line. This line through the joint centers is referred to as the parasagittal line.

Normally, the flexion and extension axes of the

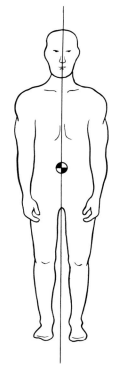

Fig. 6-22. Midsagittal line bisects the space between the knee and ankles. (From Lehneis, H. R.: Orthop. Prosth. Appl. J. **18**:110, 1964.)

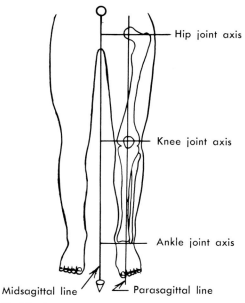

Fig. 6-23. Flexion-extension axes of the ankle, knee, and hip joints in the frontal plane are normally perpendicular to the midsagittal and parasagittal lines. (From Lehneis, H. R.: Orthop. Prosth. Appl. J. **18**:110, 1964.)

hip, knee, and ankle are essentially perpendicular to the midsagittal and parasagittal lines (Fig. 6-23). For orthotic alignment purposes, however, the parasagittal line cannot be used since in the case of a deformity it will no longer follow the criteria just discussed. The midsagittal line, on the other hand, remains constant regardless of whether the extremity is in normal alignment or deformed and therefore may be used to relate the alignment of the brace to the body as a whole. This is accomplished by orienting the shoe and the brace joint axes perpendicular to the midsagittal line. As a consequence, the shoe will be flat on the floor, and the joints will be horizontal and parallel to each other as viewed in the frontal plane.

Alignment in the sagittal plane

While the actual position of the mechanical joints with regard to the anatomic joints in the sagittal plane depends to a great extent on the fit of the shoe, bands, and cuffs, various joint alignment criteria can be adduced.

Hip joint. The flexion-extension axis of the hip joint is considered to coincide with a point ¼ inch anterior and ¼ inch superior to the proximal tip of the greater trochanter. The mechanical axis of the orthotic hip joint must therefore be placed to coincide with this point.

Knee joint. As discussed earlier, the knee is a polycentric joint (Fig. 6-24), whereas nearly all orthotic knee components have a single joint axis. Accurate mechanical and anatomic joint alignment, therefore, cannot be achieved. However, since most above-knee orthoses are equipped with a knee lock,

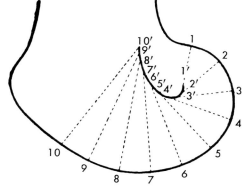

Fig. 6-24. Schematic sagittal cut through the medial condyle of the femur showing the polycentricity of the knee indicated by the evolute of the curvature of the condyle. (From Gocht, H., et al.: In Gocht, H., editor: Deutsche Orthopaedie, Stuttgart, 1920, Ferdinand Enke, vol. 2.)

this is of no consequence in walking. Accuracy in mechanical-anatomic joint alignment is much more important in a sitting position.

For orthotic considerations the flexion-extension axis of the knee joint is considered to be approximately ¾ inch proximal to the tibial plateau in the average adult and at a point that is half of the anteroposterior diameter of the knee, not including the thickness of the patella. Although the mechanical knee joint is placed in this position, accommodations for comfortable sitting must be made in the brace bands to compensate for the discrepancy produced by the anteroposterior and proximodistal shifting of the polycentric anatomic knee joint axis.

Ankle joint. The anatomic ankle joint is considered to pass through the centers of the medial and lateral malleoli at the level of the distal tip of the medial malleolus. The medial malleolus is normally found to be ⅝ to 1 inch anterior to the lateral malleolus due to tibial torsion. If congruency between anatomic and mechanical joints is to be achieved, the orthosis must exhibit an equivalent amount of torsion.

Alignment in the transverse plane

Hip joint. With few exceptions, orthotic hip joints permit motion in the sagittal plane only, controlling abduction-adduction as well as transverse rotation of the extremity. The orthotic hip joint axis is normally placed parallel to the axis of the knee joint.

Knee joint axis. The knee joint axis serves as the reference line in the transverse plane for the alignment of orthotic components. The reason for choosing the knee axis rather than the line of progression is a practical one; that is, it would be difficult to determine the line of progression and to relate all components to it, especially if there exists internal or external rotation at the hip joint. The knee axis, on the other hand, can be fairly easily determined when the knee is moved through a flexion range of about 90°. The axis is perpendicular to the plane of motion of the shank and is approximately parallel to the plane of the popliteal area with the knee flexed to 90°. The amount of tibial torsion (rotation of the ankle axis with regard to the knee axis in the transverse plane) and the degree of toe-out can now be related to the knee joint axis regardless of whether the patient is externally or internally rotated at the hip.

Ankle joint axis. As just mentioned, normal tibial torsion serves to align the anatomic joint so that its motion is compatible with the anterolateral movement of the center of gravity. If at any given instant the ankle axis is not perpendicular to the direction of

motion of the center of gravity, compensatory motion in the subtalar joint will permit movement of the leg over the foot in the direction of the center of gravity.

Since conventional braces do not provide motion corresponding to the subtalar joint, the correct location of the mechanical ankle axis is of great importance. To achieve this proper location, the mechanical ankle joint must be aligned in accordance with the amount of external rotation of the anatomic joint, that is, with the amount of tibial torsion. This is especially significant when free-motion ankle joints are used.

A common error is to relate ankle joint placement in the transverse plane to "toe-out." Toe-out may be defined as the relationship of the long axis of the foot to the line of progression. Normally, the foot exhibits approximately 15° of toe-out. However, the amount of toe-out may be influenced by several factors other than the normal torsion of the tibia, for example, rotation in the hip or knee joints, eversion and inversion at the subtalar joint, and forefoot abduction or adduction. Furthermore, the ankle joint axis is normally rotated externally 10° to 15° from a line perpendicular to the long axis of the foot (Fig. 6-25). Ankle joint placement will be inaccurate, therefore, if it is solely related to the degree of toe-out.

Toe-out. Toe-out does not bear a constant relation-

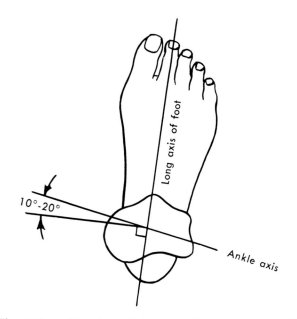

Fig. 6-25. Ankle joint axis is normally rotated externally 10° to 15° from a line perpendicular to the long axis of the foot. (From Lehneis, H. R.: Orthop. Prosth. Appl. J. **18**:110, 1964.)

ship to tibial torsion since some of the factors discussed previously may influence the degree of toe-out without affecting the position of the ankle axis. The measurement and accommodation of toe-out in orthotics, therefore, must be treated separately from that of tibial torsion.

• • •

The proper relationship of the hip, knee, and ankle joints as well as toe-out in the transverse plane can best be determined by first locating the knee axis and then relating all other factors to it.

EFFECTS OF INCORRECT ORTHOTIC ALIGNMENT
Frontal plane

If the shoe and brace joints are not perpendicular to the midsagittal reference line, the effects will be as follows:
1. Uneven floor contact will result in unequal pressure distribution on the foot with possible callus formation and rotation in the subtalar or midtarsal joints. As an example, if the brace is not aligned to accommodate a genu valgum deformity, excessive pressure on the medial surface of the foot may result.
2. Lateral instability will occur if the plantar surface of the shoe is not parallel to the floor.
3. The durability of brace joints will be decreased since sheer stresses and uneven wear of joint surfaces will occur.

Sagittal plane

Malalignment in the sagittal plane will result in relative motion and changing pressure patterns between the extremity and the brace bands. The greater the range of motion at any particular joint, the greater the magnitude of relative motion and pressure change.

Transverse plane

Hip joint. If the mechanical hip joint is internally or externally rotated, the effect will be to cause the brace and the extremity to either internally or externally rotate and/or cause undue pressure of the pelvic band on the pelvis as the hip is flexed.

Knee joint. Rotational malalignment of the mechanical knee joint is of little consequence during ambulation since the knee is ordinarily locked. In the sitting position, however, such malalignment may result in uncomfortable pressures. Fortunately this particular alignment fault is a rare occurrence. More

frequently knee axis malalignment in the transverse plane results from failure to properly accommodate the patient's toe-out, as discussed later.

Ankle joint. If the mechanical ankle joint does not accommodate the patient's tibial torsion, that is, if the mechanical ankle joint axis is parallel to the knee axis as projected in a transverse plane, the brace will tend to move in a direction parallel to the line of progression during stance phase. This, however, is inconsistent with normal locomotor patterns in which the tibia and the suprastructure move in an anterolateral direction from heel-strike to the midstance phase. The adverse results of this inconsistency may be as follows:
1. Pressure concentration on the lateral surface of the foot. This may induce valgus deformity if there is weakness in the subtalar joint or forefoot pronation if there is weakness in the midtarsal joints.
2. Patient fatigue due to binding between anatomic and mechanical ankle joints. In order for the anatomic and mechanical joints to go through the prescribed range of motion, the anatomic joint must align itself with the mechanical ankle joint axis. As the two axes, anatomic and mechanical, attempt to coincide, the resulting stresses tend to cause binding and to produce abnormal motions in the joints of the foot, possibly leading to an acquired deformity.
3. Increased wear of brace joints due to torque. The binding between the anatomic and mechanical joints from the forces exerted by the brace to make the anatomic ankle joint conform to the brace ankle axis not only results in patient fatigue but also places undue torque on the brace joints.

Toe-out. If, for instance, the patient has more than normal toe-out that is not compensated for in the brace, the effects will be as follows:
1. Sitting discomfort with the above-knee brace. The external rotation of the foot will cause a loosely fitting brace to rotate externally on the limb. As a result, the mechanical knee joint axis will be rotated externally with respect to the anatomic knee, with ensuing interference and discomfort in sitting.
2. Varus attitude of the foot. Another effect of the anatomic-mechanical knee joint incongruency caused by insufficient toe-out accommodation is that the foot is forced into a varus attitude when the patient sits. This occurs because the anatomic joint must align itself with the me-

chanical joint in order to flex. Such alignment is only possible, however, by the ankle assuming a varus attitude which, in effect, externally rotates the knee so it can align itself with the mechanical joint. In a tightly fitting brace the patient's foot is kept in varus while both standing and sitting when there is insufficient toe-out in the brace.

SUMMARY

A primary objective of bracing is to provide the wearer optimum performance with minimum technical assistance and maintenance. This objective can be realized only if the brace is compatible with the alignment of the involved extremity and of the body as a whole.

The most important aspects of providing a brace that meets this criterion are as follows:

1. Use of the midsagittal line as a reference line for brace alignment in the frontal plane
2. Proper accommodation of tibial torsion and toe-out in relation to the knee joint in the transverse plane
3. Close approximation of mechanical and anatomic joint axes within the limits imposed by commercially available orthotic components

REFERENCES

1. Inman, V. T.: Conservation of energy in ambulation, Arch. Phys. Med. **48**:484, 1967.
2. Lehneis, H. R.: New concepts in lower extremity orthotics, Med. Clin. N. Amer. **53**:585, 1969.
3. Subcommittee on Design and Development, Committee on Prosthetics Research and Development, National Academy of Sciences, National Research Council, Report of the Seventh Workshop Panel on Lower Extremity Orthotics, Washington, D. C., 1970.

Part IV
Lower extremity orthotic components: applications and indications

JOHN GLANCY, C.O.
Indianapolis, Indiana

For this discussion it is helpful to approach the bracing of the lower extremities from a somewhat different point of view than in the past. The purpose of this approach is threefold: (1) to relate this discussion of present-day brace components to the previous presentations on the biomechanics of gait and the principles of alignment; (2) hopefully, to discuss with greater clarity the very confusing subject of *brace-to-body dynamics* (that is, what does a brace do and how does it do it?); and (3) to discuss orthotic components and their applications without reference to etiologies. Thus we can confine ourselves to biomechanical defects without regard to cause and to the various mechanical solutions available to us (that is, partial or complete substitution of the human biomechanical system by mechanical means).

In order to relate directly to Fryer's discussion on the biomechanics of the lower extremity, the phases of the walking cycle will be used in their proper sequence to emphasize at which point in the cycle motion control is possible and/or necessary. Readily available orthotic components that provide motion control for a given region will be shown. Thus, during the stance phase, we will discuss components that control various motions in the foot-ankle complex, the knee, and the hip and lightly touch upon trunk control, relating these motions to a specific time in the cycle such as heel-strike, foot-flat, midstance, etc. Currently available orthotic components that provide some control of motion in the swing phase will be discussed in the same manner.

This review will be limited to orthotic components for ambulatory patients. We will not go into night bracing and other nonambulatory conditions. The list of orthotic components for the lower extremities is a long one, as the quite extensive listing provided in the Appendices at the end of this part will attest. However, it is also an extremely repetitive list in terms of specific mechanical functions—duplications are frequent. The components discussed were selected from the list as being representative of items that provide a specific control for a given region, with the emphasis on achieving a mode of ambulation as near to normal as circumstances will permit. Following the mention of each component selected and the explanation offered for its use, the reader will be referred to the items in the Appendices that offer similar control.

This discussion will be limited to components as separate entities. However, although it will not be possible to consistently combine various components into "brace systems" for this discussion, it may be helpful to think of the act of prescribing as the combining of two or more components to devise a brace, or "mechanical system" if you will, that is intended to provide a specific function or functions.

It is precisely at this point in any discussion of bracing that clarity vaporizes. What specific function or functions can a brace, any brace, be expected to provide? Traditional terms used to define brace functions such as "assistive," "supportive," "corrective," etc. all have connotations either so broad or so narrow that their individual meaning, when used for a given situation, is subject to individual interpretation. Whenever a brace and/or its function is being prescribed or discussed, the traditional terms do not lend themselves to clear mechanical interpretation. The key question to be answered is "How?" How does any brace, regardless of its design, provide the body "assistance," "support," "correction," etc? I would suggest that all braces provide but *one* function —*control* of body *motions*. As McCollough mentioned earlier, body motions can be rotary or translatory, rotary motion being defined as movement about an axis, whereas translatory motion is linear motion. Both types of motion can occur in the sagittal, coronal, or transverse planes. Translatory motion can also be vertical and is often closely related to vertical loads to which various portions of the body are subjected. The motion requiring control may be of the body as a whole as it moves in space, movements of body segments in space that change the relationship of one segment to another, and finally, motions of segments within the body. The motions to be controlled may be "wanted" or "unwanted," normal or abnormal, present or predictable. I would further suggest that any brace can provide no more than two types of motion control, either *static* or *programmed*, programmed motion control being defined as planned or allowed motion within a given brace system versus static control of every movable segment that a brace system may encompass.

FOOT MOTIONS
Stance phase

Let us begin with the principle "unwanted" motions that occur in the foot when it must sustain the weight of the body during the stance phase from foot-flat through toe-off.

Structural collapse of the longitudinal and/or metatarsal arches. Structural collapse of the arches may occur when a vertical load is applied. Regardless of the cause, the orthotic device used is expected to prevent further collapse of the foot in the future and/or restore a balanced distribution of the body's

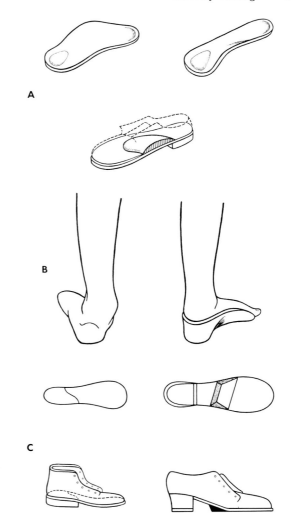

Fig. 6-26. A, Arch supporters. **B,** UCBL laminated plastic insert, which is made of polyester resin impregnated into reinforced tricot or banlon. **C,** Shoe modifications.

weight throughout the foot's structures. In this instance, abnormal motions within the foot are to be controlled. *Static control* is achieved by various types of arch supporters or inserts (Fig. 6-26, *A*), various rubber pads (navicular and metatarsal), the UCBL plastic laminated insert (Fig. 6-26, *B*), and modifications to the shoe itself (Thomas heels and metatarsal bars) (Fig. 6-26, *C*).*

Pes varus and valgus. Whatever the cause, the orthotic device must control abnormal mediolateral (ML) motion in the subtalar joint during periods of weight bearing. The key to foot balance in such conditions is control of os calcis motion. *Static control* of

---

*See Appendix G, items 17 and 18.

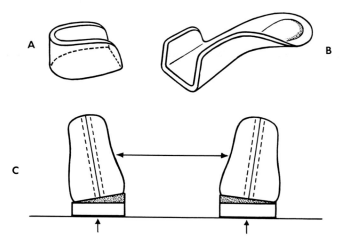

Fig. 6-27. Static control of ML motion of the os calcis. **A,** Plastic heel seat. **B,** Whitman plates. **C,** Heel wedges.

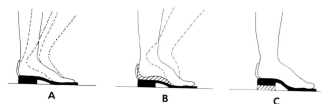

Fig. 6-28. Example of orthotic "accommodation." **A,** Normally, the tibia rotates forward of a 90° relationship to the foot prior to heel-rise. **B,** With a fixed forefoot drop, no weight can be borne by the heel during the stance phase and/or the standing position. The forefoot cannot yield and the tibia cannot rotate forward because its progress is blocked by the abnormally positioned talus. Motion is therefore limited to the MP joints. **C,** Glaubitz shoe modification.

the os calcis may be achieved by the use of plastic heel seats (Fig. 6-27, *A*), Whitman plates (Fig. 6-27, *B*), or the UCBL insert (Fig. 6-26, *B*). An intimate fitting is essential. Medial or lateral heel wedges are also used (Fig. 6-27, *C*).* It should be noted, as Lehneis pointed out earlier, that a lack of proper accommodation for tibial torsion in the alignment of either below-knee (BK) or above-knee (AK) braces can be the cause of abnormal motion in the subtalar joint.

Fixed forefoot drop. Fixed forefoot drop is the familiar condition in which the heel can be dorsiflexed to a right angle to the leg (either passively or actively) but upon weight bearing the dropped forefoot cannot yield to the vertical load of the body and therefore the metatarsal area must constantly bear the full burden since it and the toes are the only areas in

*See Appendix G, items 7 to 12.

contact with the floor. The load is excessive for the small cross section of skin that must receive it, and painful calluses develop. The Glaubitz shoe modification is a practical and efficient means of conforming a conventional shoe to this fixed deformity, enabling the heel and midfoot to share the body's weight (Fig. 6-28). It is evident that the problem here is one of "accommodation," where *fit* and *comfort* are factors—not motion control. One may ask "Are not fit and comfort also definite functions of orthotic devices?" Please permit me to defer answering this interesting question until the end of the review of orthotic components.

Swing phase

No motions occur *within* the foot during the swing phase that need command our interest. However, motions of the foot *in space* as they occur in the swing phase will be discussed under ankle motion.

ANKLE MOTIONS
Stance phase

Next, let us look at the principal motions that occur in the ankle joint during the stance phase. Motion is limited to the sagittal plane (anterior-posterior [AP] motion). These motions may be within or beyond normal ranges. Control of the foot as it moves in space from heel-strike to foot-flat is the first concern. Once foot-flat is achieved, then control of the tibia as it rotates forward over the fixed foot becomes the primary concern.

Following heel-strike. Control of plantar flexion of the foot following heel-strike (the motion that results in the position of foot-flat) may be achieved in several ways, the selection depending upon a variety of circumstances. This motion may be programmed to occur freely, partially (Fig. 6-29, *A* and *B*), or with a mechanical supplement such as springs (Fig. 6-29, *C*).* The spring-action joint can also be used as a mechanical substitute when anatomic control of plantar flexion is absent.

When plantar flexion of the anatomic ankle joint is mechanically prevented from occurring at heel-strike (for example, when a posterior stop is used to prevent foot drop), it can be mechanically simulated by adding a cushion heel to the shoe (Fig. 6-30).† The cushion heel is not applicable if a swing-to or swing-through gait is to be taught the bilaterally involved patient. It is functionally useless to such a

*See Appendix E, item 1.
†See Appendix G, item 16.

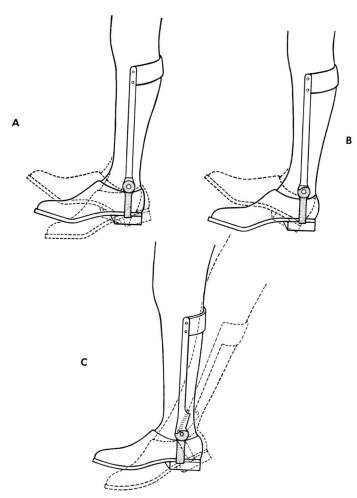

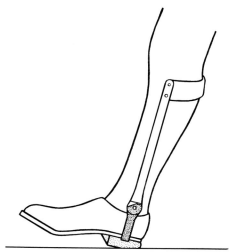

Fig. 6-30. Cushion heel (simulation of plantar flexion). At heel-strike the cushion heel absorbs the impact (15% to 20% in excess of body weight). As the body's weight is being borne forward, the cushion heel compresses in a manner that converts the heel to a "rocker," permitting a smooth "rolling" transfer similar to a heel-toe gait.

Fig. 6-29. Programmed control of AP motion of the foot. **A,** Conventional BK brace in which the free joint permits the full range of plantar flexion and dorsiflexion. **B,** Conventional BK brace in which the plantar flexion stop joint permits the full range of dorsiflexion while preventing plantar flexion. **C,** When the pretibial muscles are functioning but the triceps surae are either weak or unable to function, the springs' thrust provides the following: (1) An assistive force to gravity to overcome the out-of-phase isotonic contraction of the pretibial muscles at heel-strike facilitates the position of foot-flat and prevents the development of a calcaneal gait. (2) Once foot-flat is achieved and the foot is now a fixed pivotal point over which the tibia rotates forward, the springs become a substitute for the triceps surae by providing a resistive force to the out-of-control forward progress of the tibia; that is, the springs serve the purpose of the eccentric contraction normally provided by the triceps surae during this period of the walking cycle. (3) The position of maximum plantar flexion (dotted lines) is intended to show that the springs provide a constant stretching force to the pretibial muscles whenever they are relaxed, such as the patient seated with his legs crossed, etc. Since the pretibial muscles will fire to overcome the springs to maintain the normal degree of dorsiflexion throughout the swing phase, at no time during the walking cycle is the foot's position out-of-phase.

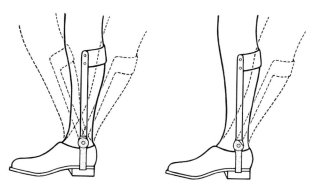

Fig. 6-31. Programmed control of AP motion of the tibia.

patient and, furthermore, would only add to their problems of standing balance.

Forward (anterior) rotation of the tibia (following foot-flat). This motion may be programmed to occur freely or it can be stopped at the midstance position (Fig. 6-31).*

When *static control* of quite normal motion of the tibia is desirable (for example, to relieve pain in an arthritic ankle joint), prevention of both plantar flexion and dorsiflexion of the foot is necessary. That is to say, in order to maintain balance in the midstance and/or standing positions, the AP angle between the foot and leg must remain fixed at ap-

*See Appendix F, items 6 and 7.

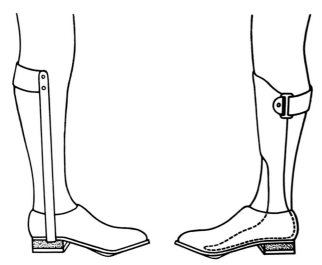

Fig. 6-32. Static control of AP motion of the tibia.

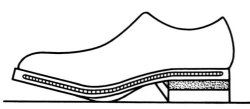

Fig. 6-33. Shoe modifications — programming motion produced mechanically. The cushion heel is the same as described in Fig. 6-30. As the body's center of gravity passes forward beyond the midstance position, the body "trips" over the rocker bar, thus *mechanically* forcing the heel to rise at its normal time in the cycle. The metal shoe plate converts the entire length of the shoe into an efficient "resistance arm" against the weight of the body's forward motion from above and the floor-reaction forces from below. It protects the laminated shell by sharing the burden of these forces. It protects and prolongs the life of the shoe.

proximately 90° throughout the walking cycle (Fig. 6-32).* For the example cited, the laminated shell would be the orthosis of choice; its intimate fit provides more efficient immobilization.

Whenever either of the BK orthoses shown in Fig. 6-32 are to be used, stresses to the anatomic joints of the ankle and foot can be further reduced by mechanically simulating the normal heel-toe gait by modifying the shoe (Fig. 6-33).†

Heel-rise. When circumstances are such that heel-rise is anatomically possible, that is, joint ranges are normal yet anatomic control is lacking (whether due to paralysis or spasticity), its occurrence will be "out-

*See Appendix E, item 6, and Appendix F, item 5.
†See Appendix G, items 15 and 16.

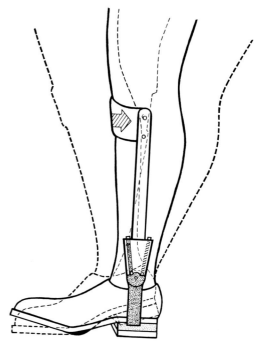

Fig. 6-34. Programmed control of AP motion of the tibia and the foot. The double-action ankle joint is very useful for conditions whose status is likely to change within short periods of time. Note that its spring action can be changed to a positive (and also adjustable) stop in either direction whenever desired without alterations to the brace frame. An anterior stop setting is illustrated.

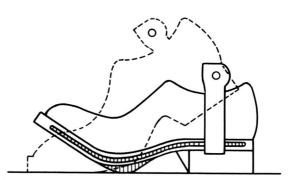

Fig. 6-35. Programmed control of AP motion of the MP joints of the foot.

of-phase" and a detriment and therefore an unwanted motion. Often, when further complications accompany the circumstances described, all that can be offered to such patients is *static control*, as shown in Fig. 6-32. However, under a substantial variety of circumstances, when the motor power is absent (paresis or flaccidity), *programmed control* of heel-rise can be provided with the use of a BK orthosis and

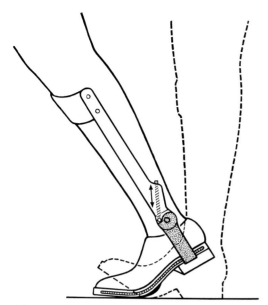

Fig. 6-36. Providing a mechanical "boost" for push-off. Note the preset toe-off metal shoe plate and rocker bar used when the spring is used as a "booster." Without the plate the spring's force would be dissipated by the uncontrolled flexion of the MP joints when anatomic control is absent. The rocker bar produces heel-rise, the prerequisite motion to the toe-off position of push-off.

the shoe modifications shown in Fig. 6-33. Programmed control of heel-rise is also possible with the use of the double-action ankle joint (Fig. 6-34) when motor power is present but anatomically uncontrolled (spasticity).* Heel-rise, then, when "untimely" in its occurrence, can be mechanically blocked and replaced with a mechanical substitute and programmed to occur at its proper time in the walking cycle.

Toe-off. Normal toe-off can be substituted for by mechanical means programmed to permit its occurrence in proper time and sequence (Fig. 6-35).†

Push-off. Although this important function occurs within the sequence of events in the normal walking cycle, it is not a motion per se of the ankle or foot. However, the body's motive power can be given a mechanical "boost" with the judicious use of spring-action joints when push-off is weak (Fig. 6-36).

Swing phase

The only motion occurring about the ankle joint during the swing phase that is of interest to us is the 3° to 5° of dorsiflexion of the foot that is normally maintained throughout the swing phase. This im-

---

*See Appendix F, items 6 and 7.
†See Appendix G, items 15 and 16.

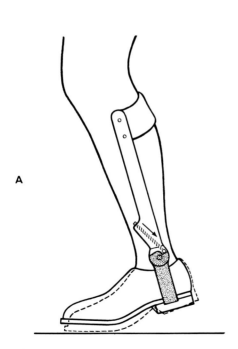

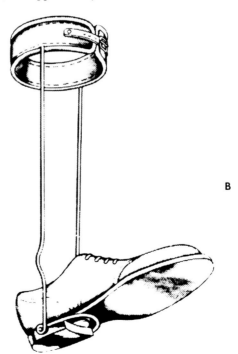

A   **B**

Fig. 6-37. Programmed control of AP motion of the foot (swing phase). **A,** The leg is in approximately midswing. The dotted outline of the shoe represents the dropped position the foot would assume without the aid of the spring to sustain the normal amount of dorsiflexion necessary for ground clearance. **B,** The coiled spring wire also provides control for this purpose. (**B** courtesy Fillauer Surgical Supplies, Inc., Chattanooga, Tenn.)

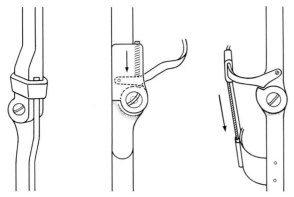

Fig. 6-38. Static control of AP motion of the knee.

portant motion, which allows clearance between the foot and the floor, can be provided and maintained mechanically throughout the swing phase when anatomic control of dorsiflexion is absent. Springs are efficient for this task, as they only need overcome the relatively light weight of the foot, shoe, and brace attachment, plus gravity's pull, as the limb moves through space. The single- or double-action spring ankle joints provide this *programmed control* (Figs. 6-34 and 6-37, *A*).* The coiled spring wire is also used for the same purpose (Fig. 6-37, *B*).†

---

*See Appendix E, items 1 and 2.
†See Appendix F, items 2 to 4.

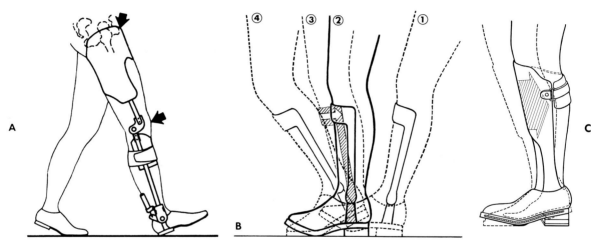

Fig. 6-39. Programmed control of AP motion of the knee. **A,** Offset knee joint as used in the UCLA functional AK brace. The arrow pointing in a downward direction at the anterior brim of the laminated thigh shell shows the direction of force at heel-strike. The force travels through the shell and down the upper bar of the knee joint unit, whose axis is 1 inch posterior to the upper bar. This placement is also posterior to the axis of the anatomic knee joint. The result to the mechanical joint is an extension moment, the line of force being forward of its axis. The magnitude of the extension force, in turn, extends the anatomic knee joint. The normal forward flexion of the trunk at heel-strike causes the pelvis and abdomen to press firmly against the high anterior brim, thus producing the force just described. **B:** (1) The foot is plantar flexing toward the foot-flat position following heel-strike. Note the impact absorption through the compressed posterior portion of the cushion heel. Free plantar flexion is permitted by the mechanical joints. (2) Midstance position. The limb in swing phase, along with the body, has rotated in the transverse plane to the lateral midline. Note the stability of the knee at this period when the magnitude of downward vertical force is high. The preset toe-off positioning of the metal shoe plate is evident. (3) Just before heel-rise. The body's center of gravity has now rotated in the transverse plane forward of the lateral midline. Note the stabilizing of the knee by the counterpressure of the anterior metal band. The 2° to 3° of forward motion allowed the tibia by the anterior stops in the ankle joints permits normal knee flexion during this period. (4) The forward rotation of the body in the sagittal plane has "tripped" over the rocker bar and placed the foot in the toe-off position in preparation for push-off. The knee is free to rotate through its normal range throughout the swing phase. **C,** This AK laminated shell and shoe modifications embody the same principles as those ascribed to the use of components in Figs. 6-32 and 6-33 with one exception — the posterior portion of the heel is made higher to force the knee into slight flexion to block the force (indicated by arrow) so it cannot push the knee into recurvatum. (**A** from Anderson M. H.: Orthop. Prosth. Appl. J. **18**:273, 1964; **B** from Glancy, J.: Orthop. Prosth. Appl. J. **24**:21, 1970.)

KNEE MOTIONS
Stance phase

"Unwanted" knee flexion. Regardless of its cause, "unwanted" knee flexion that prevents the lower extremity from supporting the body's weight must be controlled. When anatomic control is totally or functionally lacking, several joints are available that provide *static control* of the knee (Fig. 6-38).* *Programmed control* is achieved by the offset knee joint in conjunction with other components (Fig. 6-39, *A*).†

Unwanted knee flexion in the presence of spasticity in the foot-ankle complex can be mechanically controlled in a variety of ways by BK orthoses; Fig. 6-39, *B*, illustrates one example.‡

Unwanted knee flexion such as occurs in many patients with spina bifida, which is necessary to them for

---

*See Appendix C, items 8 to 10.
†See Appendix C, item 2.
‡See Appendix C, item 3, Appendix E, item 3, and Appendix G, items 15 and 16.

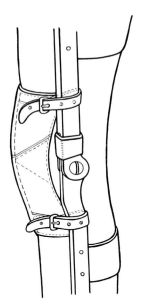

Fig. 6-40. Static control of AP motion of the knee. AP motion is prevented throughout the walking cycle.

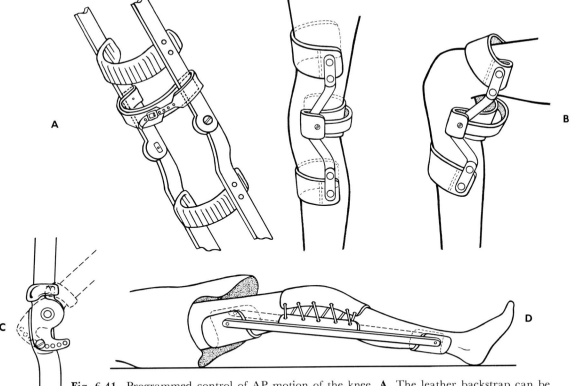

Fig. 6-41. Programmed control of AP motion of the knee. **A,** The leather backstrap can be adjusted to any desired depth to control the degree of preset flexion. **B,** Swedish hyperextension knee cage. The full range of flexion during the swing phase is permitted. This orthosis does not have joints. It is self-adjusting from the flexed to the extended positions. **C,** Adjustable knee extension joint. **D,** Engen knee contraction orthosis. (**C** courtesy Fillauer Surgical Supplies, Inc., Chattanooga, Tenn.)

purpose of balance as a means of counteracting the uncontrolled forward rotation of the tibias during periods of weight bearing, can be controlled by the BK orthosis shown in Fig. 6-39, *C*.* It should be noted that, with the orthosis shown, elevating the heel to prevent genu recurvatum cannot be divorced from other factors. As an example, crutches are recommended if the bilaterally involved patient's quadricep muscles do not permit him to stand from a sitting position without the assistance of his arms. For although the shells mechanically "fix" the tibias when standing, his quadricep muscles could not prevent his thighs from assuming a "sitting" position, with a resulting loss of balance.

Genu recurvatum. When muscular control is totally lacking in the knee, *static control* of this abnormal motion is provided by an AK brace with a locking knee joint (Fig. 6-40).† When adequate knee extension control is present, a free knee joint with a posterior stop preset in slight flexion is effective, thus providing *programmed control*, as the knee is allowed the freedom to flex during the swing phase (Fig. 6-41, *A*).‡

It should be noted that an anterior stop at the ankle joint with a 90° setting or the placing of the foot in a fixed position of equinus would be contraindicated since either induces an extension moment at the knee joint.

If functional anatomic knee extension and ankle and foot controls are present, the Swedish hyperextension knee cage provides effective programmed control (Fig. 6-41, *B*).§

Knee contractures. If ambulation is desired, a lock-knee joint with adjustable extension is used (Fig. 6-41, *C*). A lift added to the shoe to level the pelvis is gradually lowered as the contracture is reduced.‖

The Engen contraction splint is simple and effective (Fig. 6-41, *D*). It is usually prescribed for the nonambulatory patient.

Both approaches provide *programmed control* since both provide a force to produce gradual motion in a "correcting" direction of extension.

Genu varum or valgum (ML motion). If this abnormal ML motion of the tibia occurs during weight bearing but is not evident when the limb is not bearing body weight or when the tibia can be

*See Appendix F, item 5, and Appendix G, items 15 and 16.
†See Appendix C, items 8 to 10, and Appendix G, items 1 and 2.
‡See Appendix C, items 5 and 7.
§See Appendix C, items 14 and 15.
‖ See Appendix C, item 11.

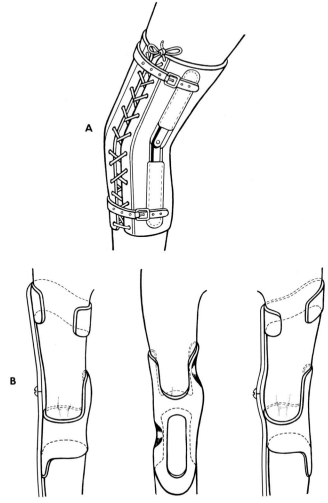

Fig. 6-42. Static control of abnormal ML motion of the knee joint. **A,** Elastic knee cage with ML hinges. **B,** Left, AK genu valgum brace. Center, Lehneis laminated knee orthosis. A genu varum shell is shown; the indented pressure points are reversed for genu valgum. Right, AK genu varum brace.

brought into normal alignment by manipulation, *static control* is provided by an elastic knee cage (Fig. 6-42, *A*),* AK braces, or the Lehneis laminated knee shell (Fig. 6-42, *B*).†

Single lateral or single medial uprights with pressure pads are used when normal alignment by "presetting" prior to weight bearing is not possible. *Programmed control* is provided; that is, external force is used to gradually achieve normal alignment or to prevent a predictable increase in the present abnormal angulation of the tibia (Fig. 6-43).†

*See Appendix C, item 14.
†See Appendix C, item 7, and Appendix G, items 5 and 6.

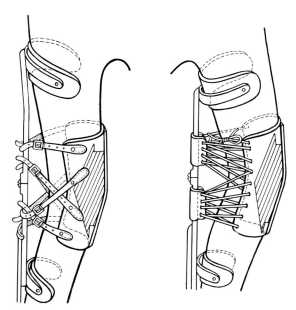

Fig. 6-43. Programmed control of abnormal ML motion of the knee.

Swing phase

Hip flexion following push-off can be used to initiate *knee flexion* during the swing phase (Fig. 6-44). Gravity's force provides the means to extend the knee.

Knee extension is maintained just prior to heel-strike by a downward pressure supplied by the abdomen and pelvis with use of the UCLA functional long leg brace (Fig. 6-39, *A*). Functional anatomic control of flexion-extension of the trunk must be present to operate this brace. The UCLA functional AK brace is not recommended for patients with bilateral involvement.

HIP MOTIONS
Stance phase

Heel-strike. When anatomic controls are present, flexion of the femur has occurred during the swing phase. The femur remains flexed at the hip from heel contact until the foot is flat upon the floor.

Foot-flat. The femur begins to gradually extend at the hip joint, while the pelvis is simultaneously rotating in the direction of extension. By the time the midstance position is reached, the relationship of the trunk to the thigh is a 180° line.

There are no components presently available that can provide *programmed control* of flexion and extension motions of the pelvis and/or femur during the stance phase when anatomic control of these motions is lacking. However, when anatomic control of trunk

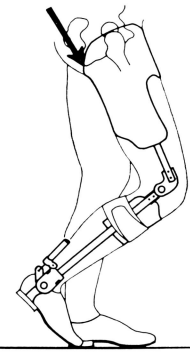

Fig. 6-44. Programmed control of AP motion of the knee. UCLA functional AK brace. When hip flexors are inadequate, the arrow gives the direction of the force and the contact point between the ischial tuberosity and the posterior brim of the thigh shell, which produce both hip and knee flexion simultaneously. To make contact at the proper phase of the gait cycle, the patient is taught to use his abdominal muscles to raise his hip on the affected side and rotate his pelvis forward, which produces the thrust indicated by the arrow. The thigh shell is not fitted to bear ischial weight during the stance phase as the downward force described would overcome the offset knee joint and cause the knee to buckle. (From Anderson, M. H.: Orthop. Prosth. Appl. J. **18**: 273, 1964.)

flexion and extension is present, programmed control of the femur is possible with the use of a free-motion hip joint. That is, flexion and extension of the hip is allowed, whereas other motions are inhibited. It should be noted that when a free AP–motion hip joint and pelvic band are incorporated into a well-fitting AK brace, transverse rotation of the femur at the hip is blocked. Such is the case whether these motions are desirable or unwanted.*

Static control of trunk AP flexion at the hips during the stance phase (which might be referred to as unwanted motion) can be provided. The cost, in terms of function, is very great indeed, for with AP flexion control of the trunk, current braces inadvertently inhibit femoral flexion, femoral adduction-

---

*See Appendix A, items 2 and 3.

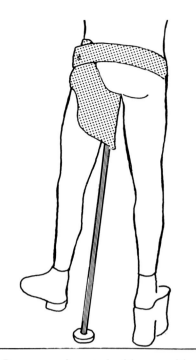

Fig. 6-45. Programmed control with prepositioning of the femur. Prepositioning of the femur in the transverse plane is accomplished by the quadrilateral shaping of the laminated cuff. Transverse slipping between the cuff and thigh is eliminated. The intimate fit ensures that the femur can be placed in the acetabulum at any desired angle and be maintained in the desired position by the alignment of the cuff to the brace frame. Motion in the AP plane is allowed in the example shown.

abduction, pelvic ML tilting, and transverse rotation of both the pelvis and the femurs, whether or not anatomic control for one or all is present.*

Programmed control may involve "prepositioning" the femur while allowing motion in several planes with the use of a quadrilateral cuff (Fig. 6-45).†

Swing phase

Programmed control of unwanted or abnormal *internal or external rotation* of the femur can be provided by the use of cable rotators without inhibiting flexion and extension of either the femurs or trunk at the hips during the swing phase (Fig. 6-46).‡ Control of internal and external rotation of the femurs is also sustained during the stance phase.

Static control of unwanted femoral *adduction or abduction* during the swing phase can be provided with the use of any metal hip joint and a pelvic band.

The motions in other planes that may be secondarily or unintentionally blocked will depend upon the joint selected (for example, free versus locking joints and their effect upon flexion and extension).

VERTICAL MOTION IN STANCE PHASE

Vertical motion in stance phase can be predicted to occur if the total weight of the body is allowed to

---

*See Appendix A, items 4 and 5.
†See Appendix B, item 1.
‡See Appendix A, item 1.

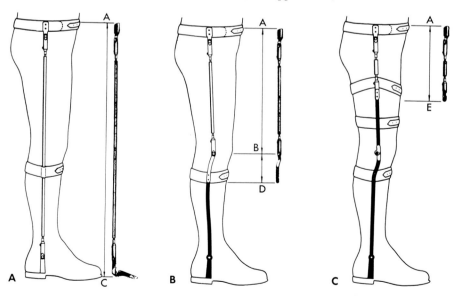

Fig. 6-46. Programmed control of transverse ML motion of the femur (femoral rotator — twister). **A,** Rotator cables attached directly to the shoes. **B,** Rotator cables used with BK brace. **C,** Rotator cables used with AK brace. (Courtesy Becker Orthopedic Appliance Co., Birmingham, Mich.)

descend upon a dysfunctioning lower extremity. Unwanted or abnormal motion between two or more segments within the limb may need control, such as at a fracture site. In *programmed control,* motion is allowed within the rest of the brace system, whereas *static control* is maintained at the site of the fracture. Unwanted normal motion of one or more segments of the limb may be the control concern. For example, unwanted knee flexion when ischial weight bearing is desired would require a locking knee joint.

If the femur is the concern, the vertical load may be reduced with the use of a thigh lacer (Fig. 6-47, *A*),* a quadrilaterally shaped Thomas ring (Fig. 6-47, *B*), or a plastic laminated quadrilateral cuff (Fig. 6-47, *C*).† The brace uprights receive the weight, making it possible to bypass the limb.

When the tibia is the concern, the vertical load may be reduced with the use of the plastic laminated

*See Appendix B, items 2 to 4.
†See Appendix B, item 1.

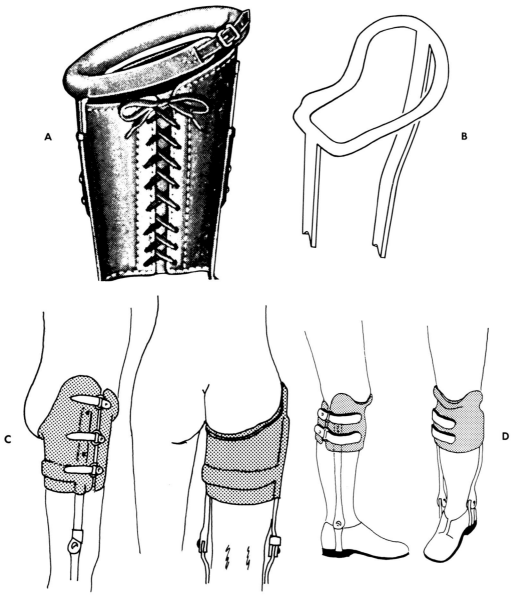

Fig. 6-47. Programmed control of vertical translatory motion. **A,** Thigh lacer. **B,** Thomas ring, quadrilaterally shaped. **C,** Laminated quadrilateral cuff. **D,** BK orthosis with a laminated PTB cuff.

PTB cuff, thus bypassing the lower portion of the tibia and foot through the brace uprights (Fig. 6-47, *D*).* It should be noted that due to the intimate fitting of either the laminated quadrilateral cuff or the PTB cuff, the alignment of the other components of these braces is especially important.

CONCLUSIONS

In the introductory remarks I suggested without reservations that all braces provide but *one* function—control of body motions. Later, in discussing the condition of fixed forefoot drop, the question arose as to whether or not factors such as "fit" and "comfort" should be categorized as functions. Perhaps the key to clarification of this thoroughly confusing area

_____

*See Appendix D, items 1 to 3.

is *purpose* or *intent*. Are such individual "components" as a heel insert with a depression, or hole, to accommodate for a calcaneal spur; the addition of an appropriate heel lift to a shoe to accommodate for a fixed forefoot drop; or the stretching of an enlarged "pocket" into the side of a shoe to accommodate for a bunion to be confused with a brace? It would seem reasonable to conclude that a brace is intended to *control*. That is, a brace is meant to arrest or to modify a situation that is unacceptable, whereas accommodation, by definition, accepts a situation as it is. Orthotic devices would appear to fall into one or the other of two distinct classifications—*control devices* or *accommodation devices*, fit and/or comfort (as with cosmesis) being considerations directly related to patient acceptance of items in either classification.

Appendices to Part IV*

APPENDIX A. HIP CONTROL

Components	Biomechanical function			Material
	Plane of function			
	Sagittal	Coronal	Transverse	
1. Hip twister with pelvic band	Permits flexion-extension	Permits abduction-adduction	Resists internal-external rotation	Coil spring housed within plastic tube
2. Hip joint with free motion and pelvic band	Permits flexion-extension	Prevents abduction-adduction	Prevents internal-external rotation	Aluminum, stainless steel, carbon steel, chrome molybdenum
3. Hip joint assembly with positive stop and pelvic band	Limits extension; permits flexion	Prevents abduction-adduction	Prevents internal-external rotation	Aluminum, stainless steel, carbon steel, chrome molybdenum
4. Hip joint assembly with drop ring lock and pelvic band	Prevents flexion-extension	Prevents abduction-adduction	Prevents internal-external rotation	Aluminum, stainless steel, chrome molybdenum, carbon steel
5. Hip joint assembly with lever lock and pelvic band	Prevents flexion-extension	Prevents abduction-adduction	Prevents internal-external rotation	Aluminum, stainless steel, carbon steel, chrome molybdenum
6. Hip joint assembly with plunger lock, abduction and/or adduction hinge, and pelvic band	Prevents flexion-extension	Limits abduction and/or adduction	Prevents internal-external rotation	Carbon steel

*The contributions of Dr. Edward Peizer and Mr. Anthony Staros of the Veterans Administration Prosthetic Center in the preparation of the Appendices are gratefully acknowledged.

APPENDIX A. HIP CONTROL—cont'd

Components	Biomechanical function			Material
	Plane of function			
	Sagittal	Coronal	Transverse	
7. Hip joint assembly with ring lock, abduction and/or adduction hinge, and pelvic band	Prevents flexion-extension	Limits abduction and/or adduction	Prevents internal-external rotation	Stainless steel
8. Hip joint assembly with hyperextension stop, abduction and/or adduction hinge, and pelvic band	Limits extension; permits flexion	Limits abduction and/or adduction	Prevents internal-external rotation	Carbon steel
9. Silesian belt	Permits flexion-extension	Resists abduction	Resists external rotation	Metal and fabric

APPENDIX B. WEIGHT-BEARING CONTROL (THIGH)

Components	Biomechanical function			Material
	Plane of function			
	Sagittal	Coronal	Transverse	
1. Quadrilateral socket	Prevents longitudinal translation and, depending on site of structural defect, may resist rotations and horizontal translation	Prevents longitudinal translation and, depending on site of structural defect, may resist rotations and horizontal translation	Depending on site of structural defect, may resist internal-external rotation	Plastic laminate
2. Ischial weight-bearing band with ischial plateau	Prevents longitudinal translation	Prevents longitudinal translation	Permits internal-external rotation	Padding with leather or plastic sheeting covering
3. Ischial ring (half) with ischial plateau	Prevents longitudinal translation	Prevents longitudinal translation	Permits internal-external rotation	Padding with leather or plastic sheeting covering
4. Ischial ring (full) with ischial plateau	Prevents longitudinal translation	Prevents longitudinal translation	Permits internal-external rotation	Padding with leather or plastic sheeting covering

APPENDIX C. KNEE CONTROL (SINGLE OR BILATERAL BAR)

Components	Biomechanical function			Material
	Plane of function			
	Sagittal	Coronal	Transverse	
1. AK socket (non-weight bearing)	Provides extension moment in early stance phase (UCLA functional long leg brace)	No significant function	No significant function	Polyester laminate
2. Knee joint (offset)	Provides extension moment in early stance phase; permits flexion-extension; prevents hyperextension (UCLA functional long leg brace)	Prevents abduction-adduction of tibia	Prevents internal-external rotation	Stainless steel

Continued.

APPENDIX C. KNEE CONTROL (SINGLE OR BILATERAL BAR)—cont'd

Components	Biomechanical function			Material
	Plane of function			
	Sagittal	*Coronal*	*Transverse*	
3. Pretibial cuff	Provides extension moment in stance phase (UCLA functional long leg brace)	Prevents abduction-adduction of tibia	No significant function	Plastic laminate
4. Hydraulic ankle joint assembly	Provides extension moment late in stance phase by resisting dorsiflexion (UCLA functional long leg brace)	No significant function	No significant function	Aluminum, stainless steel, carbon steel
5. Knee joint (polycentric)	Provides extension moment in early stance phase; permits flexion-extension; prevents hyperextension	Prevents abduction-adduction of tibia	Prevents internal-external rotation	Aluminum
6. Knee joint (single axis, free motion)	Permits flexion-extension	Prevents abduction-adduction of tibia	Prevents internal-external rotation	Aluminum, stainless steel, carbon steel, chrome molybdenum
7. Knee joint with hyperextension control	Limits hyperextension; permits flexion-extension	Prevents abduction-adduction of tibia	Prevents internal-external rotation	Stainless steel, steel, aluminum, chrome molybdenum
8. Knee joint with drop ring lock	Prevents flexion-extension	Prevents abduction-adduction of tibia	Prevents internal-external rotation	Aluminum, stainless steel, carbon steel, chrome molybdenum
9. Knee joint with plunger lock	Prevents flexion-extension	Prevents abduction-adduction of tibia	Prevents internal-external rotation	Chrome molybdenum
10. Knee joint with lever lock	Prevents flexion-extension	Prevents abduction-adduction of tibia	Prevents internal-external rotation	Aluminum, stainless steel, carbon steel, chrome molybdenum
11. Knee joint, adjustable (with turnbuckle, dial, etc.)	Provides extension moment; permits flexion or extension	Prevents abduction-adduction of tibia	Prevents internal-external rotation	Carbon steel, stainless steel
12. Single-bar joint with hyperextension stop	Limits hyperextension; permits flexion-extension	Prevents abduction-adduction of tibia	Prevents internal-external rotation	Stainless steel extension
13. Single-bar joint with lever lock	Prevents flexion-extension	Prevents abduction-adduction of tibia	Prevents internal-external rotation	Stainless steel
14. Knee joint, hyperextension control (knee cage)	Limits hyperextension; permits flexion-extension	Prevents abduction-adduction of tibia	Permits internal-external rotation	Stainless steel, aluminum uprights
15. Knee cage, hyperextension control (without joint)	Limits hyperextension; permits flexion-extension	Prevents abduction-adduction of tibia	Permits internal-external rotation	Aluminum uprights
16. Knee joint, drop ring lock (knee cage)	Prevents flexion-extension	Prevents abduction-adduction of tibia	Permits internal-external rotation	Stainless steel, aluminum uprights

APPENDIX D. WEIGHT-BEARING CONTROL (LEG OR FOOT)

Components	Biomechanical function			Material
	Plane of function			
	Sagittal	*Coronal*	*Transverse*	
1. PTB socket	Prevents longitudinal translation and, depending on site of structural defect, may resist rotations and horizontal translation	Prevents longitudinal translation and, depending on site of structural defect, may resist rotations and horizontal translation	Depending on site of structural defect, may resist internal-external rotation	Plastic laminate, posterior opening
2. PTB supra-condylar socket	Prevents longitudinal translation and, depending on site of structural defect, may resist rotations and horizontal translation	Prevents longitudinal translation and, depending on site of structural defect, may resist rotations and horizontal translation; resists abduction-adduction	Depending on site of structural defect, may resist internal-external rotation	Plastic laminate, posterior opening
3. PTB supra-condylar supra-patellar socket	Prevents longitudinal translation and, depending on site of structural defect, may resist rotations and horizontal translation; resists hyper-extension	Prevents longitudinal translation and, depending on site of structural defect, may resist rotations and horizontal translation; resists abduction-adduction	Depending on site of structural defect, may resist internal-external rotation; resists internal-external rotation	Plastic laminate, posterior opening

APPENDIX E. ANKLE CONTROLS AND UPRIGHTS (SINGLE OR BILATERAL DESIGN)

Components	Biomechanical function			Material
	Plane of function			
	Sagittal	*Coronal*	*Transverse*	
1. Leg uprights, single spring-loaded ankle joint assembly with one-piece or split stirrup	Resists plantar flexion, permitting dorsiflexion, or resists dorsiflexion, permitting plantar flexion	Inhibits abduction-adduction of subtalar joint	Prevents internal-external rotation	1. *Uprights:* Aluminum, stainless steel, carbon steel, chrome molybdenum 2. *Stirrup:* Stainless steel, carbon steel
2. Leg uprights, double spring-loaded ankle joint assembly with one-piece or split stirrup	Resists plantar flexion and dorsiflexion	Inhibits abduction-adduction of subtalar joint	Prevents internal-external rotation	1. *Uprights:* Aluminum 2. *Stirrup:* Stainless steel
3. Leg uprights, positive stop ankle joint assembly with one-piece or split stirrup	Limits plantar flexion, permitting dorsiflexion, or limits dorsiflexion, permitting plantar flexion, or limits both	Inhibits abduction-adduction of subtalar joint	Prevents internal-external rotation	1. *Uprights:* Aluminum, stainless steel, carbon steel, chrome molybdenum 2. *Stirrup:* Stainless steel, carbon steel
4. Leg uprights, positive stop ankle joint assembly with caliper	Limits plantar flexion, permitting dorsiflexion, or limits dorsiflexion, permitting plantar flexion, or limits both	Inhibits abduction-adduction of subtalar joint	Prevents internal-external rotation	1. *Uprights:* Stainless steel, carbon steel, chrome molybdenum 2. *Caliper pins and box:* Carbon steel, stainless steel

Continued.

APPENDIX E. ANKLE CONTROLS AND UPRIGHTS (SINGLE OR BILATERAL DESIGN)—cont'd

Components	Biomechanical function			Material
	Plane of function			
	Sagittal	*Coronal*	*Transverse*	
5. Hydraulic ankle joint assembly	Resists dorsiflexion; permits plantar flexion (UCLA functional long leg brace)	Inhibits abduction-adduction of subtalar joint	Prevents internal-external rotation	Stainless steel
6. Stirrup-upright combination (no joint at ankle)	Prevents plantar and dorsiflexion	Inhibits abduction-adduction of subtalar joint	Prevents internal-external rotation	Carbon steel, stainless steel
7. Single leg upright, spring-loaded ankle joint assembly	Resists plantar flexion, permitting dorsiflexion, or resists dorsiflexion, permitting plantar flexion; permits longitudinal translation	Inhibits abduction-adduction of subtalar joint	Permits internal-external rotation	Stainless steel, aluminum
8. Single leg upright ankle joint, positive stop	Limits plantar flexion, permitting dorsiflexion, or limits dorsiflexion, permitting plantar flexion, or limits both	Inhibits abduction-adduction of subtalar joint	Prevents internal-external rotation	Stainless steel, aluminum

APPENDIX F. LEG UPRIGHTS AND ANKLE JOINT ASSEMBLIES (COMPLETE BRACES)

Components	Biomechanical function			Material
	Plane of function			
	Sagittal	*Coronal*	*Transverse*	
1. Posterior upright with footplate	Resists plantar flexion	Inhibits abduction-adduction of subtalar joint	Resists internal-external rotation	Blue clock spring material
2. Posterior upright and caliper tube	Resists plantar flexion	Permits abduction-adduction of subtalar joint	Resists internal-external rotation	Carbon steel
3. Bilateral spring or wire uprights with caliper pin or tube or machine screw and nut for shoe attachment	Resists plantar flexion	Inhibits abduction-adduction of subtalar joint	Resists internal-external rotation	Music wire or stainless steel
4. Bilateral spring-loaded uprights or bars	Resists plantar flexion	Inhibits abduction-adduction of subtalar joint	Prevents internal-external rotation	Aluminum, stainless steel
5. Molded leg-ankle-foot support (fits within shoe)	Prevents plantar-dorsiflexion	Prevents abduction-adduction of subtalar joint	Prevents internal-external rotation	Polyester laminate or molded leather over plaster of Paris cast reinforced with stainless steel or carbon steel uprights and footplate

APPENDIX F. LEG UPRIGHTS AND ANKLE JOINT ASSEMBLIES (COMPLETE BRACES)—cont'd

Components	Biomechanical function			Material
	Plane of function			
	Sagittal	*Coronal*	*Transverse*	
6. Biaxial spring-loaded ankle and subtalar joint	Resists ankle plantar flexion, permitting ankle dorsiflexion, or resists dorsiflexion, permitting plantar flexion	Permits and/or resist inversion and/or eversion of foot	Prevents internal-external rotation	*Uprights:* Carbon steel, aluminum
7. Biaxial positive stop ankle and subtalar joint	Limits ankle plantar flexion, permitting ankle dorsiflexion, or limits dorsiflexion, permitting plantar flexion, or limits both	Permits and/or resists inversion and/or eversion of foot	Prevents internal-external rotation	*Stirrup:* Carbon steel, stainless steel

APPENDIX G. COMPONENT ACCESSORIES

Components	Biomechanical function			Material
	Plane of function			
	Sagittal	*Coronal*	*Transverse*	
1. Kneecap	Limits flexion	No significant function	No significant function	Leather or plastic sheeting and/or fabric
2. Under patellar strap	Limits flexion	No significant function	No significant function	Leather or plastic sheeting and/or fabric
3. Kneecap for knock-knee	No significant function	Prevents abduction	No significant function	Leather or plastic sheeting and/or fabric
4. Kneecap for bow knee	No significant function	Prevents adduction	No significant function	Leather or plastic sheeting and/or fabric
5. Pressure pad for knock-knee	No significant function	Prevents abduction	No significant function	Sponge rubber or felt covered with leather or plastic sheeting
6. Pressure pad for bow knee	No significant function	Prevents adduction	No significant function	Sponge rubber or felt covered with leather or plastic sheeting
7. T or Y strap (medial)	No significant function	Prevents foot eversion	No significant function	Leather or plastic sheeting and/or fabric
8. T or Y strap (lateral)	No significant function	Prevents foot inversion	No significant function	Leather or plastic sheeting and/or fabric
9. Ankle pressure pad (medial)	No significant function	Prevents eversion	No significant function	Sponge rubber felt covered with leather or plastic sheeting
10. Ankle pressure pad (lateral)	No significant function	Prevents inversion	No significant function	Sponge rubber felt covered with leather or plastic sheeting

Continued.

APPENDIX G. COMPONENT ACCESSORIES—cont'd

Components	Biomechanical function			Material
	Plane of function			
	Sagittal	*Coronal*	*Transverse*	
11. Heel wedge (medial)	No significant function	Prevents eversion	No significant function	Leather or neoprene
12. Heel wedge (lateral)	No significant function	Prevents inversion	No significant function	Leather or neoprene
13. Sole wedge (medial)	No significant function	Prevents forefoot eversion	No significant function	Leather or neoprene
14. Sole wedge (lateral)	No significant function	Prevents forefoot inversion	No significant function	Leather or neoprene
15. Rocker bar	Simulates dorsiflexion and resists toe extension moment	No significant function	No significant function	Leather or neoprene
16. SACH-type heel wedge	Simulates plantar flexion	Simulates inversion-eversion	Simulates internal-external rotation	Rubber or neoprene
17. Thomas heel	No significant function	Prevents eversion	No significant function	Rubber or neoprene
18. Reversed Thomas heel	No significant function	Prevents inversion	No significant function	Rubber or neoprene

Chapter 7

Advanced degenerative arthritis of the hip

Part I
Introduction

MARK B. COVENTRY, M.D.
Rochester, Minnesota

As man's longevity increases, degenerative affections of the musculoskeletal system assume a growing importance. The hip is no exception. Degenerative arthritis of the hip has been the subject of countless clinical investigations, and the surgical approach to this problem is truly exciting. Starting out in the early days of aseptic surgery with the occasional osteotomy, it has progressed through cheilectomy and acetabuloplasty, drilling, forage, denervation, cup arthroplasty, intertrochanteric osteotomy, tenomyotomy or "hanging hip," prosthetic arthroplasty, resection of the head and neck, and now total hip replacement.

The semantics are interesting. "Malum coxae senilis" and "morbus coxae senilis" are terms seldom used today except in a historic way. But we really should avoid the term "arthritis," for it is seldom that the pathologist returns to us the diagnosis of "inflammation" from the synovium in the average patient with coxarthrosis. Yet in the United States the term "degenerative arthritis" is most popular. In Europe, "coxarthrosis" is extensively used.

Robert Adams,[1] writing perhaps the first textbook of orthopaedics in the English language (circa 1836), described what he termed morbus coxae senilis, that is, the sick hip of the aged. He described the case of Patrick Mackin, a postillion and groom, who ". . . walks with great labour and pain, and now requires assistance of a stick in each hand . . . in the morning his movements are stiff and confined, but they become freer on exercise." This description is as true today as when it was written.

Early degenerative arthritis of the hip was the subject of a symposium at the American Academy of Orthopaedic Surgeons in 1966. At that time osteotomy, in particular, was discussed. We have been assigned the subject of advanced degenerative arthritis of the hip. There is a wide, overlapping border between early and advanced coxarthrosis. Is this difference in degree radiographic only? Is it subjective—does it pertain only to severity of symptoms? Or does it pertain to range of motion? Does it relate to the age of the patient? All these factors are important and together determine the degree of severity of the disease. A point system of grading hip function must be used to record the involvement of the hip according to degenerative changes. If some remaining joint space is visible by x-ray examination, and if the patient has an acceptable range of motion (perhaps 80° of flexion), then certainly for this discussion we will call it early coxarthrosis, and osteotomy should be strongly considered (Fig. 7-1). But if these factors do not pertain, and osteotomy does not seem the best procedure, then such a case falls in the range of the discussion in this chapter—namely, advanced degenerative hip disease.

One of the contributors will discuss arthrodesis; another, cup arthroplasty; and the third, total hip arthroplasty. Less commonly used methods of relieving pain in coxarthrosis than these, however, should be included for completeness, and I shall discuss them briefly.

The "hanging hip," or myotenotomy, popularized and advanced by Voss, is a useful operation in some instances of severe coxarthrosis. I do this procedure only when other methods, perhaps those more sure of success, cannot be carried out because of the impaired medical condition of the patient. "Hanging hip" surgery can be done in a brief operating time. The patient can be out of bed the next day without fear of dislocating the hip. Blood loss is minimal. It is a relatively nontraumatic operation, requiring virtually no specialized aftercare except instruction

155

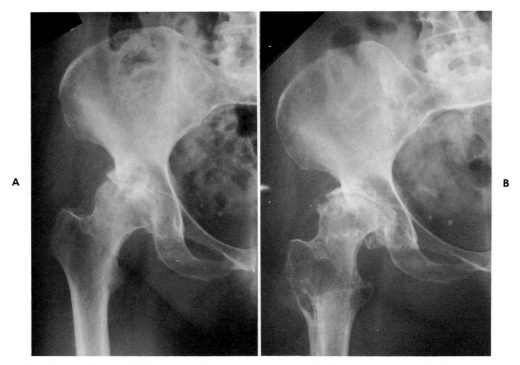

Fig. 7-1. A 57-year-old forester with early coxarthrosis. **A,** Before osteotomy. **B,** Three years after osteotomy. There is no flexion contracture, 100° of flexion, and no pain. He can walk for miles without difficulty.

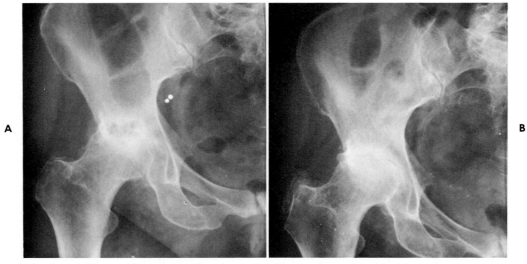

Fig. 7-2. A 73-year-old retired railroad carman. He stated that his right hip had been painful for 24 years and he had retired 10 years ago because of it. He had been on crutches for 3 years. Flexion was from 15° to 70°, there was no internal rotation, and abduction was 5°. X-ray films showed marked degenerative changes with flattening, a sclerotic head, and involvement of the acetabulum. A hanging hip operation was done. **A,** Before hanging hip surgery. **B,** Two and a half years later. Note reconstitution of the joint line and lessening of cystic changes.

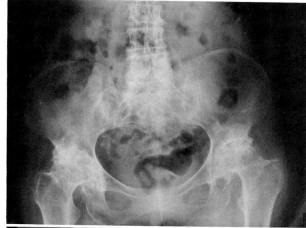

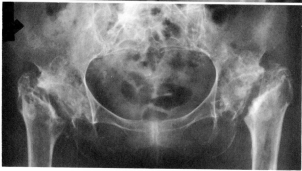

Fig. 7-3. A 76-year-old widow who was unable to walk. **A,** Before Girdlestone resection. She could not separate her knees and had only a few degrees of hip motion at 50° flexion. **B,** Two years, 8 months after surgery. Fifteen degrees of abduction was possible in each hip and there was 90° flexion of the right hip, 75° flexion of the left hip, normal rotation, normal adduction, and virtually no pain (she takes an occasional aspirin). She walks nicely with two canes.

in crutch-walking. These seem to be the chief virtues of the hanging hip procedure in advanced hip disease; of course, it does relieve pain in a significant number of patients (Fig. 7-2).

Resection of the head and neck of the femur à la Girdlestone has been helpful in severe bilateral degenerative disease. But surely there will be less need for this operation as total hip arthroplasty becomes better defined. In severely advanced bilateral coxarthrosis with "frozen hips" and pain, the Girdlestone resection gives relatively good results (Fig. 7-3). I prefer to keep these patients in traction for 4 to 6 weeks postoperatively, and then allow them up to use crutches until the pain is gone. Some patients will never get off crutches; others will be able to use canes. Rarely will a patient in the older age group ever walk without a considerable limp and without a cane after a bilateral Girdlestone procedure. About 50% of normal motion usually can be achieved. The disadvantages of this operation are the lack of really good motion afterward and the need, as mentioned, for canes or crutches postoperatively. And then, of course, not all these patients are relieved of pain.

There is no need to dwell on other less commonly used procedures such as denervation or forage; they have not withstood the test of time.

REFERENCE

1. Adams, R.: Hip-joint, abnormal conditions. In Tood, R. B., editor: The cyclopaedia of anatomy and physiology, London, 1836-1839, Longman, Brown, Green, Longmans, & Roberts, vol. 2, pp. 780-825.

Part II

Surgical management of advanced degenerative disease of the hip

ALAN DeFOREST SMITH, M.D.
New York, New York

The advantages of hip fusion in the treatment of advanced arthritis of the hip have tended to be overlooked in recent years. Attention has been focused on methods for reconstructing the joint and preserving motion such as various types of arthroplasty and

osteotomy. Were the results of these latter operations always perfect there would be no question about their use, but unfortunately this is not the case.

Hip fusion produces an absolutely painless extremity that is not subject to fatigue. It permits one to do an unlimited amount of walking or standing. Following the operation there is no need for prolonged physical therapy. With the use of internal fixation the period of confinement to bed and convalescence has been materially reduced.

It cannot be denied, however, that fusion has certain disadvantages, the chief of which is lack of motion in the joint. It makes sitting somewhat awkward, but this is not as serious as some suppose. With the hip fixed in a moderate degree of flexion, one can sit without much difficulty. A stiff hip also causes a limp, but this is not too conspicuous.

Hip fusion is best suited for a relatively young individual who, by preference or out of necessity, requires much activity, including walking and standing. One of my patients was a porter who was able to resume his work after the operation with no difficulty.

Fusion is contraindicated in cases of bilateral arthritis for obvious reasons. Nothing is more disabling than two stiff hips. An occasional exception to this may be the attainment of a successful arthroplasty on one side, with the remaining hip so severely involved as to make the outcome of arthroplasty questionable. Arthrodesis should not be done when one's occupation requires movement of the hip, as in kneeling, squatting, etc., for example, a plumber.

Fusion usually is ruled out when arthritis of the hip is combined with that of the lumbar spine because the spine must compensate to a large degree for the lack of motion in the hip.

As a rule, women object to a stiff hip, although I have had several female patients who were satisfied with the result.

There are, of course, many methods for fusing the hip, but some are better suited than others for the osteoarthritic joint. Internal fixation is most desirable in that it assures the maintenance of the correct position, gives the best assurance of fusion, and permits earlier ambulation. Probably the best means of apply-

ing this is a long Smith-Petersen nail directed upward so as to penetrate the ilium above the acetabulum and thus secure firm fixation. Before doing this, however, it is essential to dislocate the hip and denude the joint surfaces. In addition, it is well to drill the head and the ilium in several places.

Another method for using internal fixation is the use of multiple square nails, most of which are driven through the femoral head into the ilium. If there is an overhanging ridge of exostoses, one nail may be placed through it into the head. It is not difficult to expose the inner surface of the pelvis and to drive a nail through the thin part of the acetabulum into the femoral head.

If the capsule and synovia are thick and somewhat poor in blood supply, it is best to excise the greater part of them. The Hibbs operation was intended for tuberculous hips and was meant to circumvent the joint to a large extent by using the greater trochanter and part of the shaft as a graft. It is not suited for osteoarthritis but may be combined with intra-articular fusion and internal fixation. Probably a better way of doing this is to employ a bone graft from the ilium.

The Brittain procedure of doing a subtrochanteric osteotomy and placing a bone graft into the ischium also was designed to circumvent the joint in cases of

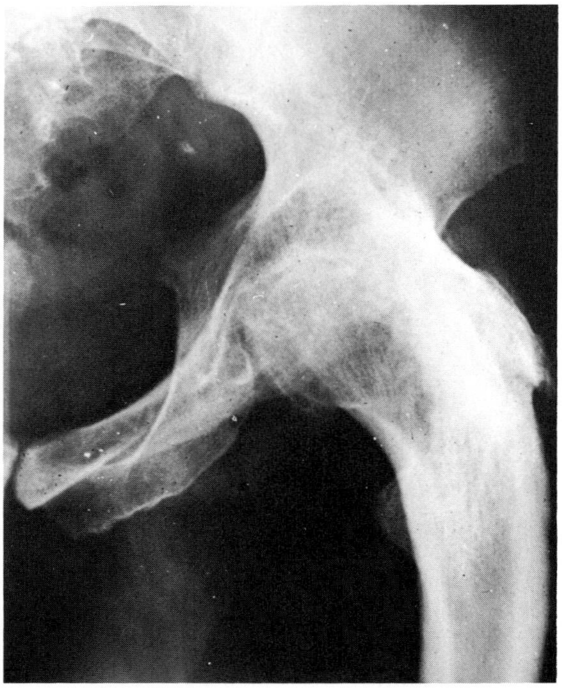

Fig. 7-4. Hibbs' type of fusion for osteoarthritic hip.

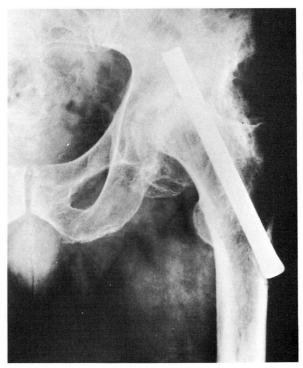

Fig. 7-5. Osteoarthritic hip fused with long triflange nail.

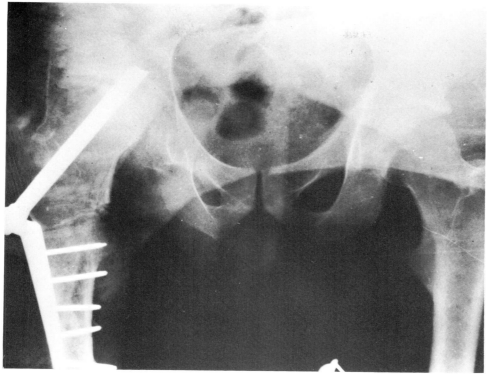

Fig. 7-6. Fusion of hip combined with subtrochanteric osteotomy fixed with a triflange nail and McLaughlin plate.

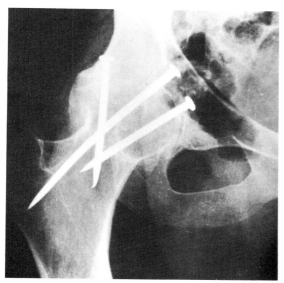

Fig. 7-7. Hip fusion for osteoarthritis using multiple nails, two from within the pelvis.

tuberculosis and is not adapted to use in osteoarthritis.

I have had no experience with Charnley's operation in which the head is driven through the floor of the acetabulum in order to obtain compression.

The combination of subtrochanteric osteotomy with hip fusion has several advantages. This was advocated by Frederick Thompson for treatment of the tuberculous hip. It allows the fusion to be carried out without changing the relationship between the femoral head and the acetabulum. Often the head is deformed and placing it in the desired position for fusion causes an incongruity between the head and acetabulum. If, instead, the fusion is done without changing the position of the head, the deformity then can be corrected by a subtrochanteric osteotomy. Fixation then can be secured with a McLaughlin nail and plate.

The position in which the hip is fused is important. It should be in about 25° of flexion in order to facilitate sitting and it should be in neutral position between abduction and adduction. Even a small degree of abduction is undesirable and results in a poor gait and bad posture. A few degrees of adduction are not harmful. (See Figs. 7-4 to 7-7.)

Part III

Use of cup arthroplasty in treatment of severe osteoarthritis of the hip

WILLIAM H. HARRIS, M.D.
Boston, Massachusetts

Smith-Petersen's innovative concept[17,18] of the *physiologic* reconstruction of the arthritic hip joint using the Vitallium mold now has a 32-year heritage. He advanced the idea of the induction of cartilaginous metaplasia after reshaping the sclerotic and distorted femoral head and acetabulum to a congruous spherical contour in cancellous bone. Long-term results are available in sizable numbers of patients from several different centers,* the average follow-up being 8 and 10 years in some series.[6,8,15] Cup arthroplasty has great versatility, demonstrated durability, and is unique in creating a biologic joint restoration.

This operation has been increasingly challenged recently, most persistently by osteotomy of the hip and by total hip replacement. It is abundantly clear that no one procedure is universally optimum for the wide spectrum of arthritic afflictions of the hip. For example, cup arthroplasty or total hip replacement is clearly preferable to osteotomy in advanced osteoarthritis. Equally clearly, cup arthroplasty is pref-

*See references 1 to 3, 7, 10 to 12, 16, 19, and 20.

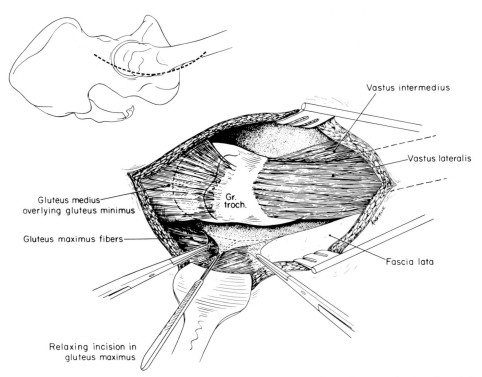

Fig. 7-8. The skin incision is a shallow curved incision that follows the posterior border of the tensor fasciae latae to the posterior superior corner of the greater trochanter. From there it goes down the lateral side of the thigh for 3 inches and then curves gently forward, duplicating the arc of the proximal half of the incision. The fascia lata is exposed through this incision and then divided along the line of the incision. The fascia lata is divided *distally* first. This enables the index finger to pass deep to the fascia lata and palpate the insertion of the gluteus maximus into the femur. This is the deep landmark. The rest of the proximal portion of the fascia lata incision must run one fingerbreadth anterior to that insertion. The posterior limb of the fascial incision is then made, beginning at the midportion of the greater trochanter and going in the direction of the fibers of the gluteus maximus for approximately 2 inches. This is a muscle-splitting incision. It is made craniad and medially into the muscle belly of the gluteus maximus. (From Harris, W. H.: Surg. Clin. N. Amer. **49:**763, 1969.)

erable to total hip replacement or osteotomy in septic arthritis.

Therefore the critical focus for our discussion is this: How is cup arthroplasty currently done and what are the results in treating severe osteoarthritis of the hip?

ADVANCES IN OPERATIVE TECHNIQUE

Great strides have been taken in the past 6 years to vastly simplify and improve the operative technique of cup arthroplasty and consequently its results. Paramount among these improvements was the development of the lateral approach for this operation.[5] Operating from the lateral approach affords several valuable assets.

In the first place, the greater trochanter is osteotomized. While this can be done through an anterior incision, it is far simpler from the side (Fig. 7-8). Trochanteric osteotomy greatly facilitates dislocation of the femoral head. Second, through the lateral approach the *posterior* capsule as well as the anterior capsule can now be excised under direct vision. Thus all of the tribulations of releasing the posterior capsule and the short external rotators from the medial side of the femoral neck, as was necessary from an anterior approach, are obviated (Fig. 7-9). Third,

the femoral head can now be dislocated both posteriorly and anteriorly. The anterior dislocation facilitates the reaming and shaping of the femoral head, whereas posterior dislocation of the femoral head behind the acetabulum provides a magnificent view of the socket (Figs. 7-10 and 7-11).

This beautiful exposure of the head and particularly the socket inspired the development of power tools for reaming and shaping the acetabulum and the proximal femur. The socket reamers are of particular value in improving and simplifying the operation because fashioning the new acetabulum is critical, and when this complex task is done by hand, great craftsmanship is required. The power reamers now make it possible to create a deeper, more concentric, and more congruous acetabulum in less time, with less skill, and less blood loss.

Finally, the combination of the deeper acetabulum and the trochanteric transfer, plus lateral transplantation of the iliopsoas, has greatly improved stability of the hip. Even more important, trochanteric transplant materially improved abductor power[4,13,14] by increasing the resting length of the abductor muscle fibers and also by increasing the length of the lever arm through which they act. The incidence of negative Trendelenburg tests has increased

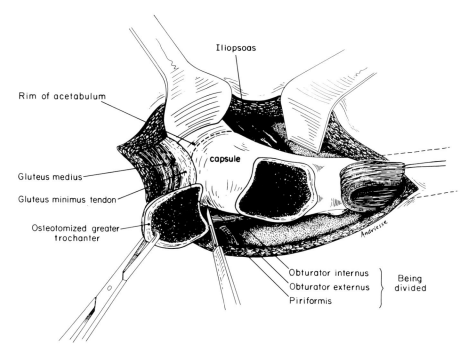

Fig. 7-9. Osteotomy of the greater trochanter greatly facilitates exposure of the hip. The freedom of the greater trochanter is enhanced by releasing the short external rotators from its deep surface. (From Harris, W. H.: Surg. Clin. N. Amer. **49**:763, 1969.)

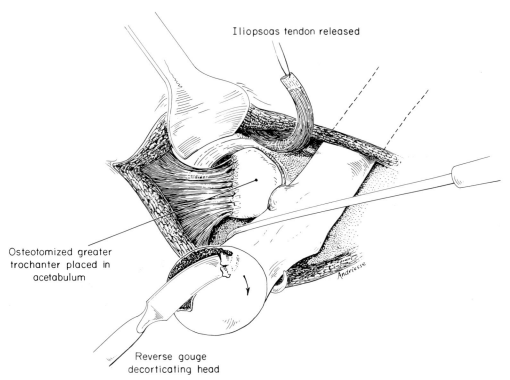

Iliopsoas tendon released

Osteotomized greater
trochanter placed in
acetabulum

Reverse gouge
decorticating head

Fig. 7-10. Visualization of the femoral head is made quite easy by dislocating the femoral head from the socket using a maneuver of adduction, extension, and external rotation. Once the greater trochanter has been placed into the acetabulum, the femoral head is well exposed. The femoral head is decorticated by hand. The final shaping and polishing can be done using a power tool. (From Harris, W. H.: Surg. Clin. N. Amer. **49**:763, 1969.)

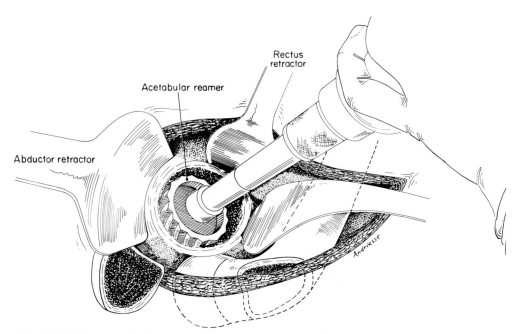

Rectus
retractor

Acetabular reamer

Abductor retractor

Fig. 7-11. Exposure of the acetabulum is distinctly improved by dislocating the femoral head posteriorly. This calls for flexion, adduction, and *internal* rotation. This wide exposure allows the use of power tools to ream and shape the acetabulum. (From Harris, W. H.: Surg. Clin. N. Amer. **49**:763, 1969.)

markedly and postoperative gait has been very much improved as a result of routine distal and lateral transplantation of the greater trochanter.

The long and extra long cup that was introduced by Aufranc in 1963 has eliminated the former problem of the cup tipping into varus and occasionally eroding the inferior femoral neck.

And very importantly, in the postoperative management the routine use of prophylactic anticoagulation with warfarin sodium (Coumadin) has virtually eliminated the number one complication of all hip surgery, namely, thromboembolic disease.[9] We have performed 1,800 consecutive cup arthroplasties using prophylactic warfarin anticoagulation without a single fatal pulmonary embolus. The data show that between 18 and 36 patients out of the 1,800 would have died from pulmonary emboli without the warfarin.[11,15,21] Approximately 180 additional patients would have had nonfatal emboli without protection of warfarin. Instead, there were only six cases of emboli, none of them fatal.

EVALUATING HIP FUNCTION

In order for any report on the results of hip surgery to be meaningful, a common language is necessary. Such a universal mode of communication has recently been provided by the Results Evaluation Committee of the Academy in the adoption of a uniform method of rating hip function, which was published in the *Journal of Bone and Joint Surgery*.[6]

In any evaluation method one must immediately recognize that *differences in severity* of the disease are vitally important in assessing relative improvement. So, too, are the compelling differences, both in result and prognosis, that arise from the *treatment of different diseases*. Osteoarthritis, for example, carries an entirely different prognosis than ankylosing spondylitis or septic arthritis, regardless of the method of therapy. It is for this reason we have limited this discussion to *osteoarthritis* of a *severe degree*. Unilateral versus bilateral involvement is another powerful determinant of the end result. This new evaluation system takes all of these items into account as well as providing a flexible method of rating the improvement.

The key features of this system are these: First and foremost, it is *patient oriented*. That means that prime consideration is given to the patient, not to the operation. It is not biased in favor of motion, which would unduly give preference to arthroplasty or total hip replacement, nor does it unduly stress stability, which would bias it in favor of hip fusion. Rather, the emphasis is on pain and function. These are the two really dominant aspects of the overall picture of hip disease from the patient's point of view.

The system is quite flexible. It is utilitarian and adapts easily to computer programming and is reproducible by the same observer at different times and different observers at the same time. The overall rating scheme is broken down as follows: pain, 44; function, 47; deformity, 4; and motion, 5—for a total of 100.

The pain categories are largely self-explanatory and are discrete enough to be very useful as well as quite discriminatory.

Function is broken down into two major headings—gait and daily activities. Analysis of gait is made both simple and effective by separating three aspects—limp, the amount of support used, and the distance walked. For example, a man who has a mild limp but refuses to use a cane loses points for his limp but is credited for the ability to forego support. Conversely, if he uses a cane and thus eliminates the limp, his scoring is the same since he has gained credit for not limping but loses points for the use of a cane.

A short list of daily activities is then assessed, providing quite an accurate profile of important functional activities.

Four points are lost if any of the really compromising deformities are present—a permanent flexion contracture greater than 30°, a fixed internal rotation contracture of greater than 10°, a fixed adduction contracture of greater than 10°, or a leg length discrepancy exceeding 1¼ inches.

Finally, motion is recorded and graded by giving special weight to those most important areas of arcs of motion, primarily flexion, abduction, and external rotation. Only 5 points in all are given for motion per se, because motion by itself is not the important item. Rather, it is the uses of that motion that are critical and this has already been rated heavily under the heading of function.

In the following review of cases, all the ratings have employed this scheme.

REVIEW OF CASES

What, then, will cup arthroplasty deliver in 1971? I have reviewed my last 200 cup arthroplasties using the lateral approach and power tools. Of this group, deep postoperative sepsis occurred in only one patient, but this was one of the ten in this group that had sepsis prior to cup arthroplasty. *Proteus mirabilis* was responsible for this recurrent sepsis, an unusual organism for hip sepsis. Two patients had wound cellulitis that responded to antibiotics but have had no subsequent difficulty over a period of 4 years in one case and 6 years in the other.

Ten revisions have been done, an incidence of 5%. Five of these were necessary because of further avascular necrosis in patients whose primary disease was avascular necrosis. One was for the recurrent sepsis, one for myositis ossificans, and two because of failure to develop cartilaginous metaplasia. The final revision was performed because of sinking of the cup. There were no operative deaths or postoperative deaths within the first 6 months.

Because of the nature of our referral practice in complicated and in unusual hip problems, only 56 of these 200 cup arthroplasties were done in a total of 52 patients with primary osteoarthritis. Thirty-six of these patients had unilateral cup arthroplasties for unilateral disease, whereas four had bilateral cup arthroplasties and twelve had a cup arthroplasty on one side with another type of hip surgery on the other side. The composition of the group is shown in Table 7-1. The sex ratio showed slightly more males than females in the group with bilateral disease.

Among the unilateral cup arthroplasties in *unilateral severe osteoarthritis*, all thirty-six patients rated below 70 preoperatively and only one did so postoperatively. The overall final ratings are shown in Table 7-2. There was a marked improvement in the ratings for pain (Table 7-3). Pain decreased in every patient but one. No patient had moderate or marked pain postoperatively and no patient took any pain medicine stronger than aspirin. The overall figures for total functional improvement are shown in Table 7-4. More specifically, the figures for distance walked showed marked improvement (Table 7-5). Limp also showed substantial improvement (Table 7-6). The need for some support definitely decreased in twenty-

five of the thirty-six patients (69%) (Table 7-7). Eleven patients continued to require some support full time.

The other parameter of daily functional activities also showed a marked improvement following cup arthroplasty. The average flexion contracture postoperatively was 4°, with twenty-three patients having none. The average range of abduction was 20°, with only four patients having less than 5° of abduction. Average postoperative hip flexion was 90°, with the range being 50° to 120°; all but eight patients had flexion of 90° or more. The average leg length discrepancy was 1.4 cm. The Trendelenburg test was negative in 11% of the patients preoperatively and 80% of the patients postoperatively. No revisions were done. No cases of sepsis developed.

In summary, for a patient of an average age of 63 years with severe unilateral osteoarthritis, cup arthroplasty done via the lateral approach can offer a high degree of relief from pain, a satisfactory but slightly restricted range of motion, and marked improvement in functional capacity. In 70% of such patients no support or at most a single cane is required for long walks and virtually all of them will be able to walk 2/3 of a mile or more.

The problems presented by the presence of *bilateral disease* are obviously far more formidable. The change in overall rating in these patients is shown in Table 7-8. In terms of pain, the improvement was great but not as impressive as in unilateral disease (Table 7-9). Limp also improved (Table 7-10). The total functional points are shown in Table 7-11. Leg length discrepancy is even less of a problem in bilateral cases, the average being 0.8 cm. There was abduction of 10° or more in all but one patient and an average flexion of 90°. Seven patients had less than 90° of

Table 7-1. Composition of group of patients with primary osteoarthritis who underwent cup arthroplasty

	Number of patients	Age		Sex		Duration of follow-up	
		Range (yr.)	Average (yr.)	Male	Female	Range (mo.)	Average (mo.)
Unilateral disease	36	38-81	63	21	15	12-39	24
Bilateral disease	16 (20 hips)	43-67	61	10	6	12-55	35

Table 7-2. Overall ratings in patients with unilateral disease

	Below 60	60 to 69	60 to 70	80 to 89	90 to 100
Preoperative	30	6	0	0	0
Postoperative	0	1	9	14	12

Table 7-3. Ratings for pain in patients with unilateral disease

	None	*Slight*	*Mild*	*Moderate*	*Marked*	*Disabled*
Preoperative	0	0	2	21	13	0
Postoperative	12	16	8	0	0	0

Table 7-4. Total points for function in patients with unilateral disease

	Range	*Average*	*Mode*
Preoperative	12-39	24	26
Postoperative	27-47	38	44

Table 7-5. Distances patients with unilateral disease could walk

	Unlimited	*6 blocks*	*2 to 3 blocks*	*Indoors only*	*Confined to bed and chair*
Preoperative	11	8	12	5	0
Postoperative	31	5	0	0	0

Table 7-6. Limp in patients with unilateral disease

	None	*Slight*	*Moderate*	*Severe*	*Unable to walk*
Preoperative	2	4	25	5	0
Postoperative	10	21	5	0	0

Table 7-7. Need for support in patients with unilateral disease

	None	*One cane for long walks*	*Cane full time*	*Crutch*	*Two canes*	*Two crutches*	*Unable to walk*
Preoperative	13	3	13	1	0	6	0
Postoperative	15	10	7	3	0	1	0

Table 7-8. Overall ratings in patients with bilateral disease

	Below 60	*60 to 69*	*70 to 79*	*80 to 89*	*90 to 100*
Preoperative	20	0	0	0	0
Postoperative	2	4	8	5	1

Table 7-9. Ratings for pain in patients with bilateral disease

	None	*Slight*	*Mild*	*Moderate*	*Marked*	*Disabled*
Preoperative	0	0	0	9	11	0
Postoperative	6	6	6	1	1	0

Table 7-10. Limp in patients with bilateral disease

	None	*Slight*	*Moderate*	*Severe*	*Unable to walk*
Preoperative	1	5	8	6	0
Postoperative	7	11	2	0	0

Table 7-11. Total points for function in patients with bilateral disease

	Range	*Average*	*Mode*
Preoperative	8-31	22	20
Postoperative	24-47	30	26

Table 7-12. Distances patients with bilateral disease could walk

	Unlimited	6 blocks	2 to 3 blocks	Indoors only	Confined to bed and chair
Preoperative	3	3	4	10	0
Postoperative	10	7	3	0	0

Table 7-13. Need for support in patients with bilateral disease

	None	One cane for long walks	Cane full time	Crutch	Two canes	Two crutches
Preoperative	6	1	6	1	1	5
Postoperative	4	2	4	1	4	5

flexion, the range being 55° to 120°. The average postoperative flexion contracture was 17°, with a range of 0° to 40°. Walking ability was enhanced (Table 7-12), but the need for support remained quite high (Table 7-13). Of the twenty hips in which cup arthroplasty was performed, seven patients were unable to put on their socks and tie their shoes independently. One patient had to have a revision because of failure to develop fibrocartilage, the only revision in the entire group. No patient had post-operative infection. There were no dislocations, sub-luxations, or pulmonary emboli.

SUMMARY

In the treatment of severe osteoarthritis, cup arthroplasty provides excellent relief of pain and good motion in a high percentage of patients. The need for revision is very low, the danger of infection is even lower, and complications are few. The results in unilateral disease are distinctly superior to those in bilateral disease.

The results using cup arthroplasty and total hip replacement are of such a high caliber that fusion is less and less frequently done in this country in the treatment of severe osteoarthritis. While enthusiastically acknowledging the excellent early results with total hip replacement, two major concerns persist relative to the uncritical use of total hip replacement. The first is sepsis. The second is the long-term effect. Not only is the incidence of sepsis high in several series but the magnitude of the disaster that results when a total hip replacement becomes septic is, in some cases, overwhelming. The concern about the long-term effect deals with both wear and late toxic potential. Since data on total replacement cover only a period of 9 years, these concerns are paramount in deciding what therapy should be used in patients with a life-span of 20 years or more.

Orthopaedics has suffered through the trials of the acrylic prosthesis, through the disaster of ostamer, and through the failure of the Teflon total hip replacement. Good judgment is mandatory to avoid adding another chapter to that list.

For the aforementioned reasons I have confined the use of total hip replacement to patients 50 years or older or to younger patients who have a limited life-span. Patients with bilateral disease and those with a marked leg length discrepancy are sometimes exceptions to this rule, since the solution to their problem by cup arthroplasty is not as effective as in a patient with unilateral disease who has full leg length.

REFERENCES

1. Aufranc, O. E.: Constructive hip surgery with Vitallium mold: a report on 1000 cases of arthroplasty of the hip over a fifteen-year period, J. Bone Joint Surg. **39-A:** 237, 1957.
2. Aufranc, O. E.: Constructive surgery of the hip, St. Louis, 1962, The C. V. Mosby Co.
3. Aufranc, O. E., and Sweet, E. B.: The study of patients with hip arthroplasty at Massachusetts General Hospital, J.A.M.A. **170:**507, 1959.
4. Charnley, J., and Ferreira, A. de S. D.: Transplantation of the greater trochanter in arthroplasty of the hip, J. Bone Joint Surg. **46-B:**191, 1964.
5. Harris, W. H.: A new lateral approach to the hip joint, J. Bone Joint Surg. **49-A:**891, 1967.
6. Harris, W. H.: Traumatic arthritis of the hip after dislocation and acetabular fractures: treatment by mold arthroplasty. An end result study using a new method of results evaluation, J. Bone Joint Surg. **51-A:**737, 1969.
7. Harris, W. H., and Aufranc, O. E.: Mold arthroplasty —its use in the treatment of sepsis following hip nailing, J. Bone Joint Surg. **47-A:**31, 1965.
8. Harris, W. H., and Hamblen, D. L.: Septic arthritis of the hip in the adult: management using mold arthroplasty, Proc. Roy. Soc. Med. **62:**14, 1969.

9. Harris, W. H., Salzman, E. W., and DeSanctis, R.: The prevention of thromboembolic disease by prophylactic anticoagulation, J. Bone Joint Surg. **49-A**:81, 1967.

10. Hunt, D. D., and Larson, C. B.: Treatment of residua of hip infections by mold arthroplasty. An end result study of 33 hips, J. Bone Joint Surg. **48-A**:111, 1966.

11. Ivins, J. C., Benson, W. F., Bickel, W. H., and Nelson, J. W.: Arthroplasty of the hip for idiopathic degenerative disease, Surg. Gynec. Obstet. **125**:1281, 1967.

12. Jakobsen, A.: Vitallium mould arthroplasty for osteoarthritis of the hip joint, New York, 1958, The Macmillan Co.

13. Johnston, R. C., and Larson, C. B.: A study of the abductor mechanism in patients with cup arthroplasty, J. Bone Joint Surg. **50-A**:1496, 1968.

14. Johnston, R. C., and Larson, C. B.: Biomechanics of cup arthroplasty, Clin. Orthop. **66**:56, 1969.

15. Johnston, R. C., and Larson, C. B.: Results of treat-

16. Law, W. A.: Late results of Vitallium mold arthroplasty of the hip, J. Bone Joint Surg. **44-A**:1497, 1962.

17. Smith-Petersen, M. N.: Arthroplasty of the hip: a new method, J. Bone Joint Surg. **21-A**:269, 1939.

18. Smith-Petersen, M. N., Larson, C. B., Aufranc, O. E., and Law, W. A.: Complications of old fractures of the neck of femur. Results of treatment by Vitallium mold arthroplasty, J. Bone Joint Surg. **29**:41, 1947.

19. Solomon, L., and Aufranc, O. E.: Vitallium mold arthroplasty of the hip in rheumatoid arthritis, Arthritis Rheum. **5**:37, 1962.

20. Stinchfield, F. E., and Carroll, R. E.: Vitallium cup arthroplasty of the hip joint. An end result study, J. Bone Joint Surg. **31-A**:628, 1949.

21. Tubiana, R., and Duparc, J.: Prevention of thromboembolic complications in orthopedic and accident surgery, J. Bone Joint Surg. **43-B**:7, 1961.

Part IV

Total prosthesis for severe osteoarthritis of the hip

R. MERLE d'AUBIGNÉ, M.D., M. POSTEL, M.D., and M. KERBOULL, M.D.

Paris, France

Since 1946 we have been evaluating the methods used in the treatment of nearly 2,000 patients with osteoarthritis (Fig. 7-12). The patients have been reviewed 1 month, 3 months, 6 months, and 1 year postoperatively and then yearly. The preoperative and postoperative states have been compared using a grading system we published in 1948, a grading probably imperfect but simple, easy to use, and relatively accurate (Table 7-14). We have not devised any personal technique but tried to use the methods proposed by some reliable authors. We visited Smith-Petersen in 1948 and 1952, Pauwels in 1954, received Austin Moore in 1953, and visited Charnley in 1963 and McKee in 1965.

During these 20 years our methods have changed, especially when unsatisfactory results drove us to some other technique. Apart from arthrodesis and osteotomy, which are applicable in a limited number of cases, and cup arthroplasty, to which we have remained relatively faithful, our efforts in arthroplasty varied to a large extent.

In 1965, comparing the results in severe cases of osteoarthritis, we made the following observations:

1. Arthrodesis is a sound procedure with an 82% success rate but is restricted to patients with

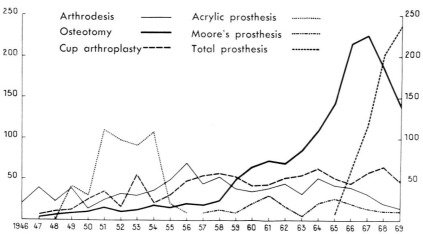

Fig. 7-12. Operations used for osteoarthritis at Hôpital Cochin since 1946.

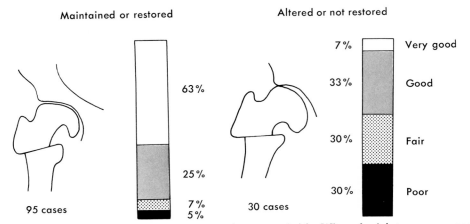

Maintained or restored   Altered or not restored

63%

25%

7%
5%

95 cases   30 cases

7%   Very good
33%   Good
30%   Fair
30%   Poor

Fig. 7-13. Results of displacement osteotomy in osteoarthritis. When the joint space appears parallel, either in neutral position, abduction, or adduction, success is frequent.

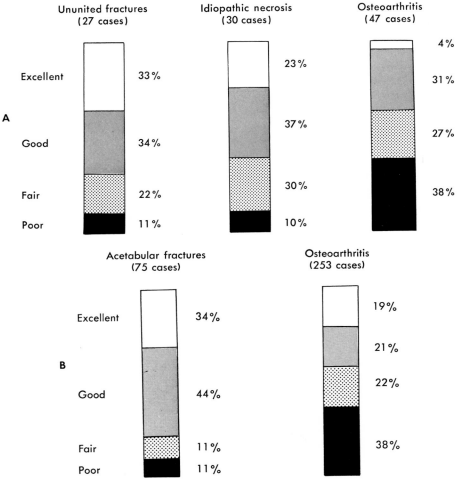

Ununited fractures   Idiopathic necrosis   Osteoarthritis
(27 cases)   (30 cases)   (47 cases)

A

Excellent   33%   23%   4%
Good   34%   37%   31%
Fair   22%   30%   27%
Poor   11%   10%   38%

Acetabular fractures   Osteoarthritis
(75 cases)   (253 cases)

B

Excellent   34%   19%
Good   44%   21%
                                         22%
Fair   11%
Poor   11%   38%

Fig. 7-14. A, Comparison of the results of Moore's prosthesis in patients with a sound acetabulum (ununited fractures or necrotic head of femur) and in those with osteoarthritis. **B,** Comparison of the results of cup arthroplasty when used as an acetabular prosthesis in patients with a sound femoral head (fracture of acetabulum) versus results in those with osteoarthritis (cup arthroplasty).

unilateral disease who have a sound vertebral column and knees.

2. Osteotomy is reliable in patients in whom pre-operative x-ray films show a parallel joint space, either in neutral position, in abduction, or in adduction, but failure is too frequent if this radiologic character is absent (Fig. 7-13).

3. As for arthroplasty, although the use of a Vitallium prosthesis did not produce bone absorption, as was observed with the acrylic prosthesis, it very rarely gave a painless hip when there was an abnormal acetabulum. On the contrary, the Vitallium head, when substituted for a necrotic head in the presence of a normal acetabulum, gave almost uniformly excellent hip results.

4. Cup arthroplasty was found to be better, but it produced really good hips in only 45% of the cases, and these results were obtained only after months and sometimes years of patient rehabilitation. However, replacement of a damaged acetabulum with a cup after fracture gave, when the head was essentially normal, a very high proportion of nearly normal hips (Fig. 7-14).

The success resulting from replacement of the head alone or of the acetabulum alone when the opposite surface was normal, contrasted with the frequent failure when both surfaces were seriously altered, as in osteoarthritis, caused many surgeons to favor the idea of complete replacement by an artificial hip.

PROSTHESES

Charnley and McKee were the real pioneers. They approached the problem in slightly different ways (Fig. 7-15). McKee, having confidence in the good tolerance of Vitallium implants, tried to protect the acetabulum against wear by the prosthetic head. Charnley's idea was clearly expressed by the title of his first publication, *Low Friction Arthroplasty*. His prosthesis was designed after very serious experimental work with engineers. Teflon was originally chosen for the acetabulum component, as it has the lowest coefficient of friction with the metallic head.

At our first visit with Charnley in Manchester we saw beautiful results. But he was having trouble with late tolerance to Teflon and was experimenting with other materials. At the present time he seems quite satisfied with high-density polyethylene, of which the coefficient of friction is between 0.021 and 0.004. This

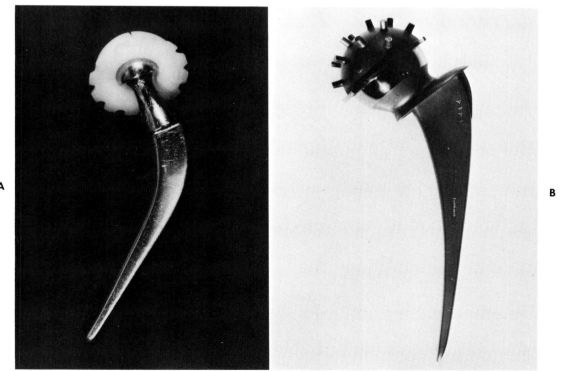

Fig. 7-15. A, Charnley's prosthesis. **B,** McKee's prosthesis.

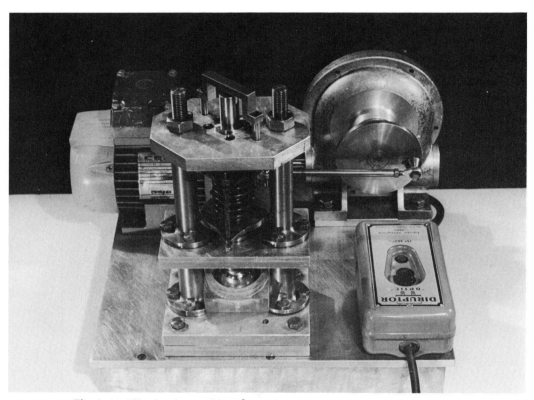

Fig. 7-16. Hip simulator with 60° angular movement and variable pressure.

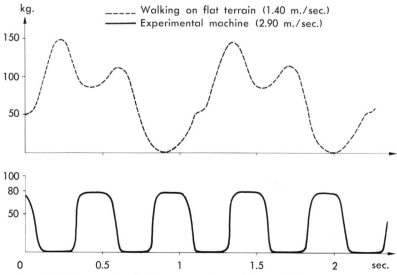

Fig. 7-17. Curve of variable pressure in machine and in normal gait.

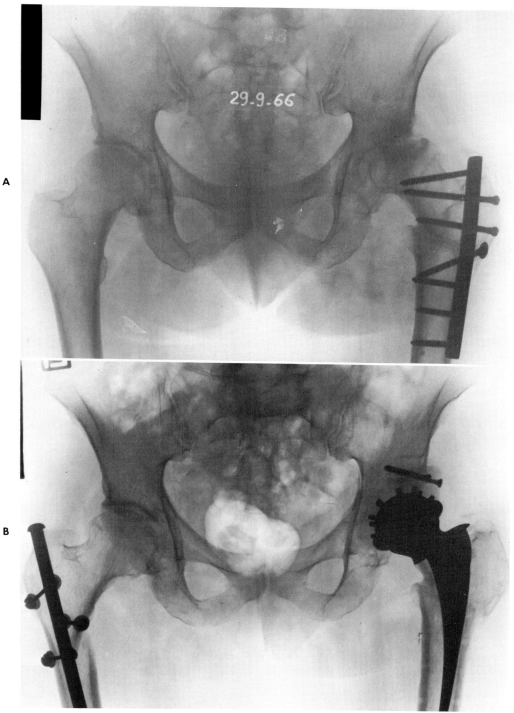

Fig. 7-18. A, A 68-year-old woman with bilateral osteoarthritis in whom displacement osteotomy of the left hip was a failure. **B,** Results were excellent 3 years after total replacement (left hip) and varus osteotomy (right hip).

is twice as much as the friction of cartilage on cartilage (0.005 to 0.010 according to Barnett) and about the same as that of a metallic skate on ice. It is difficult to obtain such low friction in mechanics, apart from ball bearings: industrial rollings with steel on bronze have a coefficient of 0.07 when lubricated with oil, ten times as much as cartilage, but 0.52 when lubricated with saline solution, 100 times more than cartilage. The coefficient of friction should diminish when the pressure increases, as is the case with normal cartilage; this is perhaps possible with steel on plastic but not with metal on metal. Moreover, it is impossible to adjust one spherical surface to another with enough accuracy to allow only a very thin, monomolecular film of liquid to come between the surfaces. For these reasons a relatively soft plastic acetabulum would be preferable to a metallic one. But however important the coefficient of friction may be, in view of the absence of proper lubrication in these artificial joints, the wearing of

the prosthesis probably has more influence on the late results. (See Figs. 7-16 and 7-17.) McKee, on the other hand, claims that although the friction is much higher, a Vitallium head in a Vitallium acetabulum is not likely to lock due to its extreme hardness.

Wearing of the surfaces may cause loosening, which is always a bad mechanical condition. But, above all, the fine particles produced may cause a foreign body reaction in the neighboring tissues, even with an apparently inert material. This happened with Teflon, and late aseptic abscesses were observed in many cases. But it has been shown that even small metallic particles may have properties entirely different from massive pieces. Solid fixation of the prosthesis to the bone seems absolutely necessary. Many of the complications observed after insertion of a prosthesis appear to be caused by progressive mobility of the implant. A methylmethacrylate cement is used by Charnley and McKee, but it is questionable whether this is the best answer. Methylmethacrylate

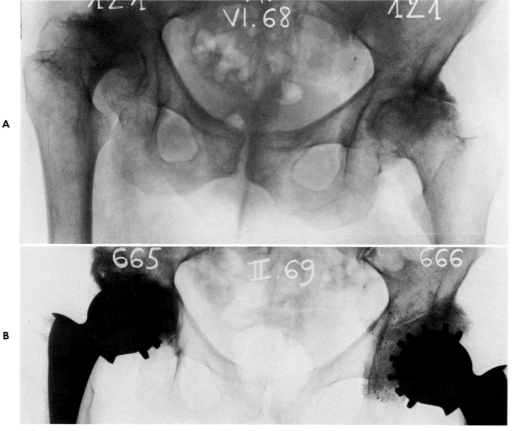

Fig. 7-19. A, A 69-year-old woman with bilateral osteoarthritis; both hips were completely stiff, she had severe permanent pain, and she was bedridden. **B,** Two years after bilateral replacement she had no pain and 90° flexion of both hips. She had a slight limp on the right side.

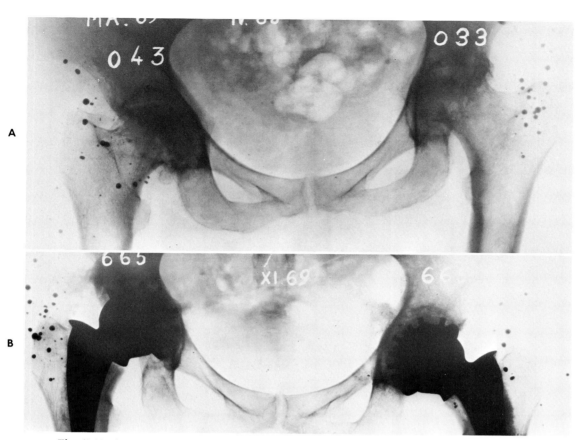

Fig. 7-20. A, A 70-year-old woman with bilateral osteoarthritis who had severe permanent pain in both hips. Mobility was less than 60° flexion. She used two canes. **B,** One and a half years postoperatively she had no pain and 90° flexion. She limped slightly but required no cane.

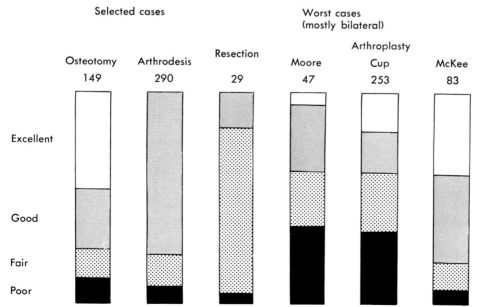

Fig. 7-21. Comparison of the results of other operations for osteoarthritis with the results in our first 83 cases using total replacement.

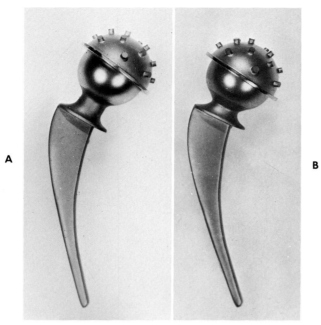

Fig. 7-22. Our modified McKee's prosthesis. **A,** Long neck. **B,** Short neck.

is an unstable, hard, and rather fragile material. It is improbable that it has a carcinogenic action in man, but the selective discovery of a cement that is as well tolerated and has better mechanical properties should be one of the aims of research.

It was clear, and it still is, that we do not have a definite answer to the problem of the artificial hip. But the clinical results obtained by Charnley in Manchester and McKee in Norwich persuaded us that the method was worth trying in the most severe cases of osteoarthritis. We started with the McKee type of prosthesis, as we feared the effects of small particles of plastic produced by wearing of the acetabulum. We now use Charnley's prosthesis also. However, we shall describe our experience at the Orthopaedic Department of the Hôpital Cochin with metallic artificial hips placed from September 1965 to the present time. It amounts to more than 900 artificial hips, of which 300 have been reviewed for 1½ to 4 years after operation. (See Figs. 7-18 to 7-21.)

The prosthesis we use is a very slight modification of McKee's prosthesis (Fig. 7-22). The acetabulum piece is identical, but the shape of the femoral component is not like Thompson's prosthesis but like Austin Moore's. We prefer its more horizontal bearing surface and its rather long stem. There are no holes

because we do not want it to "self-lock." When there is destruction of the neck we sometimes use a long straight stem comparable to the prosthesis we devised in 1952.

SURGICAL TECHNIQUE

The hip is approached by the posterolateral route. The muscles are dealt with in three ways. In a few cases the hip was opened posteriorly, behind the gluteus medius, cutting the pelvic-trochanteric muscles. However, this approach does not give a good view of the acetabulum, is more likely to endanger the sciatic nerve, and in some cases has been attended by the complication of posterior postoperative dislocation.

Some of us (Postel) cut the greater trochanter to be able to adjust the tension of the abductor muscles by raising or lowering it at the end. I (d'Aubigné) prefer to cut the gluteus medius and minimus and to leave the pyriformis and the posterior muscles intact. If the muscles appear too slack at the end, they can be overlapped and sutured. Only in cases of dislocation or protrusion, in which repair of the muscles may be difficult after reposition, is it necessary to cut the greater trochanter.

The ligaments of the hip are then exposed, cut, and in most cases removed. The head is dislocated anteriorly, and the neck is cut with an electric saw. Section is made in such a way that the prosthesis, when in place, restores as exactly as possible the normal position of the head and neck.

The acetabulum is then cleaned, shaped, and deepened with gouges and a reamer. We try to make a hemispheric acetabulum, exactly fitting the outer aspect of the prosthesis as medially as possible. Four holes, 8 mm. in diameter, are then made in the acetabulum to provide anchorage: one anterior in the pubis, two in the roof, and one posterior in the ischium. Great care must be taken to protect the vessels on the deep aspect of the ilium.

Sealing is done by pushing little pieces of acrylic cement in these holes before filling the acetabulum with the cement. The prosthetic acetabulum is then pushed in the acetabulum and held firmly until the cement takes. The position of the prosthesis should be as similar as possible to the normal acetabulum: its axis 20° anterior to the frontal plane and 45° inferior to the horizontal plane. The femur is then prepared with the rasp, filled with cement, and the femoral component put into place. The hip is reduced. If the trochanter has been cut, it is repaired with two wires. If the gluteus muscles have been cut, they are sutured with nylon while an assistant holds the limb in slight abduction and internal rotation. Suction drainage is placed behind the femur (for 24 or 48 hours) and the fascia and skin are closed.

In most cases the limb is kept for a week in suspension and slight traction using a transtibial wire.

Active flexion and extension are started on the first postoperative day. After 8 to 10 days the patient starts walking with crutches. Crutches are discarded and full weight bearing allowed at the end of the third week. At the end of the fourth week many patients can walk without a cane and without a

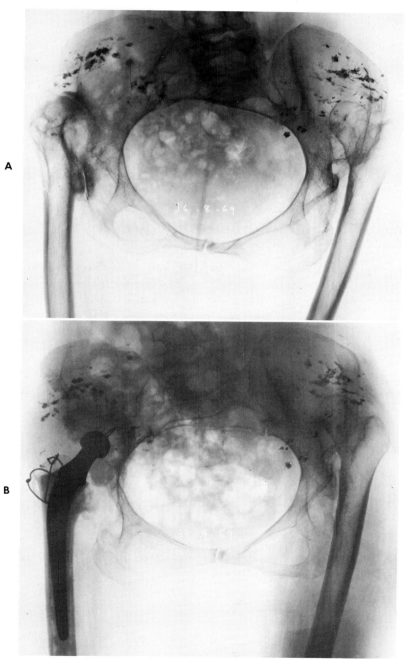

Fig. 7-23. A, A patient with a painful congenital dislocation of the right hip. **B,** One and a half years after insertion of Charnley's prosthesis results were good.

limp and are sent home after being given instructions for a program of exercise. Some patients require a longer rehabilitation period, often 6 weeks to 2 months, and cannot abandon their cane as quickly.

In patients with bilateral disease that necessitates a prosthesis on both sides, we believe it is better to perform the two operations at 2- or 3-week intervals. Rehabilitation of the first hip is not efficient if the opposite hip is painful and stiff, especially when there is contracture in adduction, abduction, or flexion.

We do not use prophylactic antibiotics except when there is a definite danger of sepsis. However, anticoagulant therapy is used routinely and eliminated gradually as the patient starts walking.

SPECIAL TECHNICAL PROBLEMS

High dislocations. In some high congenital dislocations with osteoarthritis it is possible to place the hip nearly in its normal position by enlarging the atrophic acetabulum upward and medially and fixing the femoral prosthesis at the inferior part of the neck. But one should not pull down the head with too great force because of the possible danger to the sciatic nerve. Moreover, since the iliac bone is frequently atrophic, a small prosthesis is necessary. It must be pointed out that one out of ten patients with reduced dislocations has pain (Fig. 7-23).

Osteochondritis. A small prosthesis is also convenient for patients with old reduced dislocations in whom the head and neck are reduced to a very small and deformed stump.

Hypertrophic femur. A prosthesis with a longer neck is useful when osteoarthritis develops on the large femoral heads and necks encountered bilaterally in elderly men.

Former osteotomy. Medial displacement osteotomies with only slight varus or valgus do not cause special problems when their failure necessitates a a total prosthesis. But in the old angulation osteotomies it may be impossible to place the femoral component and a deosteotomy should be performed as a first stage.

RESULTS

Since we have only twenty cases that have been followed for more than 3 years, we cannot speak of late results. Of slightly less than 1,000 operations, 300 patients have been followed for 1 to 12 years. We shall review the uncomplicated cases and discuss the troubles we have had with the complicated cases. There is a great difference between a total

prosthesis and other operations for osteoarthritis. With cup arthroplasty or osteotomy, not until perhaps 6 months later can the results be determined to be good, fair, or poor. After a total prosthesis in which there was a normal postoperative course it takes no longer than 2 months to assess whether the results are good. However, complications occur in some cases and may cause partial or complete failure.

Our first patients were over the age limit of 60 years; they had such severe conditions that the results expected from other procedures were either poor or extremely doubtful. Total prosthesis positively saved them. In practically every case a painless and mobile hip was obtained in a short time. In patients in whom osteotomy or cup arthroplasty had failed or an acrylic prosthesis had deteriorated and caused extensive bone absorption, the results were good. Fear of late deterioration was not a factor in younger patients completely crippled by bilateral painless and stiff hips, since the only alternative was resection of the head and neck, from which we could expect only instability and certainly not painlessness and movement.

The favorable results that we achieved brought to our department a great number of patients with severe involvement of both hips, many of whom had been considered impossible to treat successfully. Indications for this procedure have been widened in patients over 65 years of age since the results are regularly good and quickly obtained. In patients between 55 and 65 years of age a total prosthesis is used only when osteotomy or cup arthroplasty appears unlikely to succeed. Under 55 years of age, only patients with bilateral stiff hips are considered for total prostheses as a substitute for the Girdlestone or Milch operation.

At the present time, with 4 years of follow-up experience and a little less than 1,000 operations, we can state that in all uncomplicated cases the artificial hip eliminates pain completely, restores or maintains good mobility of the hip, and permits in a very short time (1 month to 6 weeks in unilateral cases; 3 months to 4 months in bilateral cases) the possibility of walking, very often without a cane.

Early complications

There were some early complications. Sciatic palsy occurred in five patients; it was transitory in three and one has almost completely recovered. Dislocation occurred in two patients (the posterior approach was used in both). All our patients received anticoagulant therapy. Nevertheless, we observed eleven cases of

Table 7-14. Functional grading of hip

Pain		Mobility		Gait	
None	6	No contracture, range of flexion =		Normal	6
Slight or occasional	5	90° or more	6	Slight limp or cane for distance	5
After some walk		80°-70°	5	One cane out-of-doors	4
30 min. - 1 hr.	4	70°-50°	4	One cane at all times	3
10-20 min.	3	50°-30°	3	Two canes	2
Less than 10 min.	2	Less than 30°	2	Crutches	1
Immediate	1	Contracture in flexion or external		Bedridden	0
Permanent and severe	0	rotation superior to 30°			
		Contracture in abduction, adduction, or internal rotation	⎫⎬⎭ Subtract 1 or 2		

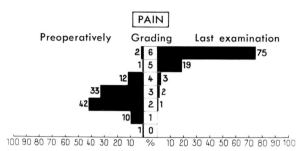

Fig. 7-24. Results of total prosthesis in regard to pain. All patients had severe pain before the operation. All patients were practically pain free postoperatively.

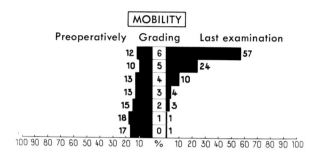

Fig. 7-25. Results of total prosthesis in regard to mobility. In all patients, mobility was reduced before the operation. Postoperatively, mobility was near normal in 57% of the patients and good in 24% of the patients.

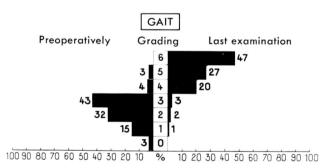

Fig. 7-26. Results of total prosthesis in regard to gait. Preoperatively, most patients used crutches, two canes, or one cane all the time. All except nine patients had a limp. Postoperatively, 74% of the patients were able to walk without a cane and did not even have a limp.

thrombophlebitis with six cases of pulmonary embolism, one of them fatal. In three patients hematomas occurred, probably due to anticoagulant therapy, but evacuation was performed without consequences. Eight cases of superficial infections were observed but they did not affect the final functional result.

Functional results

Functional results were very carefully evaluated before operation and the last examination (Table 7-14). As shown in Fig. 7-24, the pain, always present and generally severe or very severe before operation, was relieved in all but eighteen patients; most of these showed improvement, however. Postoperatively, mobility was greater than 90° of flexion in 57% of the cases and greater than 80° in 81% of the cases, regardless of the degree of stiffness present before operation (Fig. 7-25). Gait was also satisfactory, half of the patients being able to walk without a cane or limp. Twenty-seven percent of the patients had a slight limp or used a cane for long distance. Only 6% of the patients required the permanent use of a cane or crutches (Fig. 7-26).

Late complications

In spite of the excellent results, two complications occurred—infection and loosening of the prosthesis.

Infection. Although there was no acute operative infection, of the 300 cases, pain, a high sedimentation rate, and sometimes elevated temperature appeared in nine patients with delayed deep low-grade infection. This was verified at reoperation in one patient in whom removal of the prosthesis was necessary. But we must add that of the complete series of more than 1,000 cases, deep infection made the removal of the prosthesis necessary in seven patients. In one other case the prosthesis was left in place after debridement, and the patient is doing well at the present.

Loosening. Loosening of the prosthesis is the other cause of failure. Of these 300 cases, it appears probable that loosening has occurred in sixteen cases, although some of these patients are completely free of pain. Loosening has been verified by reoperation in eight cases. The prosthesis was removed and reinserted later, but at least four of the eight patients had a recurrence of pain, probably due to loosening. It is worth mentioning that the differential diagnosis of mechanical as opposed to infectious problems is very difficult. In some patients in whom we suspected low-grade infection we found loosening but negative bacteriologic tests.

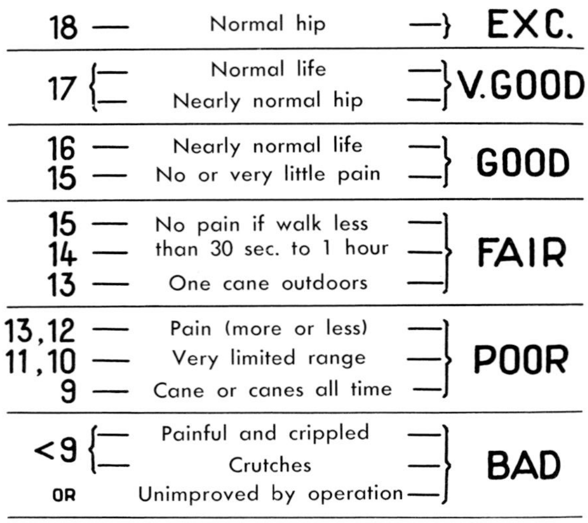

SUMMARY

To give an overall picture of the value of this operation, we have made a global evaluation of hip function (Fig. 7-27). A completely normal hip, scarcely ever seen previously after operation for osteoarthritis, is classified as "excellent." "Very good" means no pain at all and a normal gait. "Good" means very slight or occasional pain, and "fair" is still good, with use of a cane only necessary out-of-doors. Cases are classified as "bad" if the operation did not bring about improvement, even though function was acceptable.

As shown in Fig. 7-28, all the patients' conditions were poor or bad before operation; only 4% have not improved, 80% have really good function, and 93% are pain free if they limit walking to less than half an hour. The use of a cane is necessary only out-of-doors. In patients with a total prosthesis on both sides, the functional results are comparable.

Fig. 7-27. Global evaluation of hip function after insertion of total prosthesis.

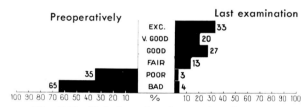

Fig. 7-28. Global results after total replacement.

Of course, we must wait some more years before this operation can really be evaluated. The danger of loosening, although it seems to nearly always occur in the first year, remains an important problem in some cases and should inspire research work on cement and fixation to bone. But in our opinion, the total prosthesis must be considered a great step forward in the treatment of painful and stiff hips.

Chapter 8

Osteotomies and muscle release operations about the hip

KARL H. MUELLER, M.D.
Milwaukee, Wisconsin

Osteoarthritis, according to Pauwels, is a biomechanical problem with tissue tolerance representing the biologic factor and structure and function of the joint the mechanical factor. In a normal joint, tissue tolerance is adequate to withstand stress from normal joint function during the individual's entire lifetime. In osteoarthritis, either one of these two factors can be altered to cause premature degeneration of the joint.

Idiopathic osteoarthritis
Normal joint structure and mechanics
Diminished tissue tolerance
Secondary osteoarthritis
Physiologic tissue tolerance
Deranged joint mechanics with increased stress

Hackenbroch has taught us the importance of the prearthrotic lesion that precedes degeneration of the joint. In secondary osteoarthritis, degeneration is due to a preexisting deformity of the joint from hip dysplasia, Legg-Perthes disease, epiphysiolysis, infectious or rheumatoid arthritis, trauma, etc. This deformity alters the mechanics of the joint. It places increased stress on the articular tissue, which exceeds its physiologic tolerance and thus leads to the well-known condition of secondary osteoarthritis. Idiopathic osteoarthritis, on the other hand, develops in a joint with originally normal structure and function. We must assume that the prearthrotic lesion is a diminished tissue tolerance that is probably generalized. The articular tissues can no longer withstand stress from normal joint function and osteoarthritic changes gradually develop.

This classification also enables us to predict the natural course of the disease and helps us to plan treatment. We know from the work of Danielsson in Sweden, Carrol B. Larsen in this country, and from our own studies that the course of idiopathic osteo-

arthritis cannot be predicted. In some patients the disease progresses rapidly; in others it progresses slowly. Sometimes it remains stationary for a long time and it may even get better without treatment. Secondary osteoarthritis, on the other hand, continues to progress after symptoms have appeared, no matter what conservative measures are employed. We cannot predict when a deformed hip joint will become painful, but once it has become painful, we know that symptoms will progress.

On the basis of this knowledge of the natural course of the disease, we can now formulate indications for treatment. Since we do not know how rapidly, if at all, idiopathic osteoarthritis will progress, conservative treatment is justified in the beginning. Weight reduction, an occasional pain pill, and support from a cane or crutches, augmented by the modalities of physical medicine, may be all the patient requires. If conservative treatment fails to retard progression of the disease, operative measures should be resorted to. When pain appears in a joint with secondary osteoarthritis, we know that the disease will progress. Conservative measures cannot prevent further degeneration of the joint but may cause us to miss the optimal time for operation. Prolonged treatment with intra-articular steroids is risky and may do more harm than good, as shown by the following case:

Case 1. R. J., a 58-year-old white woman with secondary osteoarthritis due to hip dysplasia, has had pain since 1959 (Fig. 8-1, *A*). She was treated with multiple intra-articular injections of hydrocortisone from June 1962 (Fig. 8-1, *B*) until October 1962 (Fig. 8-1, *C*), when she developed avascular necrosis of the femoral head. She should have been treated by osteotomy instead.

Patients with painful secondary osteoarthritis will require surgery sooner or later and we should not

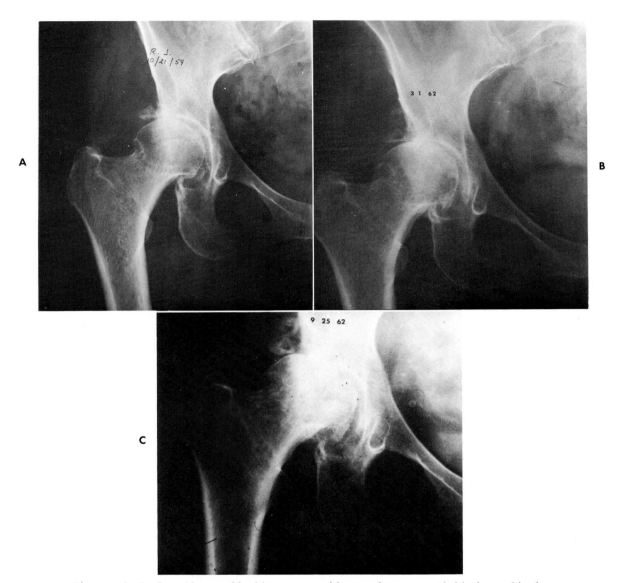

Fig. 8-1. A, R. J., a 58-year-old white woman with secondary osteoarthritis due to hip dysplasia, has had pain since 1959. Multiple intra-articular injections of hydrocortisone were administered from June 1962, **B,** until October 1962, **C,** when she developed avascular necrosis of the femoral head. Osteotomy should have been the treatment of choice.

waste valuable time with prolonged conservative treatment. The best treatment, of course, is prophylactic correction of the deformity long before osteoarthritis develops. This is especially true in patients with congenital dysplasia of the hip. Three valuable procedures are available to correct the main deformities. Valgus and anteversion deformity can be corrected very effectively by intertrochanteric varus derotation osteotomy. Innominate osteotomy, developed by Salter, corrects the fetal position of the acetabulum, whereas Chiari's pelvic osteotomy is used to deepen a shallow acetabulum. We prefer the following plan of treatment:

Intertrochanteric varus derotation osteotomy should be done in the first 3 years of life for persistent valgus and anteversion deformity of the upper femur. If done early, this operation will usually influence the development of the acetabulum enough to correct the existing dysplasia. Innominate osteotomy is reserved for those cases in which the acetabulum fails to develop adequately after correction of valgus and anteversion or in which the fetal position of the acetabulum is the main deformity. In my experience, innominate osteotomy done in the presence of marked anteversion of the femoral neck usually fails to influence this deformity significantly. When a very shallow acetabulum is present, I prefer the Chiari pelvic osteotomy. Innominate osteotomy done in the absence of adequate depth of the acetabulum may cause posterior instability of the hip joint.

SURGICAL PROCEDURES

Unfortunately, most of our patients consult us after painful arthritic changes have developed, and sooner or later we will be faced with the decision to operate. Which surgical procedures are available today for treatment of the osteoarthritic hip? We can choose from one of the following groups of operations:

1. Operations that preserve the patient's own hip joint: osteotomies, muscle release operations
2. Arthroplasties: cup arthroplasty, femoral head prosthesis, total replacement arthroplasty
3. Arthrodesis
4. Salvage procedures: femoral head resection, resection angulation osteotomy

Before we decide which operative procedure to use we must consider if the patient's own hip joint can be restored to pain-free, useful function or whether the degenerative process has done irreparable damage to the articular surfaces. If the damage is irreparable, the only possible solution is radical destruction of the existing joint by arthroplasty, arthrodesis, or one of the salvage procedures.

Total replacement prostheses such as those developed by Charnley, McKee, and Farrar in England or Maurice Mueller in Switzerland may some day be an answer to these problems. If the articular damage is less severe, one of the joint-preserving operations, preferably osteotomy, should be considered. The patient with 60° or more of hip flexion is a good candidate for osteotomy. Hip flexion of less than 50° is usually an indication that the degenerative process is too far advanced and the joint can no longer be restored to pain-free, useful function by osteotomy. Muscle release operations, arthroplasty, arthrodesis, or salvage procedures should then be considered.

An intertrochanteric osteotomy relieves pain, corrects deformity, and reverses the degenerative process. The operation is not difficult to perform, does not require extensive postoperative rehabilitation, and does not "burn any bridges." The "hanging hip" operation decompresses the joint by muscle release. The operation is done mainly for pain relief. It does not usually improve motion significantly but places it into a more functional range by correction of contractures. Osteotomy has a muscular decompression effect that is similar to that of the hanging hip procedure. In addition, it increases the weight-bearing area of the hip joint and relieves pain by cutting the bone. This pain-relieving effect from injuring the bone can be added to the hanging hip operation by osteotomy of the greater trochanter or by drilling or curetting the neck of the femur. Osteotomy and muscle release can be and in many cases should be combined, as will be discussed later.

TYPES OF OSTEOTOMIES

We distinguish two main types of osteotomies in the treatment of osteoarthritis of the hip—both are angulation osteotomies, one with angulation into varus and the other with angulation into valgus. In more advanced cases it may be necessary to correct in two or even three planes, for example, correction of valgus, anteversion, and flexion deformity in a patient with secondary osteoarthritis due to hip dysplasia. Angulation can be combined with medial displacement of the shaft of the femur, but the most effective component of the osteotomy is *angulation of the proximal fragment to increase the weight-bearing surface.* A pure displacement osteotomy is indicated very rarely and only in those cases in which the weight-bearing surfaces of the hip joint are congruous.

There has been considerable controversy as to the effect of medial displacement of the femoral shaft. Some authors maintain that medial displacement alters hip joint mechanics by moving the supporting leg closer to the center of gravity. This would be correct only if the whole hip joint were moved. A modification of a drawing by Pauwels demonstrating that medial displacement merely produces a "bend" in the support of the balance but does not alter its mechanics is shown in Fig. 8-2. Medial displacement of the femoral shaft does have effects on the hip joint, however.

1. By shortening the distance between their origin and insertion, it relaxes the adductors and iliopsoas and thus produces an additional decompression effect.
2. With a valgus osteotomy, medial displacement can be used to create a second point of support under the pelvis if the muscle strength or weight-bearing surface of the hip joint remains inadequate even after osteotomy (Fig. 8-3).

One effect of medial displacement is rarely mentioned in the literature. Medial displacement changes

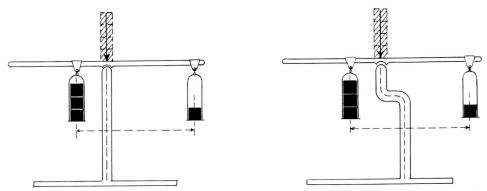

Fig. 8-2. Modification of a drawing by Pauwels showing that medial displacement merely produces a "bend" in the support of the balance but does not alter its mechanics. (From Mueller, K. H.: Clin. Orthop. **77:**117, 1971).

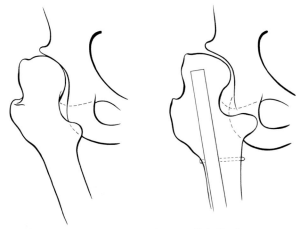

Fig. 8-3. Valgus osteotomy plus medial displacement can be used to create a second point of support under the pelvis if muscle strength or weight-bearing surface of the hip joint remains inadequate even after osteotomy.

the bending stress on the femoral shaft and the knee. This latter effect is important and should be considered when an osteotomy of the hip is done. A valgus osteotomy of the hip displaces the weight-bearing line toward the outside of the knee joint, thus producing a valgus stress on the knee. The addition of medial displacement moves the weight-bearing line even more laterally and increases valgus stress on the knee. Most patients who have had a valgus displacement osteotomy will develop a knock-knee postoperatively, which may be troublesome enough to warrant treatment, especially in those patients who have had some degree of genu valgum deformity before osteotomy (Fig. 8-4). Varus osteotomy, on the other hand, causes the weight-bearing line to fall through the medial side of the knee joint and produces varus stress on the knee. This increased

varus stress on the knee can be lessened or removed by adding medial displacement to the angulation into varus. We now recommend some medial displacement with each varus osteotomy, whereas valgus osteotomy is performed without medial displacement. Displacement should not exceed one third of the width of the femoral shaft, however, because marked medial displacement makes subsequent total hip joint arthroplasty difficult or even impossible.

What are the effects of osteotomies and muscle release operations on the hip joint? We have learned from Pauwels that two mechanical factors play an important role in achieving the improvements seen after osteotomy: (1) reduction of muscle pressure and (2) increase in weight-bearing surface. A successful osteotomy must incorporate both factors. Varus osteotomy, as shown in Fig. 8-5, increases the weight-bearing area and at the same time relaxes all three important muscle groups about the hip joint. Valgus osteotomy also increases the weight-bearing area but does not produce muscle relaxation (Fig. 8-6). Medial and upward displacement of the distal fragment, added to the angulation into valgus, will cause relaxation of the adductors and iliopsoas. The same effect can be achieved by tenotomy of these muscles, which does not add to the valgus stress on the knee.

If muscle strength or weight-bearing surface of the hip joint remains inadequate even after osteotomy, a second point of support can be created under the pelvis with marked medial and upward displacement of the femoral shaft combined with angulation into valgus (Fig. 8-3). This procedure produces considerable valgus stress on the knee and is not recommended for patients with preexisting knock-knee. It is a good procedure, however, to stabilize a paralytic hip (Fig. 8-7). Most of these patients would now be candidates for total joint arthroplasty.

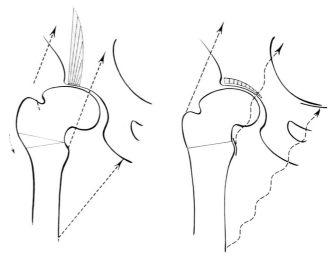

Fig. 8-6. Valgus osteotomy increases the weight-bearing area but does not produce muscle relaxation. Muscle relaxation can be obtained by tenotomy of the iliopsoas and adductors.

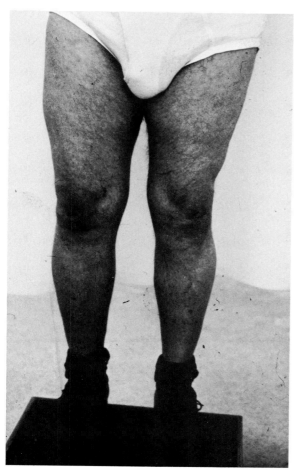

Fig. 8-4. A 58-year-old patient 3 years following valgus displacement osteotomy. Note the knock-knee deformity on the left.

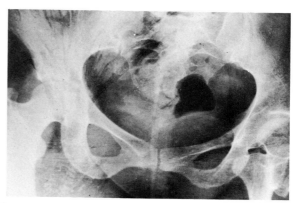

Fig. 8-7. A 43-year-old white woman with paralytic valgus deformity of the left hip following poliomyelitis. Gait and stability improved considerably after valgus displacement osteotomy.

INDICATIONS

Varus osteotomy is indicated in early or moderately advanced osteoarthritis. The patient usually has a good range of motion of the hip but should have at least 60° to 70° of flexion and 15° to 20° of abduction. Osteotomy does not always increase motion of the joint. To avoid fixed adduction deformity, angulation into varus should not exceed the patient's preoperative range of abduction. X-ray examination in abduction must either show the femoral head well centered in the acetabulum or a definite increase in congruity of the joint surfaces (Fig. 8-8). Partial avascular necrosis of the femoral head is also a good

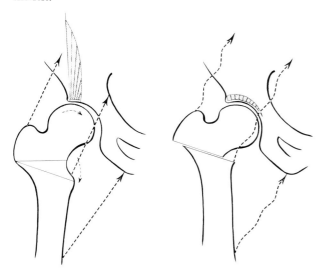

Fig. 8-5. Varus osteotomy increases the weight-bearing area and at the same time relaxes all three important muscle groups about the hip joint.

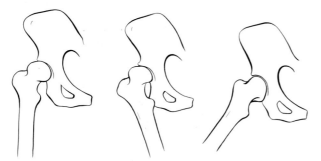

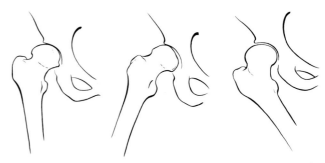

Fig. 8-8. Drawings of x-ray views of right hip in neutral, abducted, and adducted positions. Such positions are a good indication for varus osteotomy.

Fig. 8-9. Drawings of x-ray views of right hip in neutral, abducted, and adducted positions. Such positions are a good indication for valgus osteotomy. (From Mueller, K. H.: In Rütt, A., editor: Die Therapie der Koxarthrose, Stuttgart, 1969, Georg Thieme Verlag.)

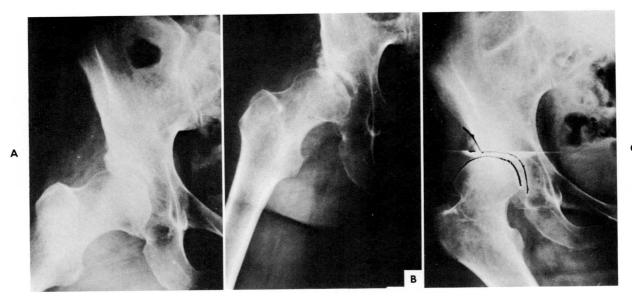

Fig. 8-10. Beginning osteoarthritis due to hip dysplasia. **A,** X-ray film taken in abduction shows considerable increase in the weight-bearing area and good congruity of the joint surfaces. **B,** Two years later an x-ray film taken in abduction shows decrease of the weight-bearing area. **C,** X-ray film taken in adduction shows increase in the weight-bearing area. Indications had changed from varus to valgus osteotomy with advancing disease. (Courtesy Dr. R. D. Ray, Chicago, Ill.)

indication for varus osteotomy provided an area of good bone can be brought into the weight-bearing area.

Valgus osteotomy is indicated in advanced osteoarthritis and arthritis due to deformity of the femoral head from Legg-Perthes disease, a slipped epiphysis, etc. The patient may have an adduction contracture or should have some adduction of the hip. Here again angulation into valgus should not exceed the patient's preoperative adduction. X-ray examination in adduc-

tion must show an increase in congruity of the weight-bearing surfaces (Fig. 8-9).

Indications for varus or valgus osteotomies can change with advancing disease. A patient who presents a good indication for a varus osteotomy today may progress to a point where varus osteotomy is no longer possible but where a valgus osteotomy is now the procedure of choice (Fig. 8-10). A small group of patients in the transition period may benefit from a pure displacement osteotomy without angulation, as

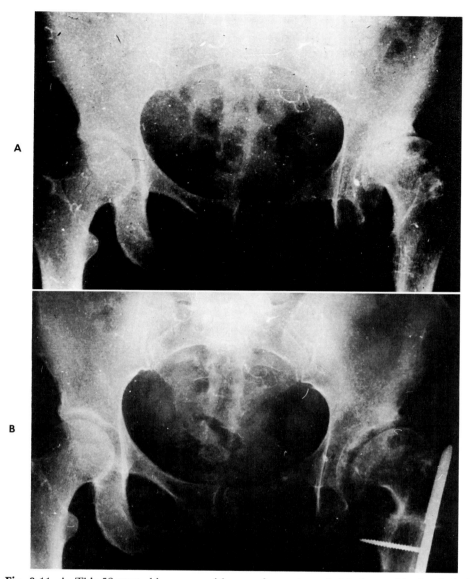

Fig. 8-11. A, This 52-year-old woman with secondary osteoarthritis due to hip dysplasia has good congruity of the weight-bearing surfaces. **B,** Three years later, a pain-free hip with good motion was obtained following displacement osteotomy.

long as the weight-bearing surfaces are congruous (Fig. 8-11).

Muscle release operations should be reserved for advanced osteoarthritis in older people. The patient usually has marked, painful limitation of motion in all directions and the weight-bearing area cannot be increased. If greater congruity of the articular surfaces can be achieved and hip motion is adequate, osteotomy is preferable. Results of muscle release operations are better and longer lasting in hips with congruous joint surfaces and concentric narrowing of the joint space. The majority of these patients belong to the group with idiopathic osteoarthritis. The hanging hip operation is usually not indicated for a patient with good range of motion or in young, active individuals. With time, these patients frequently regain their former muscle tone, the hanging hip effect is lost, and pain recurs. I have also done muscle release successfully in several patients with "tight," painful femoral head prostheses and recommend adding it to synovectomy for rheumatoid hip disease.

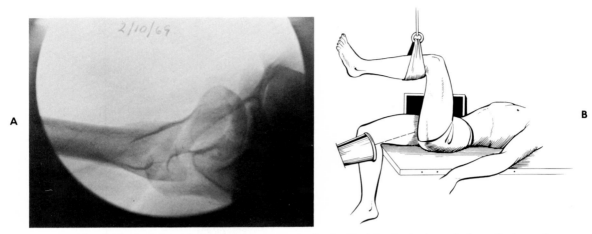

Fig. 8-12. A, A lateral view is necessary to study the hip joint in the lateral plane. It shows the weight-bearing relationships of the acetabulum and femoral head in a functional position and will give us a fairly accurate measurement of the anteversion angle. **B,** Technique used for shoot-through lateral x-ray film. (From Mueller, K. H.: Clin. Orthop. **77:**117, 1971.)

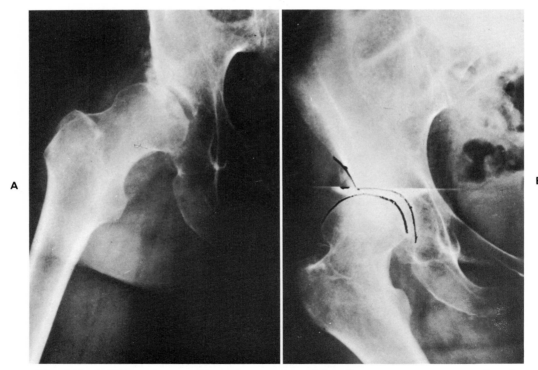

Fig. 8-13. A, This patient would not be a good candidate for varus osteotomy even though she has adequate abduction. Varus osteotomy would actually decrease the congruous weight-bearing surface. **B,** X-ray examination in adduction shows an increased weight-bearing area, which is a good indication for valgus osteotomy. (Courtesy Dr. R. D. Ray, Chicago, Ill.)

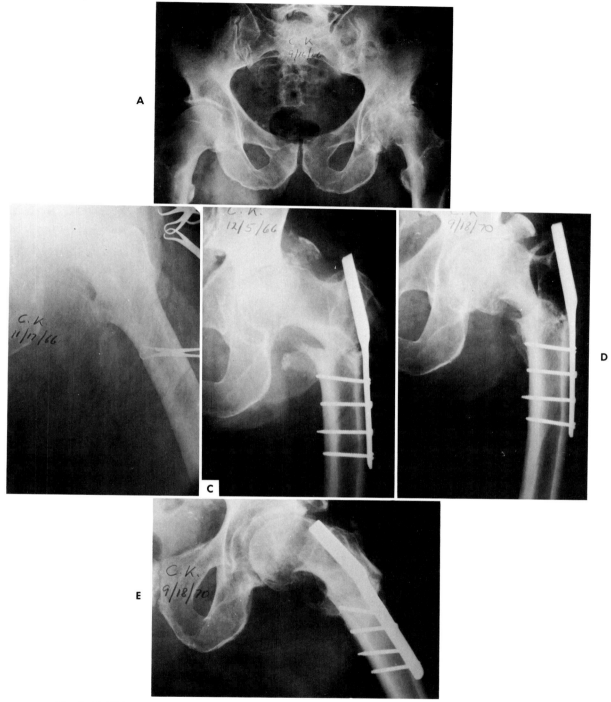

Fig. 8-14. This man had increasing pain in his left hip due to osteoarthritis and partial avascular necrosis. **A,** Maximum abduction of the left hip is seen. **B,** Reexamined under general anesthesia and following adductor tenotomy, the patient was found to have enough abduction to bring healthy bone into the weight-bearing area with a varus osteotomy. **C,** X-ray film taken following varus osteotomy. **D,** Four years later the patient has a pain-free hip. The joint space has increased and the area of avascular necrosis appears to have healed. **E,** There is excellent hip motion.

PLANNING THE OPERATION

Although we can usually decide from the clinical examination whether an osteotomy is indicated in an individual patient, the type of osteotomy should be determined on the basis of the x-ray findings. We ask for the following four x-ray views: anteroposterior views of the pelvis with the involved hip in neutral, abducted, and adducted positions (Figs. 8-8 and 8-9) and a shoot-through lateral view of the involved hip (Fig. 8-12). These views will give us adequate information about the weight-bearing relationships of the acetabulum and femoral head in different positions and we can choose the position that will produce the greatest and most congruous weight-bearing area. A lateral view is necessary to study the hip joint in that plane. The frog-leg lateral view, which can give

us valuable information in other conditions, is worthless for functional evaluation of the hip joint. It shows an anteroposterior view of the acetabulum and a lateral view of the femoral head in a position that is rarely assumed by the patient. The shoot-through lateral view shows the weight-bearing relationships of the acetabulum and femoral head in a functional position and will give us a fairly accurate measurement of the anteversion angle. Excessive anteversion should be corrected when the osteotomy is done. If correction in two or three planes is planned (for example, in a dysplastic hip with anteversion and flexion contracture), we should also obtain preoperative anteroposterior and lateral views with the hip in the position that will be produced by the osteotomy. Since an increase in the congruous weight-

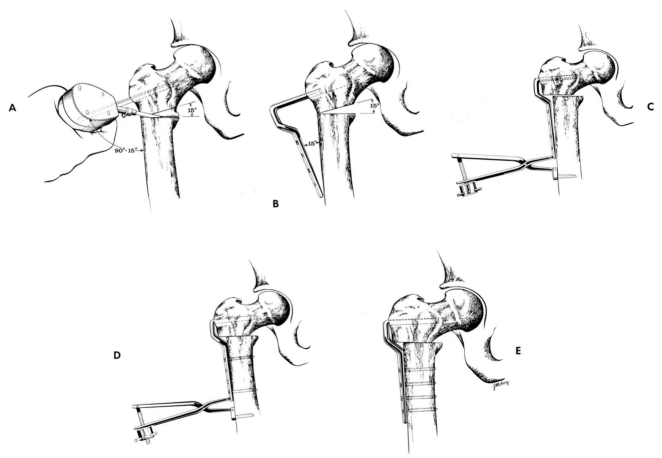

Fig. 8-15. Technique for varus osteotomy. **A,** A special chisel is inserted into the neck of the femur at the desired osteotomy angle (for example, 90° − 15° for a 15° varus osteotomy). **B,** A 15° wedge with a medial base is removed from the intertrochanteric area and the right-angle compression plate is inserted into the precut channel. **C,** The osteotomy is reduced and a compression device added. **D,** After maximal manual compression the screws are inserted and the compression device removed. **E,** Osteotomy completed. (From Mueller, K. H.: Clin. Orthop. **77:**117, 1971.)

bearing area is the most important goal of the osteotomy, we should study the x-ray films very carefully before determining which osteotomy should be done. Occasionally the patient may have adequate abduction, both clinically and on x-ray examination, but would not be a good candidate for varus osteotomy, as shown in Fig. 8-13, *A*. A varus osteotomy would actually decrease the congruous weight-bearing surfaces and would almost certainly result in eventual failure. This patient should have a valgus osteotomy, as indicated by the x-ray film taken in adduction (Fig. 8-13, *B*). If the patient has inadequate abduction for a varus osteotomy but appears to be a good candidate for this procedure according to the x-ray appearance of the hip, it may be wise to reexamine him under anesthesia and after adductor tenotomy. This may produce enough hip abduction

to make varus osteotomy the procedure of choice (Fig. 8-14).

SURGICAL PROCEDURE

After trying many different procedures, I am now satisfied with the following techniques for varus and valgus osteotomy using a right-angle compression plate* similar to that popularized by the Swiss AO group.

Varus osteotomy (Fig. 8-15)

The patient is positioned on the fracture table and the hip is placed in the position that produced the best x-ray appearance. The operative field is then prepared and draped in the usual sterile manner.

*Manufactured by Zimmer, Warsaw, Indiana.

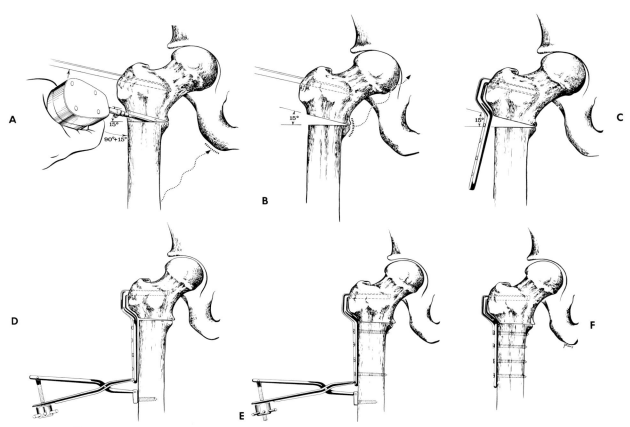

Fig. 8-16. Technique for valgus osteotomy. **A,** After preliminary adductor tenotomy, the special chisel is inserted into the neck of the femur at the desired osteotomy angle (for example, 90° + 15° for a 15° valgus angulation). **B,** A 15° wedge with a lateral base is removed from the intertrochanteric area and the iliopsoas is released from the lesser trochanter. **C,** Right-angle compression plate is inserted into the precut channel. **D,** The osteotomy is reduced and the compression device added. **E,** After maximal manual compression the screws are inserted and the compression device removed. **F,** Osteotomy completed. (From Mueller, K. H.: Clin. Orthop. **77:**117, 1971.)

The upper femur is approached through a straight lateral incision. A guide wire is then placed into the femoral neck at the desired osteotomy angle (for example, 90° − 15° for a 15° varus osteotomy). A second Kirschner wire is placed just proximal to the lesser trochanter at right angles to the femoral shaft to mark the distal cut of the osteotomy wedge. Control x-ray films confirm good placement of the wires. A special chisel is then inserted parallel to the proximal Kirschner wire to produce a channel for the right-angle compression plate (Fig. 8-15, *A*). Next an appropriate wedge with a medial base is cut out of the intertrochanteric region using either multiple drill holes and an osteotome or a bone saw. The special chisel is left in the proximal fragment and is used as a "handle." Correction of a fixed flexion deformity requires placement of the base of the wedge posteromedially. If correction in three planes is necessary, the corrective wedges should be taken from the proximal fragment to avoid loss of bone apposition when the distal fragment is rotated. The chisel is then removed and the right-angle compression plate is inserted into the precut channel (Fig. 8-15, *B*). It is not practical to divide the bone before the channel for the blade is cut. The short proximal fragment will frequently change position as soon as the bone is cut through, the bony guidelines are lost, and it becomes much more difficult to accurately insert the compression plate into the unstable proximal fragment. After insertion of the blade the osteotomy is reduced to the desired position and the compression instrument added (Fig. 8-15, *C*). Compression is then applied and the plate fixed to the femoral shaft with four screws (Fig. 8-15, *D*). After closure of the wound and application of a compression dressing the patient is returned to his regular hospital bed. No external immobilization is necessary unless the bone is very osteoporotic. Tenotomy of the iliopsoas and closed adductor tenotomy can be added to the procedure if necessary.

Valgus osteotomy (Fig. 8-16)

The patient is positioned on the fracture table and the hip placed in the position that produces the best congruity of the weight-bearing surfaces. After preliminary percutaneous adductor tenotomy the lateral aspect of the proximal femur is approached through a straight lateral incision. Two guide wires are used to mark the position of the compression plate and the distal cut of the osteotomy. The proximal wire should be inserted at the desired osteotomy angle (for example, 90° + 15° for a 15° valgus angulation). Con-

trol x-ray films confirm adequate placement of the wires. The special chisel is then inserted parallel to the proximal wire and an appropriate wedge with the base laterally is removed from the intertrochanteric region (Fig. 8-16, *A*) (or posterolaterally if a flexion deformity needs correction). The chisel is used as a "handle" for the proximal fragment. Next the distal fragment is rotated externally and the iliopsoas removed from its insertion into the lesser trochanter (Fig. 8-16, *B*). The chisel is then removed and a right-angle osteotomy plate inserted into the precut channel (Fig. 8-16, *C*). The osteotomy is reduced into the desired position and compression applied by means of the compression instrument (Fig. 8-16, *D*). The plate is then fastened to the femoral shaft by means of four screws and the compression instrument removed (Fig. 8-16, *E*). Postoperative care is the same as for a varus osteotomy.

Muscle release operation (Figs. 8-17 and 8-18)

For several years we tried to approach the individual muscle insertions from two or three different incisions. We found that the anteromedial approach to the iliopsoas and adductors had a rather high incidence of hematoma formation with subsequent infection. We are now using the following procedure: The operation is performed on a regular operating

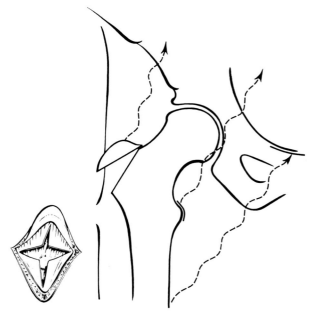

Fig. 8-17. Technique for muscle release operation. The greater trochanter is osteotomized and the iliopsoas is released from the lesser trochanter. Percutaneous adductor tenotomy is the final procedure. The insert shows crosswise sectioning of the fascia lata if it is found to be tight.

table. Both legs are draped free to permit examination of hip motion during the operation. The upper femur is approached through a straight lateral incision centered over the greater trochanter. The fascia lata is cut in a crosswise fashion if it is found to be tight. The bone is exposed and the greater trochanter osteotomized in an oblique plane and elevated approximately 1 to 1.5 cm. with the osteotome. If an adduction contracture of more than 10° is present preoperatively, release of this contracture will relax the abductor group sufficiently and osteotomy of the greater trochanter is not necessary. Next the index finger is passed around to the medial side of the femur and the lesser trochanter with the iliopsoas insertion identified. This can be facilitated by flexion and external rotation of the leg. A curved tenotomy knife or a curved scissors is then passed along the examining finger and the entire insertion of the iliopsoas released from the bone. If, after release of the iliopsoas, significant flexion contracture persists, release of the rectus femoris and the muscle attachments from the anterosuperior iliac spine should be added. This is done by extending the incision anteriorly and proximally. We do not cut the joint capsule or the Y ligament in order to avoid anterior subluxation of the femoral head in the postoperative period. The wound

is then closed. Percutaneous adductor tenotomy completes the operation. Postoperatively, the patient is placed in intermittent Buck's extension, using 6- to 7-pound weights, for a period of 2 weeks.

POSTOPERATIVE CARE
Osteotomy

The patient is allowed up in a wheelchair on the first or second postoperative day. Traction, balanced suspension, or external immobilization is usually not necessary after osteotomy. Occasionally a patient with markedly osteoporotic bone may require additional protection with balanced suspension for several weeks. Muscle reeducation and range of motion exercises are started as soon as postoperative pain has disappeared. The patient is then given a pair of crutches or a walker and allowed to ambulate without bearing weight on the leg. He progresses to partial weight bearing after a period of 6 weeks but should use his crutches for a period of 3 months. The crutches are necessary to protect the osteotomy during the healing phase and also to protect the hip joint while reversal of the degenerative process takes place. When the osteotomy has healed and the degenerative changes in the hip joint are beginning to regress, usually after approximately 3 months, the patient

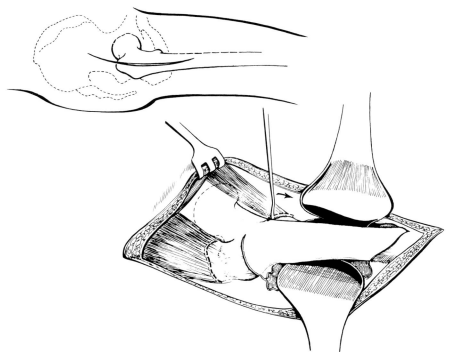

Fig. 8-18. A straight lateral approach for the muscle release operation will permit osteotomy of the greater trochanter and release of the iliopsoas from the lesser trochanter, which is facilitated by flexion and external rotation of the leg.

may be advanced to a cane, which he should use until his abductor limp has disappeared. Active muscle reeducation is extremely important following osteotomy.

Muscle release operation

Following a muscle release procedure the patient is treated with intermittent Buck's traction, using 6- to 7-pound weights, for a period of 2 weeks. He can be up in a wheelchair intermittently after the second postoperative day. After 1 week he is allowed to ambulate without bearing weight on the leg, using a walker or a pair of crutches. Partial weight bearing is permitted after 2 weeks. Range of motion exercises and muscle reeducation are begun 2 weeks after operation and are very important. After 3 months the patient may be advanced to a cane, which he should use until his abductor limp has disappeared.

• • •

Reconstructive hip surgery carries a rather high risk of thromboembolic complications and patients over the age of 45 years should be treated prophylactically with either warfarin sodium (Coumadin) or dextran until they leave the hospital.

SUMMARY

  I. Classification of osteoarthritis
    A. *Idiopathic osteoarthritis*
       Normal joint structure and mechanics
       Diminished tissue tolerance
    B. *Secondary osteoarthritis*
       Physiologic tissue tolerance
       Deranged joint mechanics with increased stress
  II. In idiopathic osteoarthritis the course of the disease cannot be predicted. Conservative treatment is justified unless progression is evident. In secondary osteoarthritis the degenerative changes progress after symptoms have appeared unless the deformity is corrected. Surgical treatment is indicated.
 III. Surgical procedures for treatment of the osteoarthritic hip can be classified into four categories:
    A. Operations that preserve the patient's own hip joint (osteotomies, muscle release operations)
    B. Arthroplasties (cup, femoral head prosthesis, total replacement)
    C. Arthrodesis
    D. Salvage procedures (Girdlestone, resection angulation)
 IV. Types of osteotomies
    A. Varus osteotomy ⎱ Correction of rotation or
    B. Valgus osteotomy ⎰ flexion deformity should be added if necessary.
    C. Valgus osteotomy with "seat" (rarely indicated)
    D. Displacement osteotomy without angulation (rarely indicated)
  V. Indications
    A. *Varus osteotomy:* Indicated in early osteoarthritis and partial necrosis of the femoral head. Sixty degrees of flexion and fifteen to twenty degrees of abduction must be present. X-ray films in abduction must show increase in congruous weight-bearing area.
    B. *Valgus osteotomy:* Indicated in advanced osteoarthritis and in arthritis due to deformity of the femoral head (Legg-Perthes disease, slipped epiphysis, etc.). Adduction contracture or some adduction and at least 60° of flexion must be present. Patients with secondary or advanced idiopathic osteoarthritis may require correction in two or three planes.
    C. *Muscle release operation:* Indicated in advanced osteoarthritis in older patients, for painful, "tight" femoral head prosthesis, and in combination with synovectomy of the rheumatoid hip. The patient usually has marked limitation of motion in all directions, all motions are painful, and the weight-bearing area cannot be increased. Osteotomy and muscle release can be, and in many cases should be, combined.

The material presented in this course is based on experience gained while I was on the staff of the Orthopedic Clinic at the University of Cologne, Germany, under Prof. M. Hackenbroch. I also wish to thank Dr. R. D. Ray, Chairman, Department of Orthopedics, University of Illinois, Chicago, for permission to study osteotomy cases in his department.

REFERENCES

1. Adam, A., and Spence, A. J.: Intertrochanteric osteotomy for osteoarthritis of the hip, J. Bone Joint Surg. **40-B:**219, 1958.
2. d'Aubigné, R. Merle, and Postel, M.: L'ostéotomie de Pauwels dans le traitement de la coxarthrose, Rev. Chir. Orthop. 45:746, 1959.
3. Auffret, M., Massias, P., and Coste, F.: Sur le rôle des dysplasies de la hanche à l'origine de la coxarthrose, Sem. Hop. Paris 15:684, 1962.
4. Bertrand, P.: Malformations luxantes de la hanche, Paris, 1962, G. Doin & Cie.
5. Bertrand, P., and Guias, H.: Osteotomie d'adduction de Pauwels dans le traitement des coxarthroses, Rev. Chir. Orthop. 45:774, 1959.
6. Blount, W. P.: Osteotomy in the treatment of osteoarthritis of the hip, J. Bone Joint Surg. **46-A:**1297, 1964.
7. Blount, W. P.: The successful high femoral osteotomy. In Rütt, A., editor: Die Therapie der Koxarthrose, Stuttgart, 1969, Georg Thieme Verlag.
8. Camera, U.: Les osteotomies dans le traitement de la coxarthrose, Rev. Chir. Orthop. 45:777, 1959.
9. Campbell, J. P., and Jackson, J. P.: Treatment of osteoarthritis of the hip by osteotomy, J. Bone Joint Surg. 38-B:468, 1956.
10. Castaing, J., LeChevallier, P. L., and Douvion, J. P.: Reflexions sur l'osteotomie inter-trochanterienne de varisation dans les coxarthroses evaluées, Ann. Chir. 15:1, 1963.
11. Cauchoix, J., Duparc, J., and Mechelany, F.: Les Osteotomies dans le traitement de la coxarthrose, Rev. Chir. Orthop. 45:762, 1959.

12. Chapchal, G.: Orthopaedische Chirurgie und Traumatologie der Huefte, Stuttgart, 1965, Ferdinand Enke.

13. Chuinard, E. G., and Logan, N. D.: Varus-producing and derotational subtrochanteric osteotomy in the treatment of congenital dislocation of the hip, J. Bone Joint Surg. 45-A:1397, 1963.

14. Coventry, M. B.: Which hip operation for which patient? J.A.M.A. 191:487, 1965.

15. Coventry, M. B.: Osteotomy of the hip for degenerative arthritis, Mayo Clinic Proc. 44:505, 1969.

16. Danielsson, L. G.: Incidence and prognosis of coxarthrosis, Acta Orthop. Scand. suppl. 66:9, 1964.

17. Delchef, J., Jr.: L'osteotomie dans la coxarthrose, Rev. Chir. Orthop. 45:771, 1959.

18. DeMarneffe, R., and Duchesne, L.: Le traitement chirurgical de la coxarthrose, Acta Orthop. Belg. 31:2, 1965.

19. Duthie, R. B., and Howe, W. B., Jr.: Displacement osteotomy for arthritis of the hip, Clin. Orthop. 31:65, 1963.

20. Endler, F.: Neuere Behandlungsmöglichkeiten der Hüftarthrose, Wien. Klin. Wschr. 73:272, 1961.

21. Endler, F.: Neuere Behandlungsmöglichkeiten der Hüftarthrose, Chir. Praxis 7:237, 1963.

22. Ferguson, A. B., Jr.: The pathological changes in degenerative arthritis of the hip and treatment by rotational osteotomy, J. Bone Joint Surg. 46-A:1337, 1964.

23. Ferguson, A., Jr.: The pathology of degenerative arthritis of the hip and the use of osteotomy in its treatment, Clin. Orthop. 77:84, 1971.

24. Francillon, M. R.: Les osteotomies dans le traitement de la coxarthrose, Rev. Chir. Orthop. 45:755, 1959.

25. Guilleminet, M., and Lapras, A.: Notre expérience de L'opération de F. Pauwels dans le traitement de la coxarthrose, Rev. Chir. Orthop. 45:726, 1959.

26. Hackenbroch, M.: Die Arthrose der Huefte, Leipzig, 1943, Georg Thieme Verlag.

27. Hackenbroch, M.: Die Arthrosis deformans des Hueftgelenks, Verh. Deutsch. Orthop. Ges. 44:28, 1957.

28. Hackenbroch, M.: Zur Frage der operativen Behandlung des formalfunktionell defekten Hueftgelenks, Z. Orthop. 92:60, 1960.

29. Hackenbroch, M.: Arthrodese, Arthroplastik, Arthrolyse, Arch. Orthop. Chir. 51:549, 1960.

30. Hackenbroch, M.: Zur normalen und pathologisch veraenderten Mechanik des Hueftgelenks. In Hohmann, G., Hackenbroch, M., and Lindemann, K., editors: Handbuch der Orthopaedie, Stuttgart, 1961, Georg Thieme Verlag, vol. 4, p. 1.

31. Harris, N. H., and Kirwan, E.: The results of osteotomy for early primary osteoarthritis of the hip, J. Bone Joint Surg. 46-B:477, 1964.

32. Harrison, M. H. M., Schajowicz, F., and Trueta, J.: Osteoarthritis of the hip: a study of the nature and evolution of the disease, J. Bone Joint Surg. 35-B:598, 1953.

33. Hirsch, C.: Intertrochanteric osteotomies in osteoarthritis of the hip, Acta Orthop. Scand. 30:129, 1960.

34. Hollander, J. L.: Treatment of osteoarthritis in the elderly patient, Geriatrics 12:394, 1957.

35. Imhaeuser, G.: Opération décompressive dans l'arthrose de la hanche. Technique de Brandes (étude critique), Rev. Chir. Orthop. 50:183, 1964.

36. Imhaeuser, G.: Technik und Ergebnisse der Muskelentspannungsoperation bei der Koxarthrose. In Rütt, A., editor: Die Therapie der Koxarthrose, Stuttgart, 1969, Georg Thieme Verlag.

37. Jacquemain, B.: Die Intertrochantere Varisierende Osteotomie. In Rütt, A., editor: Die Therapie der Koxarthrose, Stuttgart, 1969, Georg Thieme Verlag.

38. Judet, J., et al.: Indications des ostéotomies dans le traitement de la coxarthrose, Rev. Chir. Orthop. 45:735, 1959.

39. Key, J. A.: Internal and external fixation of high osteotomies of the femur, J. Bone Joint Surg. 25:737, 1943.

40. King, T.: Proximal femoral osteotomy and internal fixation for diseases and injuries of the hip, Instructional Course Lectures, The American Academy of Orthopedic Surgeons, Ann Arbor, 1957, J. W. Edwards, vol. 14, pp. 205-220.

41. King, T., and Dooley, B.: Observations on the late results of the McMurray osteotomy for osteoarthritis of the hip, J. Bone Joint Surg. 44-B:595, 1962.

42. Knodt, H.: Osteoarthritis of the hip joint. Etiology and treatment by osteotomy, J. Bone Joint Surg. 46-A:1326, 1964.

43. Knodt, H.: Pressure reducing effects of hip osteotomies, Clin. Orthop. 77:105, 1971.

44. Küntscher, G.: Die Behandlung der Coxarthrose nach Voss, Langenbecks Arch. Klin. Chir. 301:79, 383, 397, 1962.

45. Kushlick, R.: Surgical release of the psoas major in painful conditions of the hip joint, S. Afr. Med. J. 36:525, 1962.

46. Leonhardt, H.: Die Coxarthrose und ihre Behandlung mit der temporären Hängehüfte, Stuttgart, 1970, F. K. Schattauer Verlag.

47. McMurray, T. P.: Osteo-arthritis of the hip joint, Brit. J. Surg. 22:716, 1935.

48. McMurray, T. P.: Osteo-arthritis of the hip joint, J. Bone Joint Surg. 21:1, 1939.

49. Malkin, S. A. S.: Femoral osteotomy in the treatment of osteoarthritis of the hip, Brit. Med. J. 1:304, 1936.

50. Mau, H.: Idee, Indikation und postoperative Reaktionen der muskulären Entspannungsoperationen. In Rütt, A., editor: Die Therapie der Koxarthrose, Stuttgart, 1969, Georg Thieme Verlag.

51. Milch, H.: Osteotomy at the upper end of the femur, Baltimore, 1965, The Williams & Wilkins Co.

52. Mueller, K. H.: Die valgisierende Osteotomie in der Behandlung der Koxarthrose. In Rütt, A., editor: Die Therapie der Koxarthrose, Stuttgart, 1969, Georg Thieme Verlag.

53. Mueller, K. H.: Osteotomies of the hip—some technical considerations, Clin. Orthop. 77:117, 1971.

54. Mueller, K. H.: Muscle release about the hip. In Tronzo, R. G., editor: Surgery of the hip joint, Philadelphia, Lea & Febiger. (In Press.)

55. Mueller, M. E.: Die hueftnahen Femurosteotomien, Stuttgart, 1957, Georg Thieme Verlag.

56. Mueller, M. E.: 12 Huefteingriffe, A. O. Bull. suppl. 1, Sept. 1966.

57. Mueller, M. E.: Zur operativen Behandlung der Coxarthrose, Schweiz. Med. Wschr. 97:775, 1967.

58. Nicoll, E. A., and Holden, N. T.: Displacement oste-

otomy in the treatment of osteoarthritis of the hip, J. Bone Joint Surg. **43-B:**50, 1961.

59. Nissen, K. I.: The arrest of primary osteoarthritis of the hip, J. Bone Joint Surg. **42-B:**423, 1960.
60. Nissen, K. I.: The arrest of early osteoarthritis of the hip by osteotomy, Proc. Roy. Soc. Med. **56:**1051, 1963.
61. Nissen, K. I.: Un cas d'osteoarthrite primitive debutante de la hanche traité par osteotomie avec deplacement minime, Acta Orthop. Belg. **30:**651, 1964.
62. Nissen, K. I.: The early arrest of idiopathic coxarthrosis, Arch. Orthop. Unfallchir. **60:**128, 1966.
63. Nissen, K. I.: Displacement osteotomy. In Rütt, A., editor: Die Therapie der Koxarthrose, Stuttgart, 1969, Georg Thieme Verlag.
64. Nissen, K. I.: The rationale of early osteotomy for idiopathic coxarthrosis (epichondro-osteoarthrosis of the hip), Clin. Orthop. **77:**98, 1971.
65. O'Malley, A. G.: Osteoarthritis of the hip, J. Bone Joint Surg. **41-B:**888, 1959.
66. O'Malley, A. G.: The influence of flexor and adductor muscles in osteoarthritis of the hip, J. Bone Joint Surg. **44-B:**217, 1962.
67. Osborne, G. V., and Fahrni, W. H.: Oblique displacement osteotomy for osteoarthritis of the hip joint, J. Bone Joint Surg. **32-B:**148, 1950.
68. Ottolenghi, C. E., and Frigerio, E.: Intertrochanteric osteotomies in osteoarthritis of the hip, J. Bone Joint Surg. **44-A:**855, 1962.
69. Ottolenghi, C. E., Napolitano, M. F., Frigerio, E., and Nora, B.: Effects of intertrochanteric osteotomy on the hip joint, Clin. Orthop. **39:**157, 1965.
70. Padovani, P., Perreau, M., and Rainaut, J. J.: Les Osteotomies dans le traitement des Coxarthrie, Rev. Chir. Orthop. **45:**767, 1959.
71. Padovani, P., Joly, J. P., Florent, J., and Caire, H.: Cent cas d'operations de detente musculaire dans le traitement de la coxarthrie, Rev. Chir. Orthop. **50:**187, 1964.
72. Pauwels, F.: Der Schenkelhalsbruch. Ein Mechanisches Problem, Beil. Z. Orthop. Chir. **63:**entire issue, 1964.
73. Pauwels, F.: Uber eine kausale Behandlung der Coxa Valga luxans, Z. Orthop. Chir. **79:**305, 1950.
74. Pauwels, F.: Des affections le la hanche d'origine mecanique et leur traitement par l'osteotomie d'adduction, Rev. Chir. Orthop. **37:**22, 1951.
75. Pauwels, F.: Neue Richtlinien fuer die operative Behandlung der Koxarthrose, Verh. Deutsch. Orthop. Ges. **94:**332, 1961.
76. Pauwels, F.: Principles and results of treatment of coxarthrosis. In Proceedings of the Postgraduate Course of the Huitiéme Congrés de Chirurgie Orthopédique of the Société International de Chirurgie Orthopédique et de Traumatologie, Sept. 7, 1963, vol. 2.
77. Pauwels, F.: Directives nouvelles pour le traitement chirurgical de la coxarthrose, Acta Chir. Belg. **63:**1, 1964.
78. Pauwels, F.: The place of osteotomy in the operative management of osteoarthritis of the hip, Triangle **8:**196, 1968.
79. Perrot, A.: L'osteotomie varisante de Pauwels, Rev. Chir. Orthop. **45:**777, 1959.
80. Rettig, H., Eichler, J., and Oest, O.: Hüftfibel, Stuttgart, 1970, Georg Thieme Verlag.
81. Robins, R. H. C., and Piggot, J.: McMurray osteotomy. With a note on the "regeneration" of articular cartilage, J. Bone Joint Surg. **42-B:**480, 1960.
82. Rütt, A., editor: Die Therapie der Koxarthrose, Stuttgart, 1969, Georg Thieme Verlag.
83. Rütt, A., and Hackenbroch, M.: Beiträge zur Arthrosis Deformans, Z. Orthop. suppl. **89:**entire issue, 1957.
84. Schlegel, K. F.: Hängehüfte—intertrochantere Osteotomie—Resektionsarthroplastik, Arch. Klin. Chir. **301:**410, 1962.
85. Schneider, P. G.: Das Problem der Medialisierung bei intertrochangeren Osteotomien im Kindes- und Erwachsenenalter, Z. Orthop. **99:**25, 1964.
86. Shepherd, M. M.: A further review of the results of operations on the hip joint, J. Bone Joint Surg. **42-B:**177, 1960.
87. Steinhäuser, J.: Zur Frage der intertrochanteren sogenannten Reizosteotomie bei der Koxarthrose, Z. Orthop. **100:**555, 1965.
88. Steinhäuser, J.: Die Hüftnahe Femurosteotomie bei Schenkelkopfnekrose nach lateraler Schenkelhalsfraktur, Z. Orthop. **101:**508, 1966.
89. Trueta, J.: Studies on the etiopathology of osteoarthritis of the hip, Clin. Orthop. **31:**7, 1963.
90. Voss, C.: Die temporäre Hängehüfte—ein neues Verfahren zur operativen Behandlung der Koxarthrose und anderer deformierender Hüftgelenkserkrankungen, Verh. Deutsch. Orthop. Ges. **43:**351, 1955.
91. Voss, C.: Coxarthrose—die temporäre Hängehüfte, Munchen. Med. Wschr. **2:**954, 1956.
92. Voss, C.: Die Befreiung vom Hüftschmerz durch die sog. Hängehüfte, 10. Therapiewoche, p. 200, 1959.
93. Wardle, E. N.: Displacement osteotomy of the upper end of the femur, J. Bone Joint Surg. **37-B:**568, 1955.
94. Weber, B. G.: Unsere Erfahrungen mit der intertrochanteren Osteotomie nach McMurray bei der Behandlung der schmerzhaften Koxarthrose, Z. Orthop. **92:**175, 1959.
95. Weickert, H.: Spätergebnisse mit der Hängehüfte nach Voss, Z. Orthop. **99:**328, 1964.
96. Witt, A. N.: Die orthopadische Behandlung der Koxarthrose, Munchen. Med. Wschr. **2:**1191, 1956.
97. Witt, A. N.: Die operative Behandlung der Arthrosis deformans, Langenbecks Arch. Klin. Chir. **292:**493, 1959.

Chapter 9

Osteotomies of the hip—pitfalls and complications

KARL H. MUELLER, M.D.
Milwaukee, Wisconsin

In Chapter 8 the basic principles, indications, and operative techniques for treatment of osteoarthritis of the hip by osteotomy or muscle release operation were discussed. These operations are limited to patients with early and moderately advanced degenerative changes. They have no place in the treatment of hips with far-advanced changes or severe deformity of the femoral head and acetabulum. Osteotomy is expected to correct existing deformity, increase the congruous weight-bearing area, and reduce weight-bearing pressure in the hip joint. Careful study of clinical and x-ray findings preoperatively is necessary to achieve the best possible results. Some of the pitfalls and complications of hip osteotomies will be discussed in this chapter. Infection, phlebitis, thromboembolic complications, etc. are not unique to hip osteotomies and will not be dealt with.

The causes for specific osteotomy complications and failures can be classified into three categories: wrong indication, wrong osteotomy, and technical errors.

WRONG INDICATION

Osteotomy has its greatest usefulness in the treatment of early and moderately advanced coxarthrosis of both the idiopathic and secondary type. We do not consider osteotomy to be adequate treatment for the patient with far-advanced osteoarthritis. These patients should be treated by muscle release, arthroplasty, or arthrodesis, but not osteotomy. Flexion of the hip joint of less than 50° is usually an indication that degenerative changes are too far advanced for osteotomy, as shown by the following case.

Case 1. J. H. gave a history of long-standing osteoarthritis of the hip. Pain was aggravated by activity and only partially relieved by rest. At the time of surgery, hip motion in flexion was only approximately 50°. X-ray films showed severe osteoarthritis (Fig. 9-1, *A*). Intertrochanteric osteotomy was performed (Fig. 9-1, *B*). The patient had temporary relief of pain, followed by gradual reduction of hip motion and recurrence of pain (Fig. 9-1, *C*). Total hip arthroplasty was eventually performed.

A patient with advanced osteoarthritis of the hip who has less than 50° of motion in flexion is not a good candidate for intertrochanteric osteotomy.

Rheumatoid arthritis can occasionally begin in one joint and differentiation from osteoarthritis may be quite difficult. A rheumatoid hip joint does not respond well to intertrochanteric osteotomy unless synovectomy is carried out at the same time.

Case 2. J. F. F. is a 42-year-old man with a 2-year history of gradually increasing pain in his hip. X-ray findings appeared to be typical for osteoarthritis (Fig. 9-2, *A*). There was no significant involvement of other joints. The blood cell count and urinalysis were within normal limits. The sedimentation rate was slightly elevated at 22. Rheumatoid tests were not done. A valgus displacement osteotomy was performed (Fig. 9-2, *B*). Improvement of hip pain was only temporary. Other joints subsequently became involved (Fig. 9-2, *C* and *D*), and a diagnosis of rheumatoid arthritis was eventually made.

Be sure of your diagnosis. A rheumatoid hip joint rarely benefits from intertrochanteric osteotomy.

Avascular necrosis of the femoral head can occur as a complication of femoral neck fracture or as an idiopathic lesion. Involvement of the femoral head

195

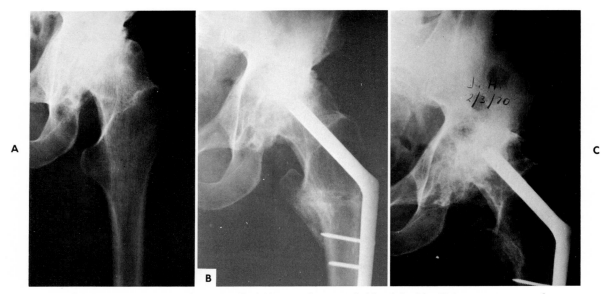

Fig. 9-1. A, J. H. had a long-standing history of osteoarthritis of the hip. Pain was aggravated by activity and only partially relieved by rest. At the time of surgery, hip motion in flexion was approximately 50°. X-ray film showed severe osteoarthritis. **B,** Intertrochanteric osteotomy was performed and his pain was relieved for 3 years. **C,** Pain then recurred, along with considerable reduction of hip motion over the subsequent years. Total hip arthroplasty was eventually performed. (Courtesy Dr. C. Hugh Hickey, Milwaukee, Wis.)

varies, depending upon the severity of the ischemia. Partial avascular necrosis quite often responds favorably to intertrochanteric osteotomy provided healthy bone can be brought into the weight-bearing area. Extensive involvement or collapse of the femoral head is usually a contraindication to intertrochanteric osteotomy.

Case 3. R. M., a 64-year-old man, had gradually increasing pain in the right hip for 2 years. X-ray films revealed avascular necrosis of the femoral head. A Phemister bone graft was performed with poor result (Fig. 9-3, *A*). The patient continued to have pain. Two years after the bone graft a displacement osteotomy was performed. Necrotic bone remained in the weight-bearing area and further collapse occurred (Fig. 9-3, *B*).

> Intertrochanteric osteotomy for treatment of avascular necrosis of the femoral head is effective only if healthy bone can be brought into the weight-bearing area. Extensive involvement and collapse of the femoral head are contraindications to intertrochanteric osteotomy.

WRONG OSTEOTOMY

Preoperative evaluation of a patient to be considered for intertrochanteric osteotomy must be thorough and exact. It is not true that cutting the

bone is the most important factor in a hip osteotomy and that the position of the proximal fragment is of secondary importance. Although we can usually expect some temporary pain relief after any osteotomy, long-term results will depend largely upon our exact preoperative evaluation and planning.

A patient with early idiopathic osteoarthritis or early arthritis due to hip dysplasia very rarely is a candidate for valgus osteotomy. If osteotomy is indicated in such a patient, it should be of the varus type.

Case 4. G. K., 44 years of age, had early secondary osteoarthritis due to hip dysplasia. Valgus displacement osteotomy relieved symptoms for a few years but then there was a gradual increase in pain and limitation of motion. X-ray examination showed progressive deterioration of the hip joint (Fig. 9-4). The osteotomy had *decreased* the congruous weight-bearing area. This patient should have had a varus not a valgus osteotomy.

Indications may change from varus to valgus osteotomy with advancing disease. Progressive loss of cartilage, fibrosis of the capsule, and osteophyte formation on the lateral edge of the acetabulum or the lateral aspect of the femoral head may prevent adequate seating of the femoral head in the acetabulum. The femoral head abuts against the acetabulum in abduction, causing further subluxation. Adduction, on the other hand, can bring the undamaged medial

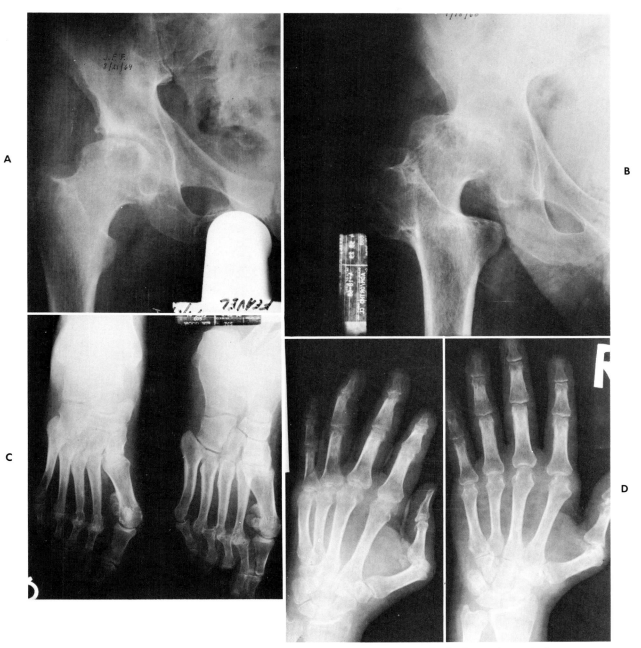

Fig. 9-2. A, J. F. F., a 42-year-old man, had a 2-year history of gradually increasing pain in his hip. X-ray film appeared to be typical for osteoarthritis. **B,** Valgus displacement osteotomy was performed. Hip pain was improved only temporarily and there was marked deterioration of the hip joint 2 years later. **C** and **D,** X-ray films of the hands and feet at that time showed the typical deformities of rheumatoid arthritis.

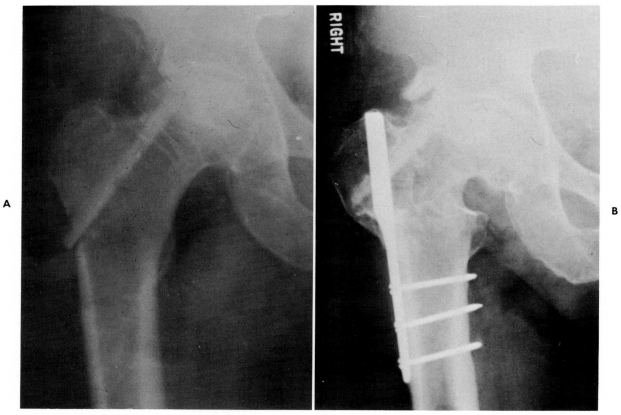

Fig. 9-3. A, R. M., a 64-year-old man, had pain in his right hip resulting from avascular necrosis of the femoral head. A Phemister bone graft was performed but caused no improvement. **B,** Two years after the bone graft a displacement osteotomy was performed. Necrotic bone remained in the weight-bearing area and further collapse occurred.

portion of the articular cartilage into the weight-bearing area and increase congruity of the weight-bearing surfaces. Careful study of abduction and adduction x-ray views is extremely important.

Case 5. B. R. had gradually increasing pain and limitation of motion from secondary osteoarthritis due to hip dysplasia. X-ray views seemed to show adequate abduction for a varus osteotomy (Fig. 9-5, *A*). The varus osteotomy (Fig. 9-5, *B*) gave only temporary relief of pain and was followed by progressive deterioration of the hip joint and recurrence of pain. Careful review of the preoperative x-ray studies would have revealed a decrease in weight-bearing area in abduction. This patient would have been a good candidate for valgus osteotomy, as shown by the postoperative x-ray films in adduction (Fig. 9-5, *C*).

> Do the right osteotomy. The osteotomy must *increase*, not decrease the weight-bearing area.

Osteotomy does not always increase motion of the hip joint. We must be careful that angulation into valgus does not exceed preoperative adduction or that

angulation into varus does not exceed preoperative abduction. If we disregard this rule, our operation may produce a bothersome fixed abduction or adduction deformity.

Case 6. A. B., a 66-year-old patient, had gradually increasing hip pain. Conservative treatment failed to retard progression of the disease and he developed an adduction deformity. Weight-bearing surfaces remained fairly congruous (Fig. 9-6, *A*). A varus osteotomy resulted in severe fixed adduction deformity (Fig. 9-6, *B*). This patient should not have been treated by varus osteotomy.

> Fixed adduction deformity is a contraindication to varus osteotomy; fixed abduction deformity is a contraindication to valgus osteotomy.

TECHNICAL ERRORS

Most complications are the result of technical errors or poor operative technique. It is extremely important to maintain this position of the osteotomy with a good

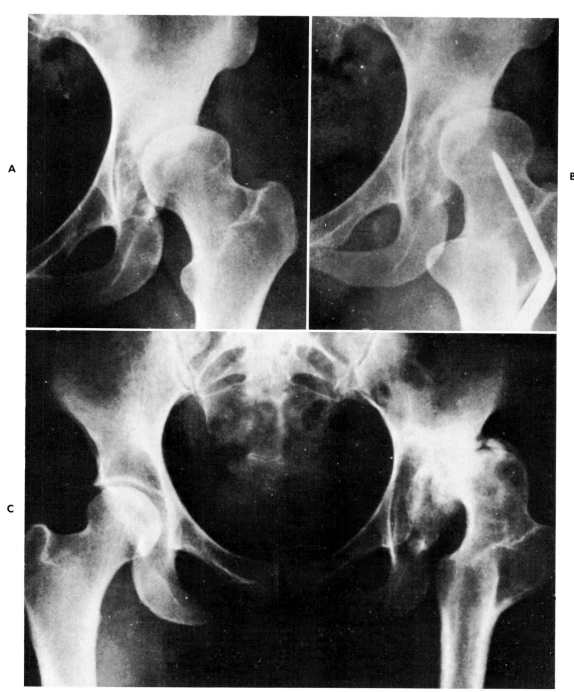

Fig. 9-4. A, G. K., 44 years old, had early secondary osteoarthritis due to hip dysplasia. **B,** Valgus displacement osteotomy relieved symptoms for only a few years. This was followed by a gradual increase in pain and limitation of motion. **C,** X-ray film showed progressive deterioration of the hip joint. (From Aufranc, O. E.: In Rütt, A., editor: Die Therapie der Koxarthrose, Stuttgart, 1969, Georg Thieme Verlag.)

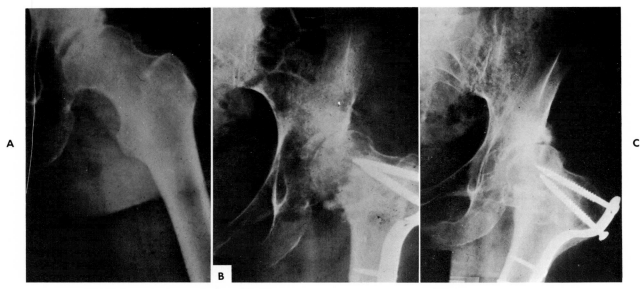

Fig. 9-5. A, B. R. had gradually increasing pain and limitation of motion from secondary osteoarthritis due to hip dysplasia. X-ray film seemed to show adequate abduction for varus osteotomy. **B,** Varus osteotomy gave only temporary relief of pain. **C,** This patient would have been a good candidate for valgus osteotomy, as shown by postoperative x-ray film taken in abduction. (Courtesy Dr. R. D. Ray, Chicago, Ill.)

fixation device. Many straight and angulated plates have been devised, but very few of them afford adequate fixation. Straight splines or V plates do not hold well against the varus stress that is placed upon the short proximal fragment by muscle pull and weight bearing. They frequently loosen in the postoperative period and allow the proximal fragment to go into more varus. This, then, results in loss of the intended valgus angulation or an excessive varus position of the proximal fragment.

Case 7. H. B. had gradually increasing degenerative arthritis of the hip. A varus osteotomy was found to be indicated and was fixed with a straight-blade plate. Postoperatively, the proximal fragment drifted into more varus, resulting in considerable shortening of the leg and an awkward abduction limp (Fig. 9-7).

Occasionally the straight-blade plate can loosen enough to permit significant motion of the proximal fragment. Nonunion of the osteotomy is not a rare complication with this type of fixation device.

Case 8. M. K. is a 71-year-old man with moderately advanced osteoarthritis of the hip. Valgus displacement osteotomy was performed and the position fixed with a straight-blade plate. Motion of the proximal fragment resulted in nonunion of the osteotomy and fracture of the straight-blade plate (Fig. 9-8).

If the straight spline is driven too vigorously, frac-

ture of the greater trochanter can occur with loss of fixation and subsequent nonunion (Fig. 9-9). An improperly inserted right-angle compression plate can also lead to loss of the osteotomy position. Care must be taken that an adequate bridge of bone remains between the blade and the osteotomy cut (Fig. 9-10).

> Stable fixation permits early motion, enhances union of the osteotomy, and prevents drift of the proximal fragment.

Angulated fixation devices with a variable angle frequently fail to resist varus stress because of loosening of the fixation screw. This allows further drift into varus, which results in excessive shortening of the leg and an awkward abductor lurch (Fig. 9-11). The development of a painful bursa over the protruding portion of the nail plate has been reported. This complication can also occur with the right-angle compression plate.

Case 9. W. H. is a 62-year-old, rather thin man with degenerative arthritis of the hip. A varus osteotomy was performed and the position fixed with a right-angle compression plate. This resulted in complete relief of pain for 2½ years (Fig. 9-12). He then began to complain of recurrence of pain in his left hip similar to the pain he had preoperatively. Examination revealed good motion of the hip joint with minimal discomfort. There was marked tenderness over the protruding fixation device. Infiltration

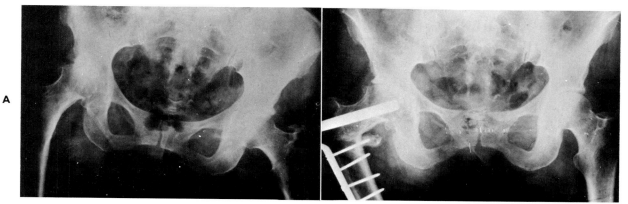

Fig. 9-6. A, M. B., a 66-year-old patient, had gradually increasing hip pain. Conservative treatment failed to retard progression of the disease and the patient developed an adduction deformity. Weight-bearing surfaces remained fairly congruous. **B,** A varus osteotomy resulted in a severe fixed adduction deformity.

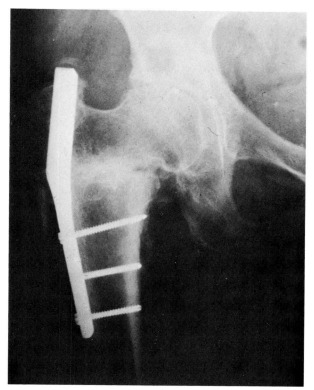

Fig. 9-7. In H. B. the proximal fragment drifted into more varus following varus osteotomy and fixation with a straight spline. This resulted in considerable shortening of the leg and an awkward abductor limp.

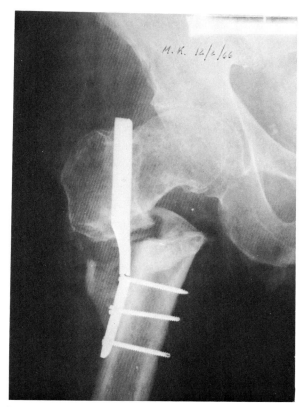

Fig. 9-8. M. K. is a 71-year-old man with moderately advanced osteoarthritis of the hip. Valgus displacement osteotomy was fixed with a straight-blade plate. Motion of the proximal fragment occurred (see x-ray markings surrounding the plate) and resulted in nonunion of the osteotomy and eventual fracture of the plate.

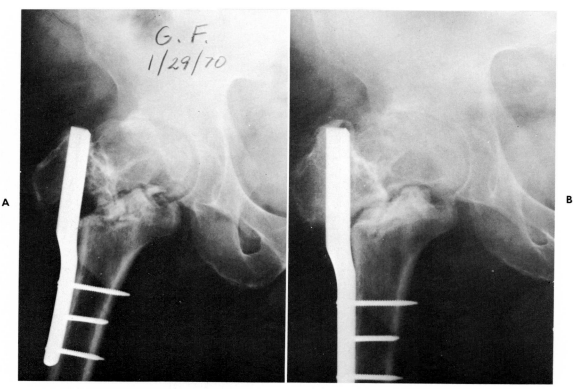

Fig. 9-9. A, The greater trochanter fractured when the straight-blade plate was driven into the proximal fragment. **B,** Loss of fixation and subsequent nonunion resulted.

of this area with 1% lidocaine (Xylocaine) gave immediate and complete pain relief. Removal of the fixation device resulted in a pain-free hip.

> Bursitis over a protruding fixation device can be painful and simulate recurrence of hip pain from arthritis. Removal of the fixation device will usually result in complete pain relief.

Two other sources of postoperative pain should be mentioned. A straight-blade plate that protrudes markedly through the cortex of the greater trochanter may cause development of a painful bursitis (Fig. 9-13). Occasional injection of the bursa during the healing phase of the osteotomy and removal of the plate after the osteotomy has healed usually result in complete relief of pain.

Another source of postoperative pain may be more difficult to treat. A medial spike left on the distal fragment may impinge on the soft tissues or even on the pelvis during weight bearing and can cause considerable pain (Fig. 9-13). This often requires repeated injections of a local anesthetic and hydrocortisone for relief of pain. Most of these spurs will eventually decrease in size and become asymptomatic, but

occasionally it may become necessary to remove a medial spike for persistent pain.

> A medial spike can cause pain.
> PREVENT IT!

SUMMARY

1. Complications and failures of intertrochanteric osteotomies can be classified into three categories: wrong indication, wrong osteotomy, and technical errors.

2. A patient with advanced osteoarthritis of the hip who has less than 50° of motion in flexion is not a good candidate for intertrochanteric osteotomy.

3. Be sure of your diagnosis. A rheumatoid hip joint rarely benefits from intertrochanteric osteotomy.

4. Intertrochanteric osteotomy for treatment of avascular necrosis of the femoral head is effective only if healthy bone can be brought into the weight-bearing area. Extensive involvement and collapse of the femoral head are contraindications to intertrochanteric osteotomy.

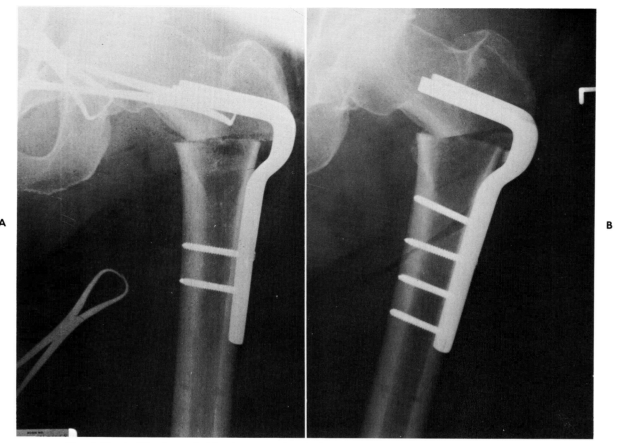

Fig. 9-10. A, The bony bridge between the blade and the osteotomy cut is too narrow and cannot withstand the varus stress on the proximal fragment. **B,** The proximal fragment promptly broke out and drifted into more varus. (From Mueller, K. H.: Clin. Orthop. **77:**117, 1971.)

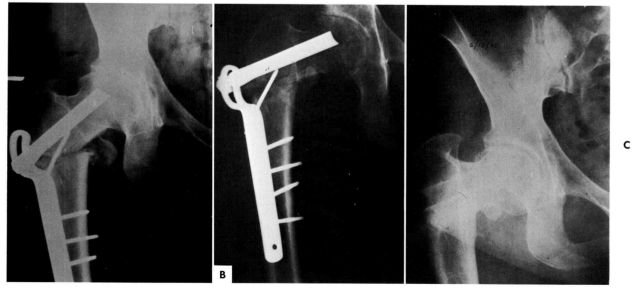

Fig. 9-11. A, Intertrochanteric osteotomy fixed with a McLaughlin nail plate. **B,** The fixation screw loosened and the proximal fragment drifted into more varus. **C,** A painful bursa over the protruding fixation device made removal of the nail plate necessary. (From Mueller, K. H.: Clin. Orthop. **77:**117, 1971.)

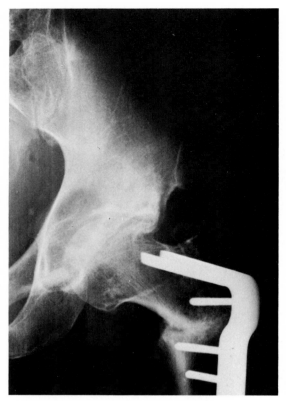

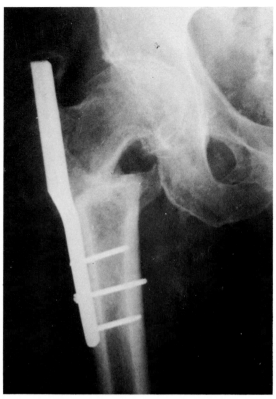

Fig. 9-12. W. H. is a 62-year-old, rather thin man with osteoarthritis of the hip. Varus osteotomy resulted in complete relief of pain for 2½ years. Pain then recurred, similar to the pain he had prior to his operation. Marked tenderness was present over the protruding fixation device. Removal of the compression plate became necessary eventually and resulted in a completely pain-free hip.

Fig. 9-13. Varus displacement osteotomy fixed with a straight spline. A medial spike left on the distal fragment impinged on the soft tissues and the pelvis and caused considerable pain. Repeated injections of lidocaine and hydrocortisone were necessary. The spur eventually decreased in size and became asymptomatic. This patient also developed a painful bursitis over the markedly protruding straight-blade plate, eventually necessitating removal of the plate.

5. Do the right osteotomy. The osteotomy must *increase*, not decrease the weight-bearing area.

6. Fixed adduction deformity is a contraindication to varus osteotomy; fixed abduction deformity is a contraindication to valgus osteotomy.

7. Stable fixation permits early motion, enhances union of the osteotomy, and prevents drift of the proximal fragment.

8. Bursitis over a protruding fixation device can be painful and simulate recurrent hip pain from arthritis. Removal of the fixation device will usually result in complete relief of pain.

9. A medial spike can cause pain—prevent it!

REFERENCES

1. Coventry, M. B.: Which hip operation for which patient? J.A.M.A. **191**:487, 1965.
2. Coventry, M. B.: Osteotomy of the hip for degenerative arthritis, Mayo Clin. Proc. **44**:505, 1969.
3. Danielsson, L. G.: Incidence and prognosis of coxarthrosis, Acta Orthop. Scand. suppl. **66**:9, 1964.
4. Endler, F.: Neuere Behandlungsmöglichkeiten der Hüftarthrose, Wien. Klin. Wschr. **73**:272, 1961.
5. Endler, F.: Neuere Behandlungsmöglichkeiten der Hüftarthrose, Chir. Praxis **7**:237, 1963.
6. Guilleminet, M., and Lapras, A.: Notre expérience de L'opération de F. Pauwels dans le traitement de la coxarthrose, Rev. Chir. Orthop. **45**:726, 1959.
7. Hackenbroch, M.: Zur Frage der operativen Behandlung des formalfunktionell defekten Hueftgelenks, Z. Orthop. **92**:60, 1960.
8. Hackenbroch, M.: Zur normalen und pathologisch veraenderten Mechanik des Hueftgelenks. In Hohmann, G., Hackenbroch, M., and Lindemann, K., editors: Handbuch der Orthopaedie, Stuttgart, 1961, Georg Thieme Verlag, vol. 4, p. 1.
9. Harris, N. H., and Kirwan, E.: The results of osteotomy for early primary osteoarthritis of the hip, J. Bone Joint Surg. **46-B**:477, 1964.
10. Jacquemain, B.: Die Intertrochantere Varisierende

Osteotomie. In Rütt, A., editor: Die Therapie der Koxarthrose, Stuttgart, 1969, Georg Thieme Verlag.

11. Knodt, H.: Pressure reducing effects of hip osteotomies, Clin. Orthop. **77**:105, 1971.
12. Mueller, K. H.: Die Valgisierende Osteotomie in der Behandlung der Koxarthrose. In Rütt, A., editor: Die Therapie der Koxarthrose, Stuttgart, 1969, Georg Thieme Verlag.
13. Mueller, K. H.: Osteotomies of the hip—Some technical considerations, Clin. Orthop. **77**:117, 1971.
14. Nissen, K. I.: Displacement osteotomy. In Rütt, A., editor: Die Therapie der Koxarthrose, Stuttgart, 1969, Georg Thieme Verlag.
15. Nissen, K. I.: The rationale of early osteotomy for idiopathic coxarthrosis (epichondro-osteoarthrosis of the hip), Clin. Orthop. **77**:98, 1971.
16. Pauwels, R.: Neue Richtlinien fuer die operative Behandlung der Koxarthrose, Verh. Deutsch. Orthop. Ges. **94**:332, 1961.
17. Pauwels, F.: Principles and results of treatment of coxarthrosis. In Proceedings of the Postgraduate Course of the Huitiéme Congrés de Chirurgie Orthopédique of the Société International de Chirurgie Orthopédique et de Traumatologie, Sept. 7, 1963, vol. 2.
18. Pauwels, F.: The place of osteotomy in the operative management of osteoarthritis of the hip, Triangle **8**:196, 1968.
19. Robins, R. H. C., and Piggot, J.: McMurray osteotomy. With a note on the "regeneration" of articular cartilage, J. Bone Joint Surg. **42-B**:480, 1960.
20. Rosborough, D., and Stiles, P. J.: Non-union after intertrochanteric osteotomy with internal fixation for osteoarthritis of the hip, J. Bone Joint Surg. **49-B**:462, 1967.
21. Schneider, P. G.: Das Problem der Medialisierung bei intertrochanteren Osteotomien im Kindes- und Erwachsenenalter, Z. Orthop. **99**:25, 1964.
22. Scott, P. J.: Non-union of oblique displacement intertrochanteric osteotomy for osteoarthritis of the hip, J. Bone Joint Surg. **49-B**:475, 1967.

Chapter 10

Surgical anatomy and exposure of the knee joint

MICHAEL HARTY, M.A., M.B., M.Ch., F.R.C.S., and
JOHN J. JOYCE, III, M.D.
Philadelphia, Pennsylvania

"There is but little room for inexactness in the field of surgery, a deviation of even a centimeter or two from the correct approach may change early success into disaster."[2] Knowledge of anatomy still forms an essential prerequisite for correct clinical diagnosis, the sine qua non of successful treatment. A clear mental picture of the changes in anatomic relationships that occur during the normal range of joint motion forms an indispensable adjunct to an accurate evaluation of symptomatology and a precise diagnosis.

The ideal surgical exposure should provide adequate access to the lesion under investigation with minimal disturbances of the structure and functions of adjacent tissue. Use of the natural cleavage planes provided by the intermuscular septa and preferably the planes between neurovascular watersheds facilitates the exposure and enhances early postoperative activity. In limb surgery the size and site of the incision will be influenced by the direction of the skin crease or wrinkle lines, by the position and course of the underlying neurovascular bundle, and by tendons, muscles, ligaments, and bone. However, when extension of the incision is contemplated, the position of these vital structures may be overlooked—their exact identification is imperative before additional exposure is performed.

The knee joint lies between the longest and strongest levers in the human body. It is exposed to severe angular and torsion strains, especially in the field of sport and athletic endeavor. The strong ligaments, reinforced by powerful quadriceps, hamstring, and gastrocnemius muscle groups, provide its main stabilizing influences. The expanded femoral and tibial condyles are designed basically for weight bearing, but they also increase the area of contact between the bones. Since many knee lesions are of traumatic origin, the anatomic and biomechanical significance of the various structures involved must be appreciated by those treating the disorder.

ANATOMIC FEATURES

Although the anatomic joint structures are discussed individually, it must be appreciated that physiologically they behave as mutually beneficial

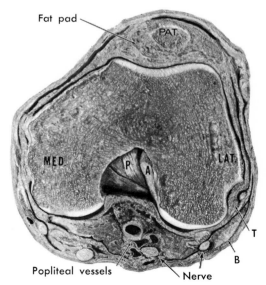

Fig. 10-1. Right knee, transverse section at level of femoral condyles. **A,** Anterior cruciate; **P,** posterior cruciate; **B,** biceps; **T,** tendon of popliteus.

206

functional units. At the knee the actual joint is superficial on the anterior, medial, and lateral aspects where it is covered only by skin, aponeurotic deep fascia, and capsule. In contrast, the flexor aspect is deeply clothed by muscles, fat, and tendons that conceal the neurovascular bundle to the leg and foot (Fig. 10-1).

Palpable structures

The patella, femoral condyles, tibial tubercle, tibial plateaus, and head of the fibula are the basic bony landmarks for orientation. In the flexed position the articular margin of the medial femoral condyle is easily palpated where it is crossed by two or more sensitive terminal twigs of the infrapatellar branch of the saphenous nerve (Fig. 10-2). The medial epicondyle, which gives attachment proximally to the tendon of the adductor magnus and at the distal margin to the medial collateral ligament of the knee joint, projects on the medial side. The tibial tubercle provides insertion for the patellar tendon. The medial and lateral tibial condyles delineating the lower margin of the knee joint are palpated most readily with the knee flexed. The joint level corresponds to

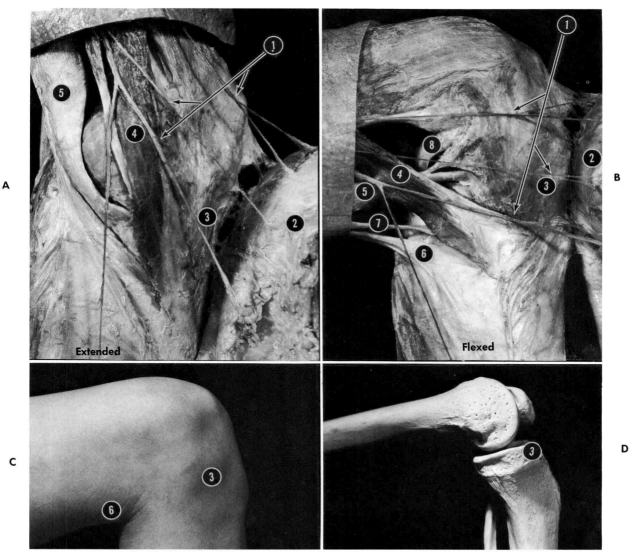

Fig. 10-2. Medial aspect of left knee. **A,** Extended. **B** to **D,** Flexed. 1, Infrapatellar branches of saphenous nerve; 2, prepatellar skin flap; 3, tibial plateau; 4, sartorius; 5, semimembranosus; 6, semitendinosus; 7, gracilis; 8, gastrocnemius.

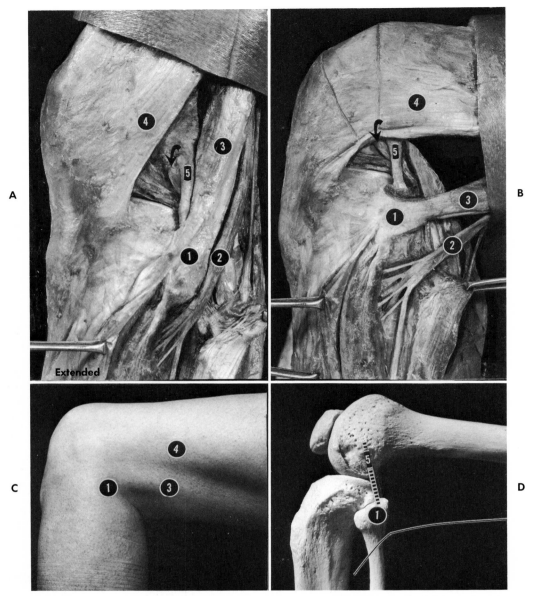

Fig. 10-3. Lateral aspect of left knee joint. The deep fascia that joins the iliotibial band to the biceps has been removed. **A,** Extended. **B** to **D,** Flexed. **1,** Fibular head; **2,** common peroneal nerve; **3,** biceps tendon; **4,** iliotibial band; **5,** lateral ligament; tendon of popliteus (arrow). (**D** from Harty, M.: Surg. Gynec. Obstet. **130:**111, 1970.)

the depressions overlying the anterior margin of the medial and lateral meniscus at the sides of the ligamentum patellae (Figs. 10-2 and 10-3). With the knee extended, these depressions are replaced by the tense fluctuant bulges of the compressed infrapatellar fat pad.

Posteriorly the medial and lateral hamstrings are identified most distinctly with the knee flexed to about 90°. When the hamstrings are tensed, the semitendinosus presents as the most superficial tendon. Slightly deeper, the gracilis tendon is also palpable (Fig. 10-2). The flat aponeurotic-like tendon of the sartorius, although not easily located clinically, is highly distinctive during surgical exposures. The tendon of the semimembranosus, which is enclosed by a bursa, joins the posterior margin of the medial tibial plateau. This tendon is made more taut and more easily palpable by flexing the hip joint. About

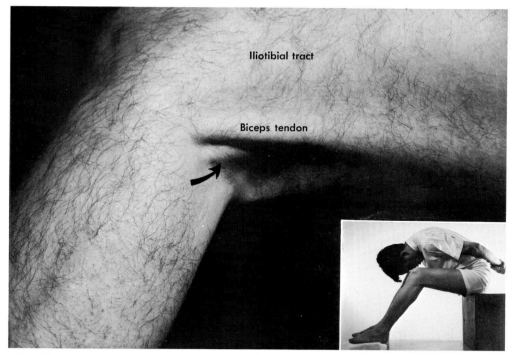

Fig. 10-4. Left common peroneal nerve (arrow). Insert: Position adapted to taut and demonstrate the nerve. (From Harty, M.: Surg. Gynec. Obstet. **130:**11, 1970.)

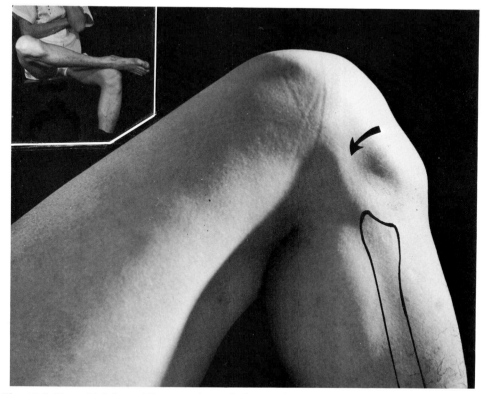

Fig. 10-5. Tensed left lateral ligament (arrow). Insert: Position adapted to put ligament under tension. (From Harty, M.: Surg. Gynec. Obstet. **130:**11, 1970.)

2 to 3 cm. anteriorly, the adductor magnus tendon gains attachment to the adductor tubercle, indicating the level of the popliteal surface of the femur.

The head of the fibula is recognized on the posterolateral aspect about 2 cm. distal to the joint line. The more prominent anterior margin of the lateral femoral condyle is concealed by the patella and vastus lateralis, except in full flexion when it protrudes through the quadriceps aponeurosis. On the posterolateral side the biceps tendon joins the fibular head and about 2 cm. distally the common peroneal nerve may be rolled painfully on the fibular neck (Fig. 10-3). This intimate neuro-osseous relationship precludes the use of tourniquets immediately distal to the level of the knee joint.

A special maneuver permits palpation of the common peroneal nerve in the popliteal fossa[5] (Fig. 10-4). With the hip fully flexed (chin on knee) and the knee flexed to about 30°, the common peroneal nerve is tensed sufficiently to make it palpable on the posterior aspect of the biceps tendon and fibular head, and in 12% of persons the nerve may be actually visible (Fig. 10-4). The iliotibial band parallels the biceps tendon anteriorly and more superficially to reach Gerdy's tubercle on the lateral tibial condyle (Fig. 10-3).

Capsule. At the knee joint the capsule is not a simple independent fibrous envelope that joins the articular margins of the adjacent bone ends. It is reinforced by aponeurotic expansions from the overlying muscles and tendons. The patella and the ligamentum patellae strengthen the capsule anteriorly. On each side the lateral and medial patellar retinacula reinforce the quadriceps attachment to the tibia. The capsule is thickened on the medial side by the deep part of the medial collateral ligament and on the lateral side by the short lateral ligament of the knee joint (see following discussion). Posteriorly the capsule is reinforced by an expansion from the semimembranosus.

Collateral ligaments. With the knee extended, the biceps tendon, which blends with the adjacent deep fascia, covers the round lateral collateral ligament. To palpate this ligament the heel must rest on the opposite knee with the hip externally rotated to its fullest comfortable extent (Fig. 10-5). In this position the biceps tendon uncovers the ligament, which is tensed by the forced distraction of the lateral condyles, and it is easily located in the line of the fibular shaft.[5] The tendon of the popliteus and the lateral inferior genicular vessels and nerve separates the lateral ligament from the underlying meniscus (Fig. 10-6).

A small but constant bursa intervenes between the lower end of the ligament and the biceps tendon. A flat fibrous condensation of the lateral capsule (the short lateral ligament) is often found in this area. It extends from the lateral epicondyle of the femur to the fibular head. Its posterior margin (arcuate ligament) arches medially over the popliteus belly to join the posterior capsule of the knee joint. The lateral collateral ligament, the iliotibial band, the biceps tendon, the tendon of the popliteus muscle, and the short lateral ligament combine to maintain stability against distraction forces on the lateral side of the knee joint.

The stronger, more extensive, and more vulnerable medial collateral ligament is divided into superficial and deep parts. Both are firmly anchored to the medial epicondyle of the femur (Fig. 10-6). The superficial component passes distally over the medial meniscus and the medial tibial condyle to gain attachment to the medial side of the tibial shaft for a distance of 4 to 6 cm. This part of the ligament, which slides on the tibial condyle, may overlie one or more bursae at the level of the tibial condyle, the medial meniscus, or the margin of the medial femoral condyle.[1] More posteriorly another bursa separates it from the insertion of the semimembranosus tendon. The deeper part of the medial collateral ligament passes distally to the medial and posteromedial

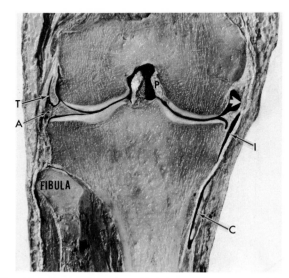

Fig. 10-6. Coronal section of left knee joint. Superficial and deep parts of medial ligament are retracted (white arrow). **P,** Posterior cruciate; **T,** tendon of popliteus; **A,** lateral genicular artery; **C,** pes anserinus bursa; **I,** intraligamentous bursa.

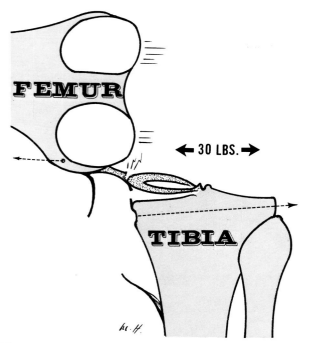

Fig. 10-7. Preparation used for applying graduated traction to deep part of medial ligament.

margin of the medial tibial condyle. En route it blends with the joint capsule and gets a strong attachment to the margin of the medial meniscus. Experimentally, a force of 30 to 35 pounds is required to separate these two structures (Fig. 10-7).

The osseous genu valgum of the normal human knee, combined with its frequent exposure to trauma from the lateral aspect, throws an enormous traction strain on the medial ligament. In the extended position of the knee joint this ligament gains additional support from the medial patellar retinaculum and semimembranosus as well as the conjoint tendinous aponeurosis of the sartorius, innervated by an extensor nerve (femoral), the semitendinosus, innervated by a flexor nerve (sciatic), and the gracilis, innervated by an adductor nerve (obturator) (Fig. 10-8). Just as the biceps reinforces the lateral ligament in extension, so this trinity reinforces the medial ligament. The pes anserinus bursa intervenes between the tendinous insertion of these three muscles and the medial ligament (Fig. 10-6). The long saphenous

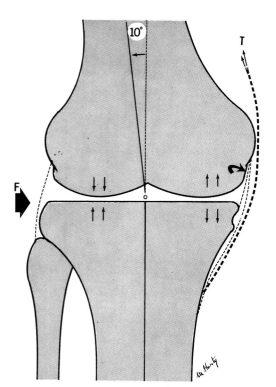

Fig. 10-8. Force, **F,** from lateral aspect produces compression of lateral condyles and traction of medial ligament (curved arrow). **T,** Pull of sartorius, gracilis, and semitendinosus.

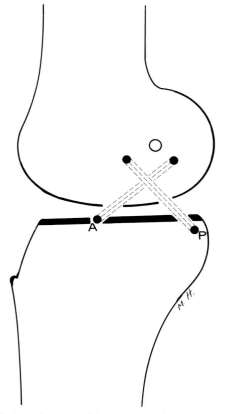

Fig. 10-9. Attachments of the anterior, **A,** and posterior, **P,** cruciate ligaments. ◯ indicates the area of the mobile axis of flexion and extension.

vein passes directly over this bursa and may present problems in the differential diagnosis of pes anserinus bursitis and thrombophlebitis in the overlying vein.

The *cruciate ligaments* form strong connections between the tibia and the intercondylar notch of the femur. They take their name from their tibial attachments and the cruciform outline is seen only on side view (Fig. 10-9). The anterior cruciate passes backward and laterally to the *posterior* margin of the lateral femoral condyle, while the shorter but thicker posterior cruciate goes in an upward anterior and medial direction to the *anterior* margin of the medial femoral condyle (Fig. 10-9). This eccentric femoral attachment ineluctably directs and regulates the glide pattern between the femur and tibia during flexion and extension. The femoral attachments may be recalled by the mnemonics A.P.EX. and P.A.IN.; the *a*nterior cruciate is attached *p*osteriorly on the *ex*ternal condyle, and the *p*osterior cruciate is attached *a*nteriorly on the *in*ternal condyle. The cruciate ligaments are intracapsular and although centrally placed in the joint they are extra- or retrosynovial. This anterior covering by synovium and subsynovial fat may obscure tears of the cruciates, especially near the femoral ends (Fig. 10-18). Due to their eccentric femoral attachments, during flexion the posterior cruciate pulls the femoral condyles posteriorly on the tibial plateau, whereas during extension the anterior cruciate pulls the femoral condyles anteriorly on the tibial plateau. The anterior cruciate restrains anterior displacement of the tibia on the femur and the posterior cruciate resists posterior displacement of the tibia on the femur. As the cruciate ligaments provide a reciprocal balanced traction between the femoral and tibial condyles during flexion and extension of the knee joint, they are not slack at any stage of motion.

The *synovial cavity* of the knee joint is the most extensive joint cavity in the body. It communicates with the large suprapatellar bursa, the bursa under the popliteus tendon, and possibly the superior tibiofibular joint. The cavity may also join the bursa on the semimembranosus tendon and occasionally presents as a cystic swelling on the medial or lateral side of that tendon.

Menisci. The menisci consist of semilunar-shaped fibrocartilaginous wedges that indirectly increase the area of contact between the convex femoral and tibial condyles. The almost flat inferior meniscal surface allows sliding and rotary movements on the articular cartilage of the tibial plateaus. The concave superior surfaces embrace the convex femoral condyles and accurately follow their ever-changing geometric out-lines. During extension the menisci slide forward on the tibial condyles, separate anteriorly by stretching of the transverse ligament, and open their curvature to accommodate the flatter anterior areas of the femoral condyles. The so-called semilunar cartilages are repeatedly exposed to vertical compression, to horizontal distraction, and to rotary and shearing forces; in order to accommodate these strains and resulting stresses, they are made up predominantly of fibrous tissue interspersed by occasional cartilaginous cells. Both menisci are attached to the intercondylar notch of the tibia by the anterior and posterior fibrous horns (Fig. 10-10). In addition, the peripheral edges of the menisci are attached (except where the popliteal tendon crosses the lateral meniscus) to the peripheral margins of the tibial condyles by the short coronary ligament (better developed and shorter on the medial side) and the synovial membrane and to the corresponding femoral articular margins by the long coronary ligaments (Fig. 10-6). One or two meniscofemoral ligaments connect the posterior margin of the lateral meniscus to the lateral aspect of the medial femoral condyle (Fig. 10-10).

The infrapatellar fat pad has a greater concentration of pain endings than any other joint structure.[4] During flexion and extension the fat pad undergoes many intrinsic alterations to accommodate the ever-changing contour of the femoral condyles and the intercondylar notch.

The named genicular arteries provide the principal blood supply to the knee joint. The typical hunterian articular vascular anastomosis is located in the subsynovial tissues at the margin of the articular cartilage and it supplies branches to the capsule, the synovial structures, and via the bony foramina, to the underlying epiphyses or condyles (Fig. 10-11). The lateral inferior genicular vessels, constantly situated on the peripheral margin of the lateral meniscus, may be injured during lateral meniscectomy[6] (Fig. 10-6).

Quadriceps. Well-developed quadriceps are indispensable for adequate knee joint activity. For maximal efficiency the total pull of the four-headed muscle mass should be perpendicular to the horizontal axis of the knee joint. Any malalignment of this pull such as that caused by genu valgum, a wasted vastus medialis, or depressed lateral tibial plateau fractures will lead to incomplete quadriceps action and eventual joint degeneration. The inferior fibers of the vastus medialis counterbalance the lateral pull that is exerted on the patella by the other three muscles. The vastus medialis arises from the trochanteric line and the medial lip of the linea aspera as far as the hiatus

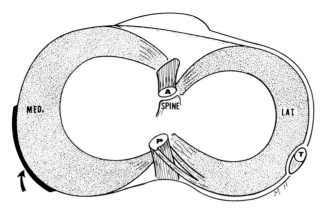

Fig. 10-10. Articular structures on superior aspect of right tibia. Anterior, **A,** and posterior, **P,** cruciate splitting the meniscofemoral ligaments into anterior (Humphrey) and posterior (Wrisberg) components. **T,** Popliteal tendon. Meniscal attachment to medial ligament is indicated by arrow.

Left lateral condyle

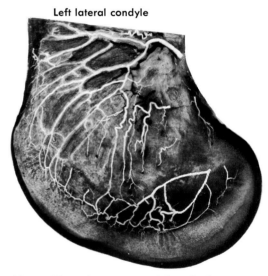

Fig. 10-11. Hunterian subsynovial articular anastomosis from the lateral superior genicular artery.

for the femoral vessels in the adductor magnus. Beyond this opening the more horizontal fibers take origin predominantly from the anterior surface and tendon of the adductor magnus muscle. Although the vastus medialis covers the medial aspect of the femoral shaft, it has no attachments to this surface of the bone. The lower vastus medialis is made up almost exclusively of muscle fibers, which may reach to the distal margin of the patella. This extension and intimate relationship of muscle fibers to the cavity and capsule of the knee joint contributes to the prompt

and rapid wasting of this muscle, which is associated with pathologic conditions of the knee joint.

Hamstrings. The deeper component of the semimembranosus tendon has a strong linear insertion to the inferior margin of the horizontal groove on both the medial and posterior aspects of the medial tibial condyle (Fig. 10-2). The superficial component of the tendon has a continuous fan- or conelike expansion that forms the oblique popliteal ligament of Winslow and the popliteal fascia, designated respectively the reflected and the direct heads by French anatomists.[9] This fascia expansion reaches the tibia in a V-shaped outline that delineates the insertion of the popliteus muscle. Cave and Porteus[3] pointed out that the superficial or direct insertions are active at all stages of knee flexion but that the reflected component pulls "only when genuflexion has attained an amplitude of 90 degrees." The deeper tendon may be surrounded in part or completely by a bursa that separates it from the upper margin of the horizontal groove, from the medial head of the gastrocnemius, and from the medial collateral ligament; it may even communicate with the joint cavity.

In posterior approaches to the knee joint the popliteal vessels and tibial nerve cross the operative field (Fig. 10-1). Slight flexion of the joint facilitates lateral retraction of these structures. This retraction may stretch the nerve supply to the medial head of the gastrocnemius, but the muscle can be detached from the medial femoral condyle and also reflected laterally.

SURGICAL APPROACHES

The following basic "ten commandments" of surgical exposure are strongly recommended.[7]

1. Orientation of the surgeon is of prime importance. Time spent in determining his precise position will spare the operator many anxious moments and will hasten recovery of the patient.
2. Easy access to the operative area is afforded by proper positioning and draping of the patient as well as by a correctly placed incision.
3. The skin cut should follow the creases or natural lines of skin tension; it should avoid bony prominences and be of sufficient length to allow performance of all required surgery. Forcible and excessive retraction with resultant maceration of skin edges is thereby avoided.
4. By following the intermuscular planes, muscle scarring is minimized and return of function is enhanced.
5. Control of hermorrhage is achieved *at operation* by use of a tourniquet, selection of a "dry" route

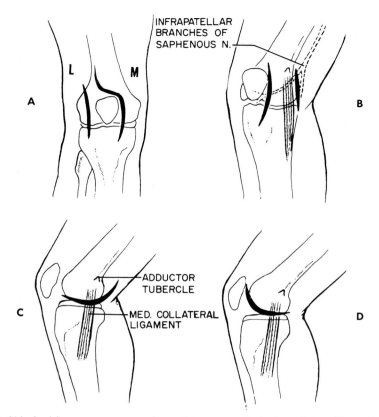

Fig. 10-12. Skin incisions more commonly used to approach the knee joint. (From Joyce, J. J., III, and Harty, M.: Orthopaedic approaches, Baltimore, 1961, The Williams & Wilkins Co.)

to visualize the operative field, isolation and ligation of vessels during the approach, use of electrocautery, and a loose closure. *Postoperatively*, control of hemorrhage is achieved by elevation of the extremity, adequate splinting when necessary, and compression dressings when indicated (the use of the so-called "Jones compression splint" for the knee is an excellent example of this principle); also, use of a small drain (preferably with suction) occasionally aids in the prevention of a postoperative hematoma.

6. Vital structures must be protected by either judicious selection of an avenue to the operative area that avoids all major structures or by visualizing them and retracting them gently out of the field.

7. Wound closure must be accurate, without tension, and contain a minimal amount of suture material.

8. Early activity of the extremity operated on prevents loss of function and enhances early recovery.

9. Adequate equipment must be available to perform the operation in question. Improvised devices at the time of surgery prolong the procedure. The patient must not be compelled to "fit the equipment."

10. Trained personnel should assist the surgeon in order to keep the operation progressing efficiently.

Since no single exposure of the knee permits access to the entire joint, anterior, posterior, medial, and lateral approaches or a combination of them may be required. Although many skin incisions have been proposed to demonstrate the knee joint, the parapatellar approaches are the most versatile and widely used (Fig. 10-12).

Medial parapatellar approach

The medial parapatellar incision, which may be combined with the posteromedial incision, is the most frequently used to explore the knee joint.

Indications. Exploration of the anterior knee compartment for mechanical derangements, drainage of infections, removal of loose bodies, arthrotomy for synovectomy, and medial meniscectomy constitute some of the more common indications for the medial parapatellar approach to the knee.

Limitations. The posterior compartment is inaccessible through the anterior route. Only an incomplete exposure of the lateral meniscus is available by the anteromedial approach; other exposures give a better view of this structure.

Landmarks. The patella, the medial femoral condyle, the tibial tubercle, the ligamentum patellae, and the joint line aid in locating the skin cut.

Danger points. Misplacement of the skin incision so that it overlies a bony prominence often results in later discomfort when the patient squats or kneels. Division of the infrapatellar branches of the saphenous nerve sometimes produces a painful neuroma or a permanent area of annoying numbness anterior to the lower knee area. Incisions placed far laterally may enter the fat pad behind the patellar tendon. Within the joint the articular cartilage may be damaged or the medial collateral ligament may be inadvertently divided, causing instability of the joint. If mobilization and visualization of the posterior meniscal horn are difficult, a second incision behind the medial collateral ligament will facilitate the procedure.

Position of patient. Many operators place the patient in a supine position with the knee flexed over the end of the table. Others prefer to place the patient on the table so that the hip is in abduction and the flexed knee slightly elevated.

Technique. The skin incision begins at a point approximately at the level of the superior patellar pole (Fig. 10-12, *B*). The knife then passes parallel to the medial patellar border, crosses the joint line parallel to the patellar tendon, and ends at about the level of the tibial tubercle. Infrapatellar branches of the saphenous nerve may be encountered in the subcutaneous tissues (Fig. 10-13). Division of the capsule (medial patellar retinaculum) will expose the synovium and medial margin of the fat pad. The synovial membrane is picked up between hemostats and opened. A wide expanse of the joint is not available with this exposure, but if seriatim retraction is used, a good view is obtained of the synovium, the notch margin of the femoral condyles, the anterior cruciate, the anterior parts of the menisci, and the fat pad (Fig. 10-13).

Posterior extension. Exposure of the posteromedial compartment is facilitated by flexion of the knee to 90°; this allows the sartorius and saphenous vein to fall posteriorly from the area of exposure. A short vertical skin incision parallel to the medial

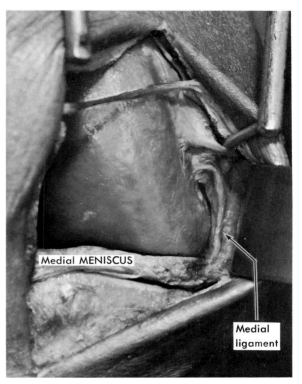

Fig. 10-13. Right knee. The medial ligament is retracted from the medial meniscus. The nerve crosses the femoral condyle.

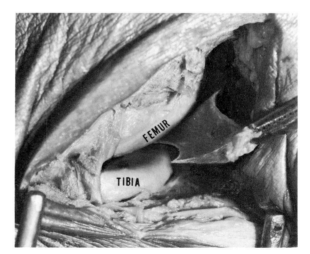

Fig. 10-14. Posteromedial exposure of right knee. Part of the medial meniscus is retracted backward.

ligament or backward prolongation of a horizontal incision exposes the capsule (Fig. 10-12, *B* to *D*). The posteromedial margin of the medial femoral condyle is a guide to the joint cavity. A curved hemostat passed through the anterior incision also helps to confirm the site for the capsule opening. The detached portion of the meniscus is passed through the posterior opening and gentle knee manipulation allows good visualization of the posterior horn (Fig. 10-14).

Lateral approaches

Of the many lateral routes to the knee joint, it is thought that the exposure described by Kaplan[8] offers many advantages over the more conventional approaches.

Indications. The Kaplan incision affords easy access to the lateral collateral ligament, the lateral meniscus, the lateral genicular vessels, and the popliteus tendon—in fact, almost the entire lateral compartment may be seen through this exposure.

Limitations. Access to the medial compartment of the joint is very limited, as is visualization of the intercondylar area.

Guideposts. In this area the patella, the fibular head, the biceps tendon, the lateral tibial condyle, the iliotibial tract, as well as the lateral femoral condyle are the guideposts. Posteriorly the lateral head of the gastrocnemius should be identified before attempting to enter that portion of the joint.

Danger points. Identification and protection of the iliotibial band, the lateral collateral ligament, and the popliteus tendon are essential (Figs. 10-3 and 10-5). The vulnerable lateral genicular vessel can be identified on the meniscus, and the common peroneal nerve, hidden behind the biceps tendon, must be remembered (Figs. 10-3 and 10-6). The lateral head of the gastrocnemius offers an intervening buffer to protect the popliteal vessels.

Technique. The patient is placed on his sound side with the knee to be operated on extended. Starting at the proximal patellar pole, the incision extends obliquely and posteriorly across the joint line, skirting the posterior margin of the superior tibiofibular joint and ending almost in the midline of the popliteal space (Fig. 10-15). After the skin edges have been retracted, the iliotibial band is identified. Through a cut extending from the superior patellar pole to the iliotibial band in the same line as the skin incision the anterior compartment of the lateral aspect of the knee joint may be visualized. Through an opening extending from the posterior edge of the iliotibial band to the biceps tendon one may find the lateral meniscus, the genicular vessel, the popliteus tendon, and the lateral collateral ligament. Wider access to the joint is afforded by Nixon's V-shaped division of the iliotibial band,[9] but every effort should be made to preserve the lateral ligament and popliteus tendon

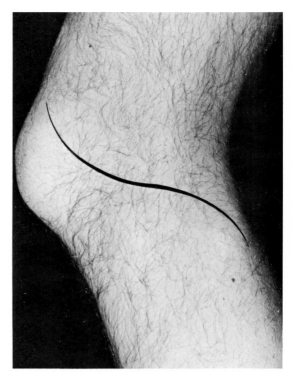

Fig. 10-15. Lateral side of left knee. Skin incision for the Kaplan approach is indicated.

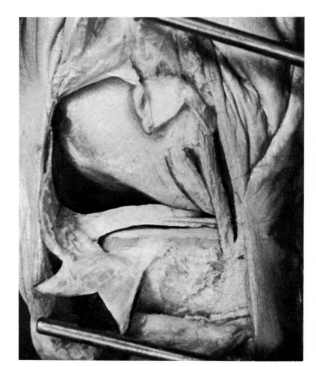

Fig. 10-16. Left lateral exposure of knee. Nixon's V incision through the iliotibial band displays most of the lateral joint. (See also Fig. 10-3, *A*.)

(Fig. 10-16). Careful repair of the iliotibial band is recommended on closure. This exposure has proved invaluable in the removal of multiple loose bodies from the lateral compartment.

Anterior approach

Although rarely required, extensive access to the entire anterior compartment of the knee joint may be obtained through a long S-shaped parapatellar incision with a plastic division of the quadriceps aponeurosis.

Indications. Lengthening of the quadriceps tendon, reduction of widely separated patellar fractures accompanied by capsular tears, extensive synovectomy, arthrodesis, insertion of prostheses, and other situations requiring extensive visualization of the entire knee joint are indications for the anterior approach. Prolonged convalesence is the major disadvantage of such a wide anterior approach.

Technique. The incision begins slightly above and medial to the tibial tubercle. The knife then sweeps proximally to parallel the patella in a line about one fingerbreadth medial to it. Upon reaching the superior patellar pole, the cut passes transversely to the lateral border of the rectus, at which point the incision is again extended proximally for 2 or 3 inches (Fig. 10-12, *A*). By careful undermining of the skin flap, the entire patella and anterior capsule are available for inspection. Division of the quadriceps aponeurosis with both parapatellar retinacula (Fig. 10-17) allows distal rotation of the patella and exposure of all the anterior joint cavity (Fig. 10-18). A meticulous repair of the soft tissues is essential. The patient should be advised that he is likely to have a permanent region of numbness in the area supplied by the infrapatellar branch of the saphenous nerve.

Posterior approach

Although not commonly utilized because the joint is deeply placed and covered by the neurovascular bundle to the leg and foot, the posterior approach is sometimes needed (Fig. 10-1).

Indications. Removal of loose bodies in the knee's posterior compartment, exposure of the popliteal face of the femur, repair of certain ligamentous tears, removal of popliteal cysts, and exposure of the neurovascular bundle constitute the more frequent indications.

Limitations. Although the exposure may not be extended easily to either side of the knee or distally, it can be extended proximally. Careful and precise dissection is required to protect the vulnerable neurovascular structures.

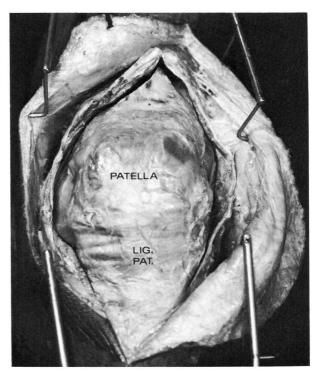

Fig. 10-17. Aponeurosis and parapatellar retinacular incision for anterior approach.

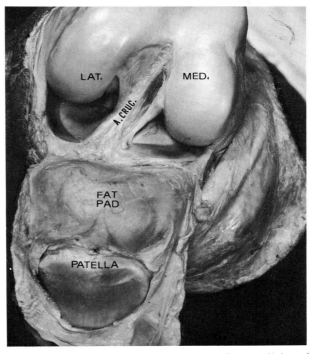

Fig. 10-18. Distal reflection of patella. The medial and lateral menisci diverge from the tibial end of the anterior cruciate.

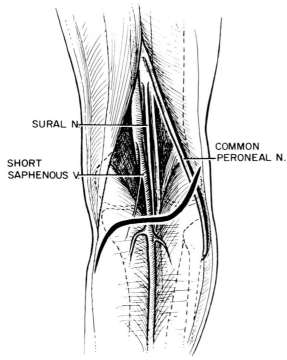

Fig. 10-19. Posterior view of right knee joint with the incision indicated. (From Joyce, J. J., III, and Harty, M.: Orthopaedic approaches, Baltimore, 1961, The Williams & Wilkins Co.)

Landmarks. The flexor crease, fibular head (lying one fingerbreadth below the joint line), hamstrings, and the heads of the gastrocnemius are important landmarks aiding the surgeon in the correct placement of the skin incision (Fig. 10-19). Immediately under the skin the short saphenous vein on the deep fascia and the sural nerve just beneath the deep fascia may be found in the groove between the heads of the gastrocnemius. Both of these structures are helpful guides in leading the operator safely to the neurovascular bundle.

Technique. An S-shaped incision is used, the horizontal portion passing parallel to the flexor crease. The two ends are extended a handsbreadth proximally and distally (Fig. 10-19). By starting the dissection in the lower portion of the wound, the short saphenous vein (Henry's "blue line") may be located in the fat overlying the gastrocnemius heads. After the deep fascia is opened, the sural nerve is located in the same manner. Gentle separation of the gastrocnemius heads will usually permit visualization of the tibial nerve and popliteal vessels (Fig. 10-19). Careful blunt dissection allows one to mobilize the neurovascular bundle so that it may be displaced sufficiently to open the joint capsule, which is often

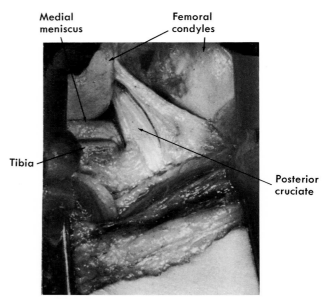

Fig. 10-20. Posterior exposure of right knee.

divided by an L-shaped cut. Careful retraction of the capsular edges discloses the posterior compartment and its contents (Fig. 10-20).

SUMMARY

Some functional and clinical aspects of the anatomy of the knee joint are presented and illustrated. The areas of the more important structures encountered during surgical exposures are emphasized. Some basic axioms of technique are reinterated.

The more commonly used surgical approaches to the knee joint and their problems are discussed.

REFERENCES

1. Brantigan, O. C., and Voshell, A. F.: The tibial collateral ligament, J. Bone Joint Surg. **25-A:**121, 1943.
2. Brock, Rt. Hon. Lord: The anatomy of the bronchial tree, London, 1946, Oxford University Press.
3. Cave, A. J. E., and Porteus, C. J.: A note on the semimembranosus muscle, Ann. Roy. Coll. Surg. Eng. **24:**251, 1957.
4. Freeman, M. A. R., and Wyke, B.: The innervation of the knee joint, J. Anat. **101:**3, 505, 1967.
5. Harty, M.: Anatomical features of the lateral aspect of the knee joint, Surg. Gynec. Obstet. **130:**11, 1970.
6. Harty, M., and Kostowiecki, M.: Vascular injuries in limb surgery, Surg. Gynec. Obstet. **121:**339, 1965.
7. Joyce, J. J., III, and Harty, M.: Orthopaedic approaches, Baltimore, 1961, The Williams & Wilkins Co.
8. Kaplan, E. B.: Surgical approach to the lateral side of the knee joint, Surg. Gynec. Obstet. **104:**346, 1957.
9. Nixon, J. E.: Lateral approach to the knee joint, Surg. Gynec. Obstet. **116:**126, 1963.
10. Rouviere, H.: Anatomie humaine, Paris, 1962, Masson & Cie, vol. 3, p. 360.

Chapter 11

Osteoarthritis of the knee and its early arrest

ARTHUR J. HELFET, B.Sc. (Capetown), M.D., M.Ch. Orth. (Liverpool), F.R.C.S. (Eng.), F.A.C.S.
Bronx, New York

A great deal of research, both clinical and experimental, is in progress to elucidate the problems of osteoarthritis. While the degenerative process is being studied at the biochemical level, a detailed macroscopic and microscopic examination of joints would improve our understanding of the condition and our ability to deal with clinical problems of the aging joint. The knee joint has proved particularly appropriate to such an investigation. It lends itself to precise clinical examination and simple surgical access.

WHAT IS OSTEOARTHRITIS OF THE KNEE?
Clinical syndrome

Recurrent effusions, pain, stiffness, and wasting of the quadriceps muscle characterize osteoarthritis of the knee. The syndrome may start insidiously, but often the symptoms appear suddenly. Even with a sudden onset, however, the situation is quite different from that following trauma to a young healthy knee, for it is superimposed on a groundwork of degenerative changes (which have followed often minimal, sometimes neglected trauma in aging tissues); these changes have not yet caused symptoms.

Repeated exacerbations follow: the capsule stretches and the joint gradually becomes unstable, with increasing pain and decreasing function. The patient may label it as "just old age" and accept it. The physician, having diagnosed osteoarthritis, consigns the patient to gradual reduction of function.

It has been my observation, over many years, that in most instances the condition we call osteoarthritis is seldom more than a mechanical derangement of the knee joint, modified in its manifestation by the qualitative process of aging that we call degeneration.

Aging of articular cartilage

With aging the matrix of articular cartilage loses its resilience. Any abnormal stress, especially if repeated, results in erosion of the articular cartilage. The patterns of erosion faithfully mirror the eroding agent (Figs. 11-1 and 11-2).

Osteoarthritis of the knee seldom begins as a generalized phenomenon: usually it is restricted to one compartment. In most instances, as will be shown, the patterns of erosion and the sequence of change may be traced to derangement of a single meniscus and to the consequent interference with normal joint movement.

Examination of a joint in which there is irregularity of part of the joint surface (for example, in chondromalacia patellae or an old osteochondral fracture) reveals a specific pattern of wear in the opposing surface. However, similar patterns of erosion are commonly found on one or other femoral condyle even without previous bony abnormality.

Bauer and Smith[2] used a focusing collimator for the detailed study of isotope uptake to determine the metabolic activity in juxta-articular bone. They confirmed the localized nature of osteoarthritis (Fig. 11-3). Not only is the increased metabolic activity confined to one condyle, but it is restricted to a part of that condyle. It is interesting that the increased metabolism corresponds to the areas of increased bone sclerosis shown on x-ray examination, which also may

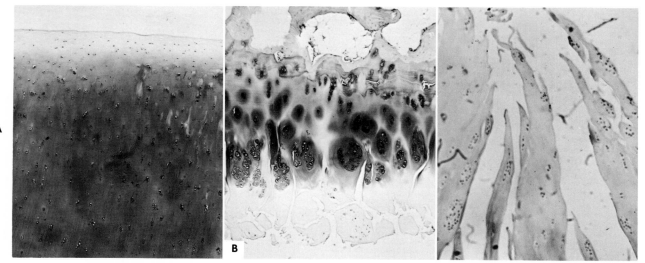

Fig. 11-1. A, Normal human articular cartilage. The surface is smooth and cells are regularly dispersed. The cartilage at the surface contains no mucopolysaccharide, whereas the deeper zones are positive for mucopolysaccharide. **B,** Human articular cartilage with moderate degenerative changes. The cartilage is diminished in height, there is fissuring of the articular surface, and fissured areas are devoid of mucopolysaccharide. Clumps of chondrocytes in the deeper zones are surrounded by halos of increased mucopolysaccharide content. **C,** Human articular cartilage with advanced degenerative changes. The cartilage is fissured throughout and devoid of mucopolysaccharide. Clumps of chondrocytes also lack a mucopolysaccharide halo. (Safranine O stain; taken with green filter at original magnifications of 56× for **A,** 90× for **B,** and 112× for **C.**

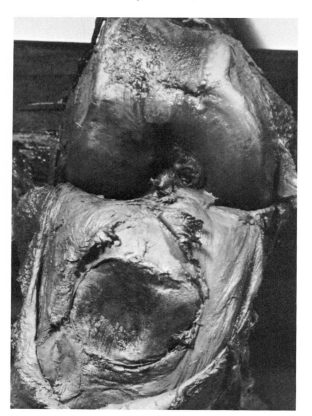

be limited to one area on one condyle (Fig. 11-4). In the majority of cases the eroding agent is the meniscus, and it would seem that the increase in isotope activity occurs in the area so irritated.

The aging meniscus

The young meniscus is white, elastic, and firm but pliable (Fig. 11-5, *A*). It is avascular except where it is attached to the capsule of the joint. When cut, it is fibrous, the fibers all running in its longitudinal axis. In cross section it is elongated, with a thin edge extending into the joint. Microscopically, it consists of fibrocartilage cells lying in a collagen matrix (Fig. 11-5, *B*). There are no blood vessels except at its base.

As it ages, the meniscus gets harder, until finally all elasticity has been lost. It changes in color, becoming yellowish and translucent, especially at its thin free border, and it contracts until it is triangular in cross section (Fig. 11-6, *A*). Microscopically there is a

Fig. 11-2. Specimen showing "minor" erosions on opposing articular surfaces of the patella and femoral condyle, a typical example of the pattern of erosion expected after recurrent dislocation of the patella. (From Helfet, A. J.: The management of internal derangements of the knee, Philadelphia, 1963, J. B. Lippincott Co.)

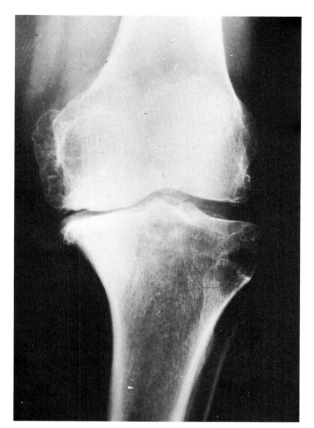

Fig. 11-3. The localized nature of osteoarthritis.

gradual loss of the cellular element; the intercellular material becomes more abundant and is gradually replaced by fibrous tissue. Finally, it is invaded by blood vessels (Fig. 11-6, *B*). We call this process degeneration. Such a degenerate meniscus is unable to stand up to the abnormal stresses to which it may be subjected. In the end the hard inelastic lump of fibrous tissue makes the complaint of some old people that "It feels as though there is a pebble in my knee," quite understandable.

Injury to the degenerate meniscus

The hardened, degenerate meniscus tears in a different manner than the younger meniscus. A minor injury is enough and causes detachment of the anterior horn. This results in aching, recurrent swellings, and buckling. Typically a middle-aged housewife, with a history of pain and swelling, kneels on the ground; if in turning she interrupts the synchrony of movement, she will rupture the attachment of the anterior horn. As a result of aging, increasing fibrosis occurs in the substance of the meniscus that causes it to contract in each direction. This is the "retracted" meniscus (Fig. 11-7, *A*), which may be separated by ½ inch or more from the anterior tibial spine.

Often the patient can straighten the knee and has

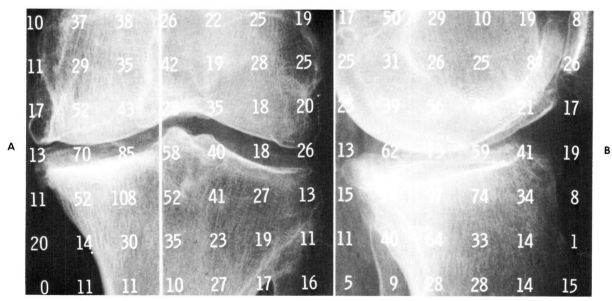

Fig. 11-4. ^{85}Sr scintimetry in a 78-year-old woman with osteoarthritis of the medial femorotibial articulation of the left knee. Note high values at involved part of knee joint. **A,** Frontal projection. **B,** Lateral projection showing low values at patellofemoral articulation in spite of presence of large osteophytes that were probably secondary to osteoarthritis of the femorotibial articulation. (From Bauer, G. C. H., and Smith, E. M.: J. Nucl. Med. **10:**109, 1969.)

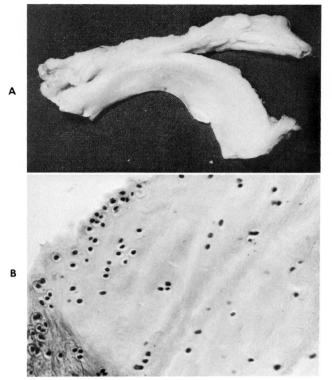

Fig. 11-5. The young meniscus. **A,** Gross specimen. **B,** Histologic specimen.

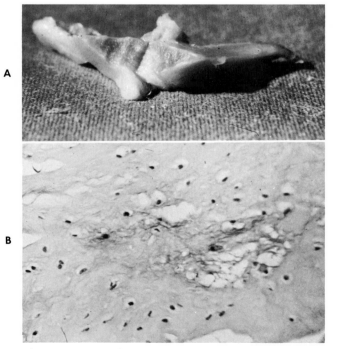

Fig. 11-6. The older meniscus. **A,** Gross specimen. **B,** Histologic specimen.

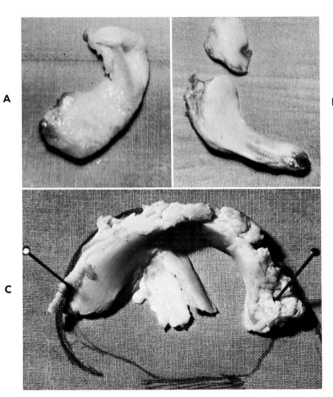

Fig. 11-7. Injuries to the degenerate meniscus. **A,** "Retracted" meniscus. **B,** "Fractured" meniscus. **C,** "Fishtail" meniscus. (**C** from Helfet, A. J.: The management of internal derangements of the knee, Philadelphia, 1963, J. B. Lippincott Co.)

no immediate pain (just as complete rupture of a ligament is painless). Within a few weeks she may complain of swelling and an ache on walking, symptoms that are present in any joint with a block to movement—in this case, limitation of external rotation and extension. The gap between the anterior horn and anterior cruciate ligament is the same as the gap of the bowstring tear in young people (approximately half the width of the patella). With time the anterior end of the retracted meniscus becomes thickened and shortened. There may be a full-blown block to rotation at this stage, but usually symptoms and signs are mild and recurrent.

In weight bearing the retracted meniscus continues to be subject to stress at the junction of the contracted anterior two-thirds and the flatter posterior third. It is incapable of bearing such stress. Following recurrent pain and swelling there is a crisis in the knee, often while the patient is walking. The joint suddenly becomes so painful that no weight can be placed on it. It is now "locked" in flexion and internal rotation. What has happened is that the retracted meniscus has "fractured" transversely at the junction of the thickened anterior two-thirds and the more normal flatter posterior third (Fig. 11-7, *B*). This is the most common finding when there has been a crisis in the knee of the older patient. The clinical findings are unequivocally those of a block due to an internal derangement.

As a variable in this series of events, a posterior segment of the immobile, contracted, thickened meniscus continues to be subjected to abnormal compression. It becomes squashed and shows a typical "fishtail" appearance at operation (Fig. 11-7, *C*). At this stage the meniscus is easy to remove because it is hard, detached at both ends, and the repeated effusions have caused capsular laxity.

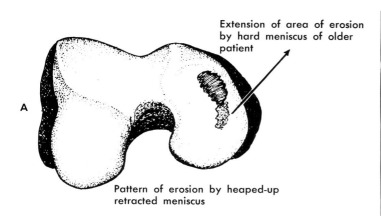
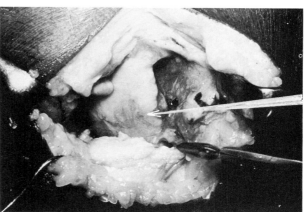

Fig. 11-8. Erosive pattern from a retracted meniscus. **A**, Diagram. **B**, Operative photograph.

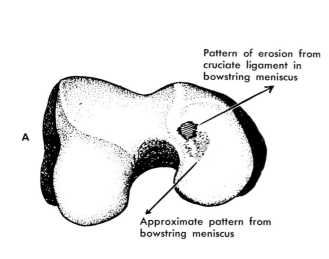
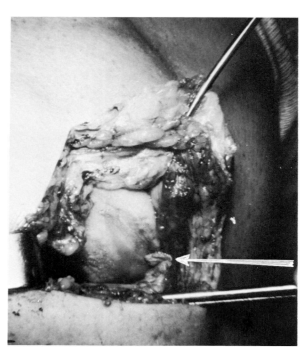

Fig. 11-9. Erosive pattern from a bowstring meniscus. **A**, Diagram. **B**, Operative photograph. (**A** from Helfet, A. J.: The management of internal derangements of the knee, Philadelphia, 1963, J. B. Lippincott Co.)

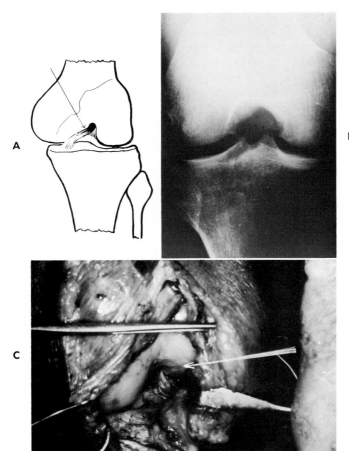

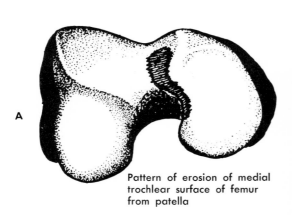

Even in the older patient, however, meniscal degeneration need not be excessive; if so, there is no reason why injury should not follow the pattern of that in the younger patient. Consequently, we occasionally find examples of bowstring, parrot-beak, and grossly degenerate menisci, in addition to the anterior or posterior detachments. They are, however, much less common.[6]

Patterns of erosion

1. An injured meniscus rubs continually against the same segment of femoral condyle so that each type of meniscal derangement produces its own specific pattern of erosion (Figs. 11-8 and 11-9). It is confined to the portion of the condyle opposite the affected meniscus and differs only with the site of the meniscal injury—front, back, or both. Because of the incongruous fit of the femoral and tibial condyles, a ridge of osteophytes forms along the medial rim of the condyle. The block to external rotation of the tibia causes the anterior cruciate ligament to impinge directly against the nonweight-bearing lateral side of

Fig. 11-10. Mechanics of cruciate erosion. **A,** Diagram. **B,** X-ray appearance. **C,** Operative photograph. (**A** from Helfet, A. J.: The management of internal derangement of the knee, Philadelphia, 1963, J. B. Lippincott Co.)

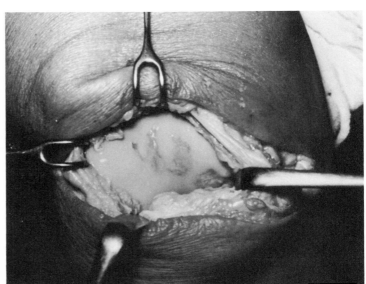

Pattern of erosion of medial trochlear surface of femur from patella

Fig. 11-11. Erosion of medial femoral condyle following loss of synchronous patellar movement. **A,** Diagram. **B,** Operative photograph. (**A** from Helfet, A. J.: The management of internal derangements of the knee, Philadelphia, 1963, J. B. Lippincott Co.)

the medial femoral condyle. An erosion therefore develops in this region also and may be visible on the radiograph (Fig. 11-10). It is high in the intercondylar notch and well away from the weight-bearing area of the condyle. (The erosion is in exactly the same place as the lesion in osteochondritis dissecans, a fact that may well throw some light on the mysterious condition.) At the same time as the cruciate ligament is stretched across the edge of the medial condyle, repeated effusions, plus the block to external rotation of the tibia, stretch the medial capsule and so explain the gradual development of the anteroposterior and medial laxity in the osteoarthritic knee.

2. The loss of external rotation with extension

means that the patella cannot follow its normal course in the trochlear groove, and a localized pattern of erosion therefore develops on the superior portion of the lateral surface of the medial femoral condyle and extends to the medial trochlear slope (Fig. 11-11). Chondrophytes and osteophytes grow on the medial edge of the erosion. The lateral slope of the trochlear groove is rarely abraded. A similar pattern of erosion and osteophyte formation occurs on the medial surface of the patella for the same reason (Fig. 11-12). Osteophytosis of the medial edge of the patella is much greater than of its femoral counterpart, probably because of the capsular and synovial attachment here.

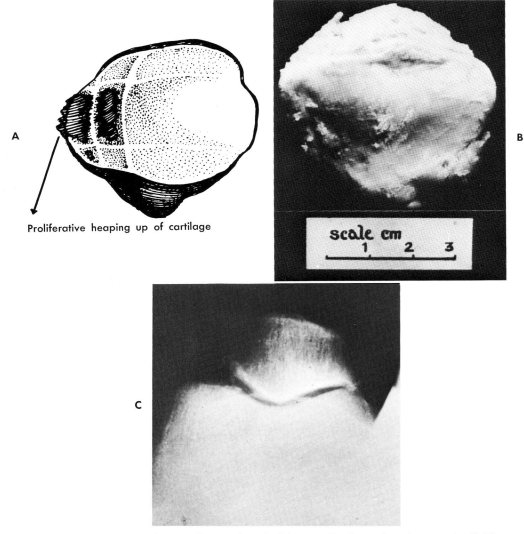

Proliferative heaping up of cartilage

Fig. 11-12. Corresponding patellar erosion. **A,** Diagram. **B,** Operative photograph. **C,** X-ray appearance. (**A** and **B** from Helfet, A. J.: The management of internal derangements of the knee, Philadelphia, 1963, J. B. Lippincott Co.)

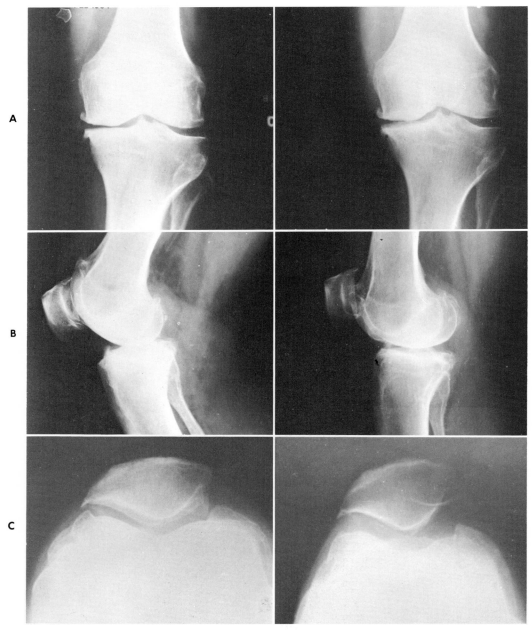

Fig. 11-13. X-ray films show arrest of osteoarthritis of knee between February 1964 and January 1966 following operative correction of mechanical derangement. **A,** Anteroposterior view. **B,** Lateral view. **C,** Skyline view of patella. Note localization of osteoarthritis to the medial compartment, resolution of subchondral sclerosis and recovery of normal trabeculation, and marked clarification of bone structure.

We now have the full-blown lesion we call osteoarthritis.

MECHANICAL DERANGEMENT AND THE CONCEPT OF EARLY ARREST

Any block to the meniscal guide mechanism converts the helical movement of the normal knee into a hinge or roller movement.[5] There is a consequent loss of the extreme of extension and/or flexion, depending upon the site of injury to the meniscus. Because of the block to tibial rotation, the medial femoral condyle cannot reach rotational alignment with the tibia; instead it projects in front of the medial tibial condyle and the prominent transverse bony protrusion can be felt on the medial side of the knee joint. The medial border of the patella, forced to rub against the lateral surface of the medial femoral condyle, becomes tender. The McMurray and "reducing" clicks may be present.[6] Repeated effusions occur in the joint from local inflammatory response in the synovium. The quadriceps muscle becomes wasted even more quickly than in the younger patient.

When derangement is overcome surgically, the symptoms are relieved and the joint no longer continues on its path of increasing deformity and loss of function. The joint becomes comfortable and resumes movement in a normal pattern, that is, synchronous rotation with flexion and extension. In time, x-ray studies show resolution of juxta-articular sclerosis and restoration of normal bone trabeculation (Fig. 11-13).[7]

If the degenerate joint with superadded mechanical derangement is left untreated, further changes invariably develop (Fig. 11-14). One can thus arrive at the concept of *arrest* of osteoarthritis of the knee and that the *earlier* the arrest, the better. When articular erosion is complete, the underlying bone becomes thickened and sclerotic. The increase in such sclerotic subchondral bone provides a radiologic indicator of progress. Isotope studies by Bauer and Smith[2] show that the sclerosis denotes increased metabolic activity. The presence of sclerosis opposite a displaced or

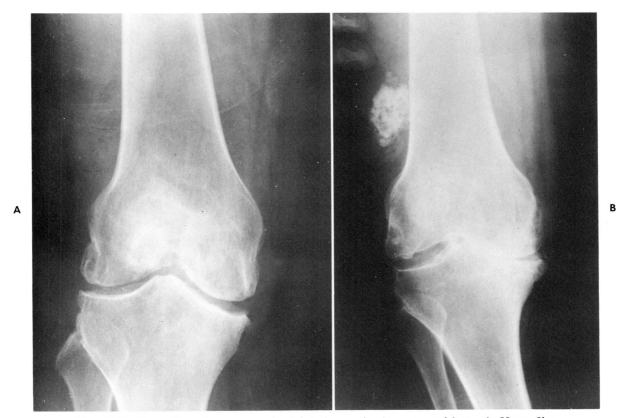

A

B

Fig. 11-14. X-ray films show progressive joint changes in the untreated knee. **A,** X-ray film taken in April 1957. **B,** X-ray film taken in March 1964.

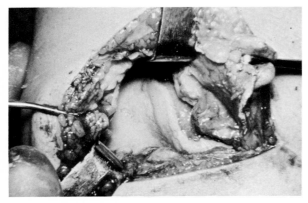

Fig. 11-15. Operative photograph shows osteophytes that must be removed before joint reduction can be obtained.

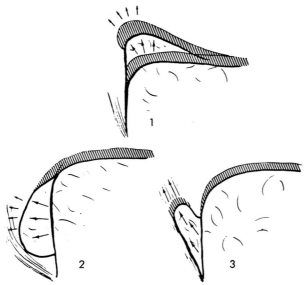

Fig. 11-16. Diagram shows the remodeling processes that occur in an osteoarthritic knee joint. **1,** Upward and lateral cartilage growth. **2,** Local periosteal new bone formation. **3,** Chondrification followed by ossification of a tendon or capsule. (From Johnson, L. C.: Lab. Invest. **8:**1223, 1959.)

distorted meniscus suggests that this is a reaction to abnormal tissue tension when movement is attempted.

Correction of the derangement by removal of the soft tissue block alone may be sufficient to correct the deformity, but when the osteoarthritis has eroded bone, removal of the offending meniscus is no longer adequate. Capsular fibrosis adds to the deforming process, and in areas adjacent to the erosions and at the joint margins where the capsule is attached, osteophytes form. They may, at first, be of

little significance, but if a joint has been left blocked for any length of time, this osteophytosis becomes so large that it acts as a bony block to reduction of the joint. These osteophytes must be removed before reduction can be obtained (Fig. 11-15). Finally, the adaptive thickening of the subchondral bone fails. Deformity now becomes structural and can be corrected only by a bone operation. Johnson's studies[8] suggest the process of resorption and replacement of bone and cartilage by which this new shaping of articular surfaces develops (Fig. 11-16).

The invariable outcome of neglect of such a knee underlines the value of early operation. Provided synchronous movement of the joint is restored in time, the process comes to a halt and further degeneration does not occur. By calling the process osteoarthritis, we are doing our patient a disservice. If we label the condition "mechanical derangement with a degenerative meniscus," we instantly take a step in the direction of early treatment. A similar philosophical point of view in relation to the hip joint (where analysis of the patterns of wear and tear are more difficult) has led us to focus our attention on early surgery to correct the abnormal mechanical dysfunction.

PAIN IN OSTEOARTHRITIS

Articular cartilage has no sensory nerve endings and erosions of cartilage do not, in themselves, give rise to pain. The damaged inelastic meniscus, however, is subjected to deforming stress when movement is attempted. The meniscus is attached to the capsule, which is itself undergoing fibrosis; this fibrotic capsule is stretched on movement and gives rise to the sensation of pain on weight bearing. Restoration of correct mechanical function of the joint overcomes the pain.

Retropatellar pain on climbing and especially on descending stairs is often an early symptom of osteoarthritis of the knee. Because of the block to synchronous external rotation of the tibia during extension, the patella is prevented from following its normally sinuous course into the trochlear groove. Instead the strong contraction of the quadriceps on stairs causes abnormal impingement of the medial facet of the patella on the corresponding slope of the trochlear groove with increasing erosion, sensitivity, and pain.

Pain may also derive from weakness and fatigue of the muscles—in which case an "achy tiredness" is felt in the thigh. Wardle,[9] Helal,[3] Apley,[1] and others consider that venous congestion in the tibia may be a potent cause of pain and indeed of the whole arthritic process. They suggest that the success of infra-articular osteotomy of the tibia in relieving pain is due to blocking of the dilated venous systems in the medulla, comparable to the effect of tying off varicose veins.

SURGERY OF THE OSTEOARTHRITIC KNEE

Successful treatment depends on exact preoperative diagnosis, gentle well-planned surgery, and adequate reablement. The operation is usually easier in the older than in the young patient (although recovery is more arduous). The extent of surgery depends upon the stage of involvement of the joint. If the meniscus alone is responsible for the internal derangement, meniscectomy will arrest the condition. The usual transverse incision with anterior extension parallel to the patella is recommended (Fig. 11-17). This extension permits examination of the medial surface of the patella and debridement when necessary. After meniscectomy any loose tags of articular cartilage that are present at the edge of the erosions are removed. If osteophytes prevent adequate reduction of either the tibiofemoral or patellofemoral joints, they are removed with a rongeur or osteotome.

Patellectomy is to be deprecated. Invariably in older patients it leaves a weaker knee with extension lag. Usually all that is required is debridement of the eroded or abraded articular cartilage of the medial facet and excision of obstructing osteophytes. If the synovium is grossly inflamed or fibrosed, such areas are excised. If there is marked laxity of the medial collateral ligament and thus instability of the joint, the operation is completed by transposing the semitendinosus tendon to an appropriate groove formed in the medial surface of the femoral condyle.[4] After operation the patient soon learns to contract his muscles actively and stability is restored. Patients who were unable to bear weight without crutches before the operation are able to bear weight on the flexed knee without assistance following this procedure.

If structural deformity has developed, and this is usually the result of collapse of the lateral tibial condyle, soft tissue operations are no longer adequate and tibial osteotomy is required as well. This is done above the tibial tubercle and must include correction of the rotational deformity. To avoid excessive strain on the superior tibiofibular joint, the fibula requires osteotomy as well.

Finally, in a very small number of patients, the process has progressed so far that arthrodesis may be considered, provided only one knee is involved. The

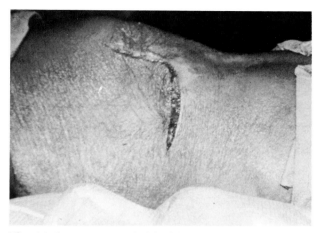

Fig. 11-17. Recommended incision for exploration of the knee, that is, transverse along joint line with vertical parapatellar extension.

operation will gradually be used less often as earlier and more accurate diagnosis is made. It cures the pain but at the expense of a great loss of function. It is the treatment for the hopeless joint and is rarely necessary. In most instances the osteoarthritic knee requires only removal of the deranged meniscus or menisci plus debridement of the medial border of the patella and sometimes of the edge of the medial femoral condyle. If full external rotation and extension of the tibia on the femur is regained on the table, all that is necessary has been done. That night the patient will sleep.

CONCLUSION

The pattern of movement of the knee is helical; lateral rotation of the tibia occurs during extension of the joint and medial rotation during flexion. Synchrony of these movements is controlled by the thigh muscles and guided by the rotator mechanism of cruciate ligaments and menisci.

Injury to this rotator mechanism leads to loss of the normal synchronous pattern of movement of the knee joint. Each type of meniscus injury produces its own particular symptoms and signs, which are no less important in the aging person than in the young adult, and this study leads to the inescapable conclusion that osteoarthritis of the knee is usually the sequel to derangement of one or both degenerating menisci.

With careful physical examination, a precise diagnosis of the mechanical derangement can be made, and if this is corrected surgically and normal synchronous movement of the joint is restored, the prognosis in the "osteoarthritic" knee is no longer hopeless—and the earlier the correction, the better the prognosis.

I wish to thank Mr. David Groebel-Lee, Mr. Clive Whalley, and Mr. Robert Jackson for their help in the preparation of this chapter.

REFERENCES

1. Apley, A. G.: Personal communication, 1965.
2. Bauer, G. C. H., and Smith, E. M.: 85Sr scintimetry in osteoarthritis of the knee, J. Nucl. Med. **10:**109, 1969.
3. Helal, B.: Pain in primary osteoarthritis of the knee, Postgrad. Med. J. **41:**172, 1965.
4. Helfet, A. J.: Function of the cruciate ligaments of the knee joint, Lancet **1:**665, 1948.
5. Helfet, A. J.: Mechanics of derangement of the medial semilinear cartilage and their management, J. Bone Joint Surg. **41-B:**319, 1959.
6. Helfet, A. J.: The management of internal derangements of the knee, Philadelphia, 1963, J. B. Lippincott Co.
7. Helfet, A. J.: The concept of arrest of osteoarthritis in the hip and knee. In Apley, A. G., editor: Recent advances in orthopaedics, London, 1969, J. & A. Churchill, Ltd.
8. Johnson, L. C.: Kinetics of osteoarthritis, Lab. Invest. **8:**1223, 1959.
9. Wardle, E. N.: Osteotomy of the tibia and fibula, Surg. Gynec. Obstet. **115:**61, 1962.

Chapter 12

Synovial fluid and synovial membrane abnormalities in arthritis of the knee joint*

EDGAR S. CATHCART, M.D., and ALAN S. COHEN, M.D., F.A.C.P.
Boston, Massachusetts

Most disorders of the knee joint, whether traumatic, degenerative, or inflammatory, are accompanied by an increased volume of synovial fluid—commonly referred to as a joint effusion. The presence of a joint effusion not only draws attention to the affected joint but affords the examining physician an opportunity to carry out certain procedures that are helpful in arriving at the proper diagnosis. It is the purpose in this chapter to describe these procedures—arthrocentesis and closed synovial membrane biopsy—and to discuss the findings that occur within the joint space when there is a detectable effusion.

ARTHROCENTESIS

Following the discovery of a joint effusion there are no absolute contraindications to synovial fluid aspiration. Furthermore, the procedure may be carried out with ease and safety in the physician's examining room or at the bedside provided aseptic conditions are maintained. It is recommended, however, that joint aspirations be carried out only after the patient has been fasting for at least 6 and preferably 12 hours, particularly if simultaneous blood and synovial fluid glucose estimations are required.

With a No. 18 or larger bore needle, the joint space is entered under the medial or lateral margins of the patella when the knee is extended or through the patellar ligament when the knee is flexed. On the other hand, if the effusion is relatively large, it is preferable to remove joint fluid directly from the suprapatellar bursa, a maneuver that is relatively painless and may be completed with or without administration of a local anesthetic. Whenever possible, a minimum of 10 to 15 ml. of synovial fluid should be withdrawn from the affected knee for diagnostic purposes, but 5 ml. or even less may suffice when more is not obtainable.

SYNOVIAL FLUID ANALYSIS

After a brief notation as to whether the synovial fluid clots and is clear, cloudy, or blood tinged, the specimen should be divided into four test tubes for routine analysis as follows:

First tube (sterile)
    Culture (aerobic and anaerobic)
Second tube (heparin or EDTA)
    Total white cell and differential count
Third tube (without anticoagulant)
    Mucin clot test
    Examination of fluid and cells for inclusions
    Examination of fluid and cells for crystals
    Test for rheumatoid factors
    Test for antinuclear antibodies
    C_3 (complement) determination
Fourth tube (calcium oxalate)
    Glucose determination (blood and synovial fluid)

The first test tube is kept sterile and should be brought as soon as possible to a bacteriology laboratory for gram stains and both aerobic and anaerobic cultures. If gonococcal infection is suspected, heated chocolate agar or a specially enriched medium should be used. If the diagnosis of tuberculosis is seriously entertained, guinea pig inoculation is also necessary.

The second test tube, which contains heparin or

*Supported in part by grants from the National Institute of Arthritis and Metabolic Diseases, United States Public Health Service, Grant Nos. AM-04599 and T1-AM-5285, and from the Arthritis Foundation and the Massachusetts Chapter of the Arthritis Foundation.

EDTA, is used to perform a total white blood cell count and differential count. After the tube has been thoroughly shaken, fluid is drawn up to the 0.5 mark in a standard white blood cell counting pipette. This is then diluted to the 1.1 mark with normal (0.85%) saline solution containing 0.1% methylene blue. (The diluting fluid normally used for performing white cell counts on whole blood cannot be used for accurate synovial fluid analysis since it contains acetic acid. This latter reagent causes hyaluronate-protein complexes in synovial fluid to precipitate and may lead to a falsely low total white cell count.) Red and white blood cells are counted in a standard hemocytometer chamber under high power ($\times 40$) and calculations are made by adding the total number of cells contained in the four large corner squares of the counting chamber and multiplying that number by 50. If the total nucleated count (white cell count) exceeds 5,000 cells/mm.^{3}, one should proceed by making a cover slip smear directly from the anticoagulated synovial fluid. On the other hand, if the nucleated cell count is less than 5,000 cells/mm.^{3}, a suitable smear may be prepared by spinning the joint fluid in a clinical centrifuge for 10 minutes at 2,000 rpm, re-

moving the supernatant and resuspending the sediment in approximately 10 drops of the anticoagulant or supernatant. Smears should be air dried and are stained with Wright's stain. Polymorphonuclear leukocytes, small lymphocytes, and large mononuclear cells are readily visualized by this technique, although fragmentation of cell membranes sometimes leads to vacuolization or the appearance of extracellular homogenized nuclear debris (Fig. 12-1).

The third test tube contains no anticoagulants and provides samples for the mucin clot test and a search for inclusion body cells and crystals. Rheumatoid factors, antinuclear antibodies, and complement components may also be measured using this sample. For the mucin clot test, 1 ml. of the joint fluid is added to 4 ml. of distilled water in a 10 ml. beaker or large test tube. After the addition of 1 drop of 7N acetic acid the appearance of the resultant precipitate is recorded according to the following criteria: a tight ropy mass contained in a clear solution indicates a *good* mucin clot; a less compact mass with some shreds in suspension is a *fair* mucin clot; a fragmented mass in a turbid solution is recorded as a *poor* mucin clot; and a few clumped flecks of mucin suspended in a cloudy

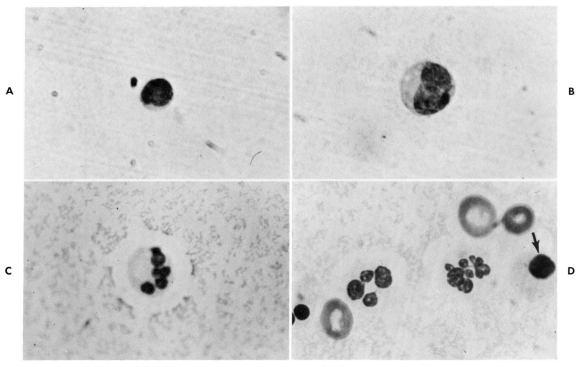

Fig. 12-1. Synovial fluid leukocytes. **A,** Lymphocyte. **B,** Monocyte. **C,** Polymorphonucleocyte with multilobed nucleus. **D,** Red blood cells and polymorphonucleocytes. The arrow points to extracellular nuclear material.

solution denotes a *very poor* mucin clot. In general the description of the mucin clot matches the duration and degree of inflammation within the joint space, although the precise mechanisms governing mucin clot precipitation by acetic acid are poorly understood.

In order to determine the presence of intranuclear inclusions and crystals, a drop of joint fluid is placed on a microscope slide and carefully scanned under low and then high power. Urate crystals exhibit a long needlelike appearance and strong negative birefringence when viewed under polarized light; calcium pyrophosphate crystals may also have a needlelike appearance but more frequently have a squat or rhomboidal configuration and manifest weak positive birefringence when viewed with a polarizing microscope. Possible confusion in the diagnosis of crystal-induced arthritis may arise if talc from the gloves of the examining physician or other crystalline materials such as calcium oxalate are inadvertently mixed with the joint fluid under study.

Finally, in order to complete the joint fluid analysis, a fourth test tube containing calcium oxalate or EDTA may be utilized to perform glucose determinations. This procedure is of most value in the diagnosis of infectious arthritis in which a synovial fluid–serum difference of over 50 mg./100 ml. glucose is not unusual.

Classification of arthritis based on synovial fluid findings

Noninflammatory joint effusions. Noninflammatory joint effusions are easily differentiated from those due to inflammatory and infectious forms of arthritis by their clear, noncloudy appearance, fair to good viscosity, good mucin clot formation, and low total white cell count (less than 1,000 cells/mm.³). As in normal synovial fluid, a fibrin clot does not form when noninflammatory effusions are left standing unless recent injury has caused a rupture of adjacent blood vessels and a resultant hemarthrosis. The most common causes of noninflammatory joint effusions are trauma and degenerative joint disease (osteoarthritis). Other less common causes of noninflammatory joint fluids include neuroarthropathy (Charcot's joints), osteochondromatosis, and osteochondritis dissecans. Patients with interval gout and pseudogout have also been encountered in whom the total white cell count is normal and the mucin test good. However, despite the absence of inflammation, rare intracellular and extracellular crystals have been observed in the joint fluids of these patients.

Mild inflammatory joint effusions. Knee joint effusions with elevated but relatively low total white cell counts (1,000 to 5,000 cells/mm.³) are commonly accompanied by fair or good viscosity and fair or good mucin clot formation. Based on the differential white cell count, a deficiency of leukocytes is more suggestive of systemic lupus erythematosus and helps differentiate this condition from other causes of mild inflammatory joint disease such as scleroderma, hemorrhagic villonodular synovitis, sarcoma, sarcoidosis, and hypertrophic pulmonary osteoarthropathy. It should also be noted that patients with rheumatoid arthritis and its variants (psoriatic arthropathy, ankylosing spondylitis, arthritis associated with ulcerative colitis and regional enteritis, intermittent hydrarthrosis, etc.) sometimes demonstrate relatively low total white cell counts.

Severe inflammatory joint effusions. A large variety of conditions may lead to joint effusions with moderate to high total white cell counts (more than 5,000 cells/mm.³), poor viscosity, and poor mucin clot formation. Counts exceeding 50,000 cells/mm.³ are relatively uncommon in noninfectious arthritis, but on occasion, patients with rheumatoid arthritis, gout, and pseudogout will manifest joint effusions that appear grossly purulent (more than 100,000 cells/mm.³).

The diagnosis of acute infectious arthritis cannot be made with certainty unless the affected knee joint has been aspirated and positive cultures obtained. Once the diagnosis has been established, joint fluid aspiration and joint fluid analyses should be repeated at daily intervals in order to determine whether the prescribed antibiotic therapy is producing the desired effect, that is, resolution of inflammation within the joint space. As a rule, antibiotics should not be injected directly into infected joints since they may cause a secondary rise in the total white cell count and make it difficult to ascertain whether bacterial resistance has developed. In uncomplicated cases one can generally assume that infection has been arrested when the synovial fluid total white cell count falls and the cultures become negative.

Gout, pseudogout, and rheumatoid arthritis are probably the most common causes of severe inflammatory effusions in the knee joint. Fortunately the two former conditions are easily recognized following inspection of joint fluid samples under polarized light (Fig. 12-2). The synovial fluid findings in rheumatoid arthritis are less specific and even the inclusion cell (ragocyte, RA cell) is no longer considered pathognomonic of this disease. By immunofluorescent studies and other techniques, synovial fluid cells from patients

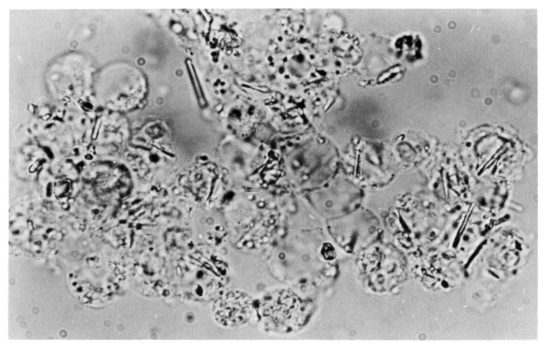

Fig. 12-2. Calcium pyrophosphate crystals in synovial fluid of patient with pseudogout.

with rheumatoid arthritis have been shown to contain rheumatoid factors, nucleoprotein, and C_3 component of complement. The pathogenic significance of these findings has not been elucidated. More recently, it has also been noted that total hemolytic complement as well as many of the individual components of complement, that is, C_2, C_3, and C_4, are quantitatively depressed in rheumatoid synovial fluid, suggesting the presence of immune complexes.

Less common forms of arthritis associated with severe inflammatory arthritis of the knee joint include Reiter's syndrome, acute rheumatic fever, bacterial endocarditis, and hypersensitivity angiitis (for example, penicillin reactions). Once again, no specific joint fluid abnormalities characterize any of these conditions, although complement levels are apparently elevated in effusions due to Reiter's syndrome. Certain viral syndromes, including rubella, mumps, and infectious hepatitis may also be accompanied by inflammatory knee joint disease, although it is still not clear whether their pathogenicity for synovial membrane is based on infection or hypersensitivity. Joint fluids from patients with viral syndromes have only infrequently been analyzed, but it would appear that a relative lymphocytosis helps to differentiate them from other types of severe inflammatory disease.

CLOSED SYNOVIAL MEMBRANE BIOPSY

Synovial membrane biopsy is indicated in those patients in whom the etiology of arthritis is obscure or in whom histologic examination of the synovial membrane may provide information that cannot be derived from examination of the joint fluid alone. Studies of synovial membrane pathology have been greatly facilitated in recent years, first by the introduction of the Polley-Bickel needle and later by the introduction of the Parker-Pearson needle, which has a cross-sectional diameter approximately one fifth that of its prototype (Fig. 12-3). The technique for closed synovial membrane biopsy is simple and relatively free of complications. Furthermore, it is possible during a single procedure to obtain four or five specimens for histologic examination plus synovial fluid specimens for routine analysis.

With the knee fully extended, 1% procaine or lidocaine (Xylocaine) is used to infiltrate the skin, the joint capsule, and finally, after a sample of synovial fluid has been withdrawn, the joint space itself. A Parker-Pearson needle is introduced either medially or laterally into the retropatellar space through a special wide-bore trocar. Multiple specimens of synovial membrane are taken from both the suprapatellar and retropatellar spaces by changing the position of the biopsy needle during the proce-

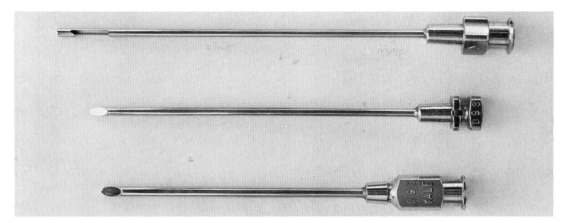

Fig. 12-3. Parker-Pearson biopsy set.

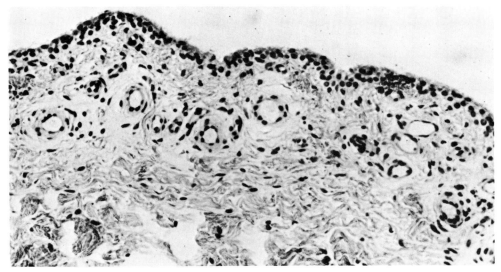

Fig. 12-4. Synovial membrane biopsy specimen from patient with traumatic arthritis.

dure. Biopsy specimens are immediately fixed in buffered formalin and in absolute alcohol when crystalline-induced arthritis is suspected.

Classification of arthritis based on synovial membrane abnormalities

Noninflammatory
    Traumatic
    Degenerative joint disease
    Neuroarthropathy (Charcot's joint)
    Osteochondromatosis, osteochondritis dissecans
    Hemachromatosis, amyloidosis
Mild inflammatory
    Rheumatoid arthritis
    Systemic lupus erythematosus, scleroderma
    Hemorrhagic villonodular synovitis, sarcoma
    Sarcoidosis
    Hypertrophic pulmonary osteoarthropathy

Severe inflammatory
    Acute infectious arthritis
    Rheumatoid arthritis
    Gout, pseudogout
    Reiter's syndrome
    Acute rheumatic fever, bacterial endocarditis
    Hypersensitivity angiitis
    Viral syndromes

Noninflammatory synovial membranes. The synovial membrane is normally composed of synovial intimal cells that form an interlacing network one to three cells thick. Mast cells, endothelial cells (lining blood vessels), and other connective tissue cells lie beneath the intimal layer and are adjacent to fibrous, fatty, or areolar tissue. In traumatic arthritis (Fig. 12-4) and degenerative joint disease the synovial membrane is usually grossly normal

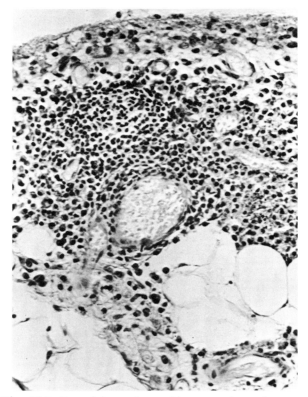

Fig. 12-5. Synovial membrane biopsy specimen from patient with rheumatoid arthritis.

apart from a notable increase in vascularity. However, noninflammatory conditions in which synovial membrane biopsy has led to a definitive diagnosis include chondrocalcinosis, hemachromatosis, and amyloidosis.

Mild inflammatory synovial membranes. In knee joint effusions in which the total white cell count is between 1,000 and 5,000 cells/mm.[3], the corresponding synovial membranes usually show a similar degree of inflammation. Biopsy has been most helpful in those cases of mild or latent rheumatoid arthritis in which the synovial fluid analysis has been unremarkable (good mucin clot, low total white cell count) but pockets of inflammation have been observed in the synovial membrane specimen (Fig. 12-5). When these findings are found in association with abundant deposits of hemosiderin, the diagnosis of villonodular synovitis may first become apparent. Although the synovial membrane abnormalities associated with systemic lupus erythematosus and scleroderma are not always diagnostic, vasculitis and hematoxylin bodies are more prone to occur in the former condition (Fig. 12-6), and marked fibroblastic proliferation may be found in the latter. Other mild inflammatory disorders in which synovial membrane biopsy has led to a definitive diagnosis include sarcoidosis and indolent fungal infections.

Severe inflammatory synovial membranes. It is well known that the synovial fluid of patients with

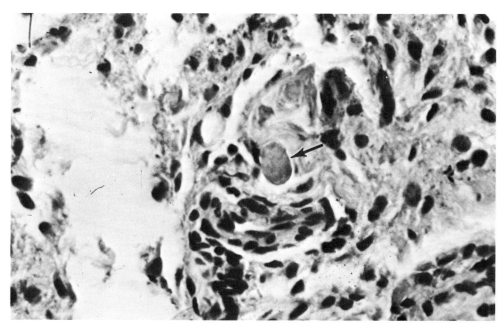

Fig. 12-6. Synovial membrane biopsy specimen from patient with systemic lupus erythematosus. The arrow points to a hematoxylin body.

rheumatoid arthritis may contain numerous polymorphonucleocytes, whereas the corresponding synovial membrane demonstrates a remarkable absence of these cells. On the other hand, the membrane in these cases is usually many cell layers thick and the resultant pannus will show some of the following abnormalities: marked villous hypertrophy; proliferation of superficial synovial cells, often with palisading; marked infiltration of chronic inflammatory cells (lymphocytes or plasma cells predominating) with a tendency to form lymphoid nodules; deposition of compact fibrils, either on the surface or interstitially; and foci or cell necrosis. If the fluorescent antibody technique is used, the synovial membrane may demonstrate numerous intracellular and extracellular deposits of immunoglobulins and complement as well as nucleoprotein, changes that closely resemble those observed in the synovial fluid.

Synovial membrane biopsy may provide a definitive diagnosis in gout and pesudogout when microcrystalline deposits are visualized. However, in these conditions, abundant crystals should also be apparent in the joint fluid. Acute bacterial infections also show a marked polymorphonuclear infiltration and necrosis of the synovial membrane. On the other hand, when the infectious organism is *Mycobacterium tuberculosis*, the resultant membrane is usually infiltrated with lymphocytes, giant cells, plasma cells, and caseating granuloma.

SUMMARY AND CONCLUSIONS

This paper is intended to be no more than a brief introduction to certain aspects of synovial fluid analysis and closed synovial membrane biopsy. Since both procedures can be performed easily and rapidly at the bedside, it is hoped that they will become part of the routine work-up of patients with arthritis. For more detailed information on these and related topics refer to standard rheumatology textbooks.[1-6]

We wish to acknowledge the expert photographic assistance of Mr. David Feigenbaum.

REFERENCES

1. Cohen, A. S., editor: Laboratory diagnostic procedures in the rheumatic diseases, Boston, 1967, Little, Brown & Co.
2. Cohen, A. S., and Cathcart, E. S.: Arthritis and connective tissue diseases. In Keefer, C. S., and Wilkins, R. W., editors: Medicine, Boston, 1970, Little, Brown & Co.
3. Copeman, W. S. C.: Textbook of the rheumatic diseases, ed. 4, Baltimore, 1969, The Williams & Wilkins Co.
4. Hollander, J. E.: Arthritis and allied conditions, ed. 7, Philadelphia, 1966, Lea & Febiger.
5. Parker, R. H., and Pearson, C. M.: A simplified synovial biopsy needle, Arthritis Rheum. 6:172, 1963.
6. Ropes, M. W., and Bauer, W.: Synovial fluid changes in joint disease, Cambridge, 1953, Harvard University Press.

Index